Univ
Subje

ht

DESIGNING AND CONDUCTING
HEALTH SURVEYS

DESIGNING AND CONDUCTING HEALTH SURVEYS

A Comprehensive Guide

THIRD EDITION

Lu Ann Aday
Llewellyn J. Cornelius

Foreword by Steven B. Cohen

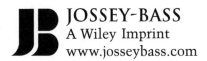

JOSSEY-BASS
A Wiley Imprint
www.josseybass.com

Published by Jossey-Bass
A Wiley Imprint
989 Market Street, San Francisco, CA 94103-1741   www.josseybass.com

Jossey-Bass books and products are available through most bookstores. To contact Jossey-Bass directly call our Customer Care Department within the U.S. at 800-956-7739, outside the U.S. at 317-572-3986, or fax 317-572-4002.

Jossey-Bass also publishes its books in a variety of electronic formats. Some content that appears in print may not be available in electronic books.

Library of Congress Cataloging-in-Publication Data

Aday, Lu Ann.
    Designing and conducting health surveys : a comprehensive guide / Lu Ann Aday and Llewellyn J. Cornelius; foreword by Steven B. Cohen.—3rd ed.
        p. ; cm.
    Includes bibliographical references and index.
    ISBN-13: 978-0-7879-7560-9 (cloth)
    ISBN-10: 0-7879-7560-5 (cloth)
    1. Health surveys.   2. Health surveys—Statistical methods.
    [DNLM: 1. Health Surveys.   2. Research Design.   3. Data Collection—methods.
WA 20.5 A221d 2006]   I. Cornelius, Llewellyn Joseph, 1959-   II. Title.
    RA408.5.A33   2006
    614.4'2—dc22   2005036447

Printed in the United States of America
THIRD EDITION
HB Printing   10 9 8 7 6 5 4 3 2 1
PB Printing   10 9 8 7 6 5 4 3 2 1

CONTENTS

FIGURES, TABLES, AND EXHIBITS

Figures

Tables

Exhibits

FOREWORD

Steven B. Cohen

Health surveys serve as a critical resource to measure the health status, risk factors, and health behaviors of the population and to assess the level of quality of the health care received. They also permit the identification of disparities in health care associated with access, use, cost, and insurance coverage and serve to identify related patterns and trends over time. The descriptive and analytical findings they generate are key inputs to facilitate the development, implementation, and evaluation of policies and practices addressing health and health care. To ensure their utility and integrity, it is essential that these health surveys are designed according to high-quality, effective, and efficient statistical and methodological practices, and optimal sample designs. It is also important that subsequent applications of estimation strategies to the survey data, as well as analytical techniques and interpretations of resultant research findings, are guided by well-grounded statistical theory.

Over the past two decades, both the first and second editions of *Designing and Conducting Health Surveys* by Lu Ann Aday have served as core references that provide a comprehensive framework to help guide survey planners, health services researchers, and the ultimate users through the major processes that are

The views are those of the author, and no official endorsement by the Department of Health and Human Services or the Agency for Healthcare Research and Quality is intended or should be inferred.

characteristic of well-designed surveys. While the large majority of the guiding principles identified in the earlier editions continue to hold, several recent technological advances have visibly modified the paradigm for the design and conduct of health surveys in the twenty-first century. This most recent revision, which now reflects a collaborative effort between Aday and Llewellyn Cornelius, gives additional attention to advances in computer-assisted data collection efforts and the advent of Web-based surveys. The book also covers recent enhancements in sophisticated statistical software to facilitate appropriate estimation, variance estimation, and imputation techniques, in addition to the application of more appropriate analytical techniques tailored to specific analyses.

Beginning with the need for a clear set of survey objectives that defines the core purpose of a given health survey, attention is given to issues of survey content, questionnaire design, cost considerations, and mode of data collection. The book also features important sample design considerations, with coverage given to topics that include frame development, sample size specifications, precision requirements, and sample selection scheme. Adhering to a total survey error framework, the authors identify the challenges that characterize well-designed health surveys and reinforce the need for informed choices by survey designers and sponsors among the available options at each stage of survey development.

Readers will benefit from the breadth of experience Aday and Cornelius convey in helping guide design decisions that bear on the accuracy, reliability, clarity and relevance, timeliness, and accessibility of survey findings. They provide effective guidelines for minimizing survey errors for each phase of the life cycle of a health survey, which go hand in hand with their informative discussion of the related trade-offs that have an impact on the quality and cost-efficiency of the design. An added feature of this updated edition is the inclusion of new, more current studies based on international, national, and state and local surveys that serve as good vehicles to illustrate both the unique and shared design challenges and to identify effective strategies to solve them.

A well-designed health survey imposes an interdependence of the survey sponsors, the survey designers, the associated statisticians and methodologists, the survey operations, field and management staff, the data processing staff, and the end users, who are primarily the health researchers, policymakers, and the public. This book provides the essential road map to help realize and strengthen these connections. When all the essential health survey contributors work in concert, following the sound practices covered in this book, the overall survey quality and utility that is achieved should be much greater than the sum of the individual successful components. As in the past, this book should continue to serve as a valuable resource to both practitioners and researchers alike, helping to provide a greater respect for the methodological and operational challenges that health surveys present and the substantive and technical expertise necessary for their effective resolution. Students engaged in health survey research should also substantially benefit from this comprehensive book by gaining an enhanced understanding of the underlying complexities inherent in the design and conduct of health surveys.

July 2005   Steven B. Cohen
Rockville, Maryland   Agency for Healthcare Research and Quality

PREFACE

Designing and Conducting Health Surveys has been a classic guide for many years for institutions and individuals interested in conducting or using health surveys. The first (1989), second (1996), and now the third (2006) editions of the book draw on methodological work on surveys in general and health surveys in particular to illuminate and illustrate the principles and approaches that should be applied in designing high-quality surveys.

The number, complexity, and scope of both privately and governmentally funded health care surveys—on the institutional, local, state, national, and international levels—have increased dramatically in response to the need for information about the sources, magnitude, and impact of health problems, and the roles of programs and providers in addressing these problems. Many hospitals, managed care organizations (MCOs), and other health care businesses are struggling for their share of the consumer market. HIV/AIDS and sociomedical morbidities such as stress-related illness place a substantial strain on the health care system as a whole. The issue of how to provide reasonable access to quality medical care in cost-effective ways with limited resources is a major problem in the United States and other countries. Health surveys have been and will continue to be important sources of information about the impact of these dynamic and complex changes underway in the health care marketplace.

This book is intended to strengthen the preparedness of survey developers in taking on these and related challenges in designing high-quality health surveys.

This third edition draws on the most recent methodological research on survey design in general and the rich storehouse of insights and implications provided by cognitive research on question and questionnaire design in particular. The evolution and application of Internet technologies for gathering survey data are also elaborated. A total survey error framework and survey quality is presented as a useful compass for charting the dangerous waters between the Scylla and Charybdis of systematic and random errors that inevitably accompany the survey design enterprise. In this edition, the specific types of errors that can occur in the design and implementation of surveys and the means that can be used for addressing them are explicitly delineated and discussed within each of the chapters.

In addition, three new studies based on national, international, and state and local surveys—the UNICEF Multiple Indicator Cluster Surveys, California Health Interview Survey, and National Dental Malpractice Survey—are used to illustrate the range of design alternatives available at each stage of developing a survey and what might be a sound basis for choosing among them.

Audience

This book is intended to be a reference for health care marketing personnel, strategic planners, program designers, agency administrators, and health professionals charged with conducting or contracting for health studies. It will also serve as a resource for academics and researchers who are interested in collecting, analyzing, and evaluating health survey data and as a text for teaching students in public health, medical sociology, health administration, health education, medicine, nursing, dentistry, allied health, health program evaluation, social work, and related fields how to design and conduct good surveys.

The issues in designing high-quality surveys parallel those to be considered in evaluating the quality of medical or nursing care. Norms of practice are taught during clinical training, based on research and experience in the profession. The precise relationship of these norms to whether the patient lives, or at least improves, is not always clear or systematically documented. What clinical researchers discover in the laboratory and what works for practitioners on the wards do provide the practical basis for training new professionals in sound medical practice. Doing good surveys is, similarly, a combination of science and practical experience.

Overview of the Contents

Chapter One introduces a framework for identifying and classifying the major topics addressed by health surveys. It lays the groundwork for thinking about what topics could be the focus of a health survey and what related studies to review before beginning one's own study. This chapter also looks ahead to the topics, technologies, and methodological and ethical challenges that are likely to affect the way health surveys are designed and conducted in the future. An approach to identifying the major types of survey errors that will be elaborated in the chapters that follow is also introduced in Chapter One.

The fundamental starting point for a study is the definition of survey objectives. The process begins with the specification of the health topics to be addressed in the survey. Deciding on the basic research questions to be addressed requires determining when, where, who, and what the focus of the study will be. Chapter Two describes major survey designs for addressing different research questions and presents guidelines for formulating detailed study objectives or hypotheses based on those questions. The research questions and study hypotheses and objectives are usually phrased in general (or conceptual) terms—for example, "Are patients of higher socioeconomic status more likely to engage in preventive self-care practices?" During the survey preparation, these concepts are translated into more directly measurable indicators—for example, "Are patients with more education and higher family incomes more likely to exercise regularly?"

Chapter Three reviews the techniques for developing working definitions of the topics or issues addressed in health surveys. It also provides two important criteria for evaluating just how useful these working definitions are: (1) Do they seem to mean the same thing all the time and to different people? (that is, are they reliable?) and (2) Are they accurate translations of what the investigators originally had in mind? (that is, are they valid?). Techniques are also discussed for reducing the number of variables produced by many different survey questions to a more economical set of indicators through the use of summary typologies, indexes, and scales.

Chapter Four reviews the logic and methods to use in formulating the analysis plan for a survey. Analyzing the data is one of the last steps in the survey process. Having an idea of the analysis plan for the study can, however, help guide decisions made at every subsequent stage of the survey. Survey researchers, like good scouts, should be prepared and know before setting out what they want to accomplish.

Chapter Five explains the advantages and disadvantages of different ways of collecting data in general—and data on health topics in particular. Methods of data collection considered here include face-to-face interviews, telephone interviews, and self-administered questionnaires. These can be either recorded on paper copy questionnaires or input directly into a computer or adapted for e-mail or Web-based surveys. Combinations of these data-gathering approaches can also be used, depending on the funding and technical capabilities at the researcher's disposal.

All of the decisions made to this point, especially those relating to the method of data collection, influence the process of sampling or selecting the people or organizations to be included in the study. Chapter Six reviews the basic types of sample designs used in surveys and presents examples of each from major health studies. Chapter Seven introduces approaches to estimating the sample size required for a study. It also discusses the problems or errors that can arise in the sampling process and ways to deal with these, both in the course of the study and later, in data analysis using a particular sample design.

The heart of the survey is generally a questionnaire containing questions designed to elicit the information the investigator wants from study participants. Although rules for asking these questions are not always clear-cut, methodological research, particularly the applications of cognitive psychology in designing survey questions, has yielded useful guidelines for composing valid and reliable questions. Chapter Eight provides a general overview, based on the emerging research, of some of the issues to consider in formulating questions in general—regarding both the form of the question itself and the possible response categories to use with it. Similarly, Chapters Nine, Ten, and Eleven present guidelines for developing particular types of questions—objective questions about the respondents' characteristics or behavior, subjective questions about their attitudes toward or knowledge about certain health issues, and questions about their perceived or clinically evaluated health status. Examples of each type of question, drawn from health surveys, are also presented.

Individual questions represent the building blocks of the survey questionnaire itself. The order or context in which questions are placed in the questionnaire and the form and clarity of the questionnaire have been found to influence the quality of data obtained in surveys. The type of data collection method chosen (face-to-face, telephone, self-administered, or computerized or Internet adaptations of these) can also significantly influence the phrasing of individual questions and the form and format of the questionnaire itself. Chapter Twelve presents general rules of thumb to consider in designing questionnaires and the adaptations required for different modes of data collection.

The issue of quality control during data collection is discussed in Chapter Thirteen. The way the survey is actually conducted is shaped by all the prior decisions about study design, as well as the dress rehearsals (pilot studies or pretests) to see how well the questionnaires and procedures are performing, the training and experience of the data collection staff, and the management and monitoring of the data-gathering process.

Coding the data entails assigning numbers to answers so that they can be processed by computers. Before the data can be analyzed, adjustments may have to be made to correct for missing or incomplete data from certain types of respondents on certain questions. The method of data collection (especially if computerized) can directly affect the ways the data are subsequently coded, processed, and cleaned. (Cleaning refers to the process of identifying and correcting errors.) Chapter Fourteen discusses these preparations.

Chapter Fifteen reviews the major univariate, bivariate, and multivariate methods for analyzing survey data. The methods the researcher uses will depend on the analysis plan chosen for the study (Chapter Four), the research question being addressed, the design of the study, and the measurement of the survey variables to be used in the analysis.

The final step in designing and carrying out a survey is writing up what has been learned in a report to interested audiences. The report may be addressed to the funder, as evidence of fulfillment of grant or contract objectives; to an operating agency's administration or board of directors, as part of their strategic planning process; or to legislative committees, task forces, or staff, as background research on a particular piece of pending legislation. The survey may also be the basis for a thesis, book, or journal article. This final chapter describes what the form and content of a basic research report based on the survey might be and presents a framework for evaluating the overall quality of the study. A summary table highlighting the major types of survey errors that have been reviewed in the previous chapters is introduced to serve as a checklist for identifying what might be particular strengths or limitations of a survey in the context of a total survey errors and survey quality framework.

Major survey examples cited throughout the book and highlighted in the resources at the end of the book include face-to-face, telephone, and mail surveys. Key sources of information on health surveys and an inventory of health survey archives are also provided. Many specific examples of health surveys at the international, national, state, and local levels are presented.

In summary, this book provides an overview of the basic tenets of good health survey design for those who have a role in gathering, analyzing, or interpreting health survey data.

Acknowledgments

We gratefully acknowledge the contributions of a number of people to this book.

We thank the mentors and colleagues who first contributed to our understanding of how to design and conduct high-quality health surveys: Ronald M. Andersen, Odin W. Anderson, and Robert L. Eichhorn.

We acknowledge the important contributions that our health survey research colleagues as well as private sector survey organizations and public agencies make to the development and testing of survey methods. It is their dedication to the field of survey research that supports the design and implementation of high-quality surveys.

Special thanks go to Anne D. Wiltshire, who helped to compile and edit the extensive set of references for the book. Her hard work, patience, and attention to detail were invaluable.

We gratefully acknowledge the contributions of Manish Aggarwal, Yu-Chia Chang, Rebecca Toni, Erin Gilbert, and Kieva Bankins in locating and compiling sources for the manuscript, as well as the helpful administrative support provided by Regina Fisher and Elizabeth S. Brown.

Particular thanks go to the colleagues who contributed the sample surveys for which questionnaires are presented in Resource A, B, and C and that are used as examples throughout the book: E. Richard Brown, California Health Interview Survey; Peter Milgrom and Danna Moore, National Dental Malpractice Survey; and Edilberto Loaiza, UNICEF Multiple Indicator Cluster Survey.

We also thank Helena M. von Ville, librarian at the University of Texas School of Public Health, and her staff who facilitated access to state-of-the-art sources on surveys.

We are grateful for the supportive environment at our home institutions, the University of Texas School of Public Health and the University of Maryland School of Social Work, which allowed us the flexibility to write this book, and to the students in our Health Survey Research Design courses, who challenged us to strengthen the clarity and relevance of the manuscript.

Our appreciation is also extended to Cielito Reyes-Gibby and Sarah A. Felknor, who assisted in teaching the course upon which the book was based.

We especially thank our families and close friends, particularly Katherine V. Wilcox and Lydia M. Cornelius, who have provided the support and inspiration for us to pursue our dreams.

We enjoyed and learned from writing this book. Our hope is that others will learn from and enjoy reading it.

October 2005   Lu Ann Aday
                                                                 Llewellyn J. Cornelius

THE AUTHORS

Lu **Ann Aday** is Lorne D. Bain Distinguished Professor in Public Health and Medicine at the University of Texas School of Public Health–Houston. She received her bachelor's degree in economics (agricultural economics, with high honors) from Texas Tech University and her master's and doctoral degrees in sociology (with a specialization in health services research) from Purdue University. Aday was formerly associate director for research at the Center for Health Administration Studies of the University of Chicago. Her principal research interests have focused on indicators and correlates of health services utilization and access. She has conducted major national and community surveys and evaluations of national demonstrations and published extensively in this area, including numerous books dealing with conceptual or empirical aspects of research on access to health and health care for vulnerable populations. Her recent books, a number of which have been published in second or third editions, include *Reinventing Public Health: Policies and Practices for a Healthy Nation* (2005); *At Risk in America: The Health and Health Care Needs of Vulnerable Populations in the United States* (2nd ed., 2001); and *Evaluating the Healthcare System: Effectiveness, Efficiency, and Equity* (3rd ed., 2004). Aday's excellence in teaching and mentoring was acknowledged when she received the University of Texas at Houston Health Science Center Excellence in Scholarship Award, the John P. McGovern Outstanding Teacher Award, the Committee on the Status of Women Distinguished Professional Woman Award, the President's Award for Mentoring Women, and the statewide Minnie Stevens Piper Foundation Award for Excellence in Teaching. Dr. Aday's scholarship is recognized nationally through her election to membership in the Institute of Medicine of the National Academy of Sciences and in receiving an honorary doctorate of social sciences, *honoris causa,* from Purdue University.

Llewellyn J. Cornelius is a professor at the University of Maryland School of Social Work. He received his B.A. degree from Syracuse University, majoring in psychology and sociology, and received a master's degree in social science as well as master's and doctoral degrees in social service administration from the University of Chicago. Cornelius has extensive research experience in examining access to medical delivery and the outcome of care for African Americans and Latinos. He has taught a doctoral research practicum where he assisted students in the development, pilot testing, and fielding of surveys. In addition to teaching survey research, he has participated in the design and implementation of a multitude of studies, including the fielding of a statewide survey that examined the cultural competency of mental health providers; the development and implementation of surveys that assessed the use of technology in social work; the design and implementation of a statewide survey on minority physicians' attitudes toward managed care; and the coordination of portions of a data management contract for a federal survey of fifteen thousand households (the 1987 National Medical Expenditure Survey). Cornelius was the recipient of the University of Chicago's 1996 Elizabeth Butler Young Alumni Award for his contributions to health care research on African Americans and Latinos.

DESIGNING AND CONDUCTING
HEALTH SURVEYS

CHAPTER ONE

THINKING ABOUT TOPICS
FOR HEALTH SURVEYS

Chapter Highlights

1. Surveys systematically collect information on a topic by asking individuals questions to generate statistics on the group or groups that those individuals represent.
2. Health surveys ask questions about a variety of factors that influence, measure, or are affected by people's health.
3. Health survey researchers should review the major international, national, state, and local health surveys relevant to their interests before undertaking their own study.
4. Good survey design is basically a matter of good planning.
5. The total survey error and survey quality framework alerts researchers to ways to identify and mitigate both bias and variable errors in surveys.

This book provides guidance for designing and conducting health surveys. These surveys systematically collect information on a topic of interest (such as state health care reform legislation) by asking individuals questions (about whether they and their family members have insurance coverage) to generate statistics (percentage who are uninsured) for the group or groups those individuals represent (noninstitutionalized residents under sixty-five years of age).

This chapter addresses (1) the topics, techniques, and ethical issues that will characterize the design and conduct of health surveys in the future; (2) the defining features of surveys compared with other data collection methods; and (3) the reasons for studying health surveys. It also provides (4) a framework for classifying the topics addressed in health-related surveys, (5) illustrative examples of health surveys used in this book, and (6) an overview of the total survey design and survey quality approach to designing and conducting health surveys.

Future Health Surveys

Health surveys have been and will continue to be important sources of information for health care policymakers, public health professionals, private providers, insurers, and health care consumers concerned with the planning, implementation, and evaluation of health-related programs and policies. The design and conduct of health surveys in the future will be shaped by changes in the diversity, complexity, and sensitivity of the topics addressed in these studies; the innovative techniques and technologies that are being developed for carrying them out; and the new or intensified ethical dilemmas that are a result of these changes.

Topics

The topics addressed in health surveys have been and will continue to be sensitive and complex. Such sociomedical morbidities as HIV/AIDS, child abuse, sexual dysfunction, drug and alcohol addiction, and family violence, among others, are now encompassed in definitions of public health and medical problems. The issue of access to medical care focuses on vulnerable and hard-to-locate populations differentially experiencing these sociomedical morbidities: gay/lesbian/bisexual/transgendered (GLBT) persons, drug abusers, the homeless, medically fragile children and the elderly, and undocumented migrant and refugee populations. Health care program designers are concerned with the number of people in these vulnerable groups; the particular health problems they experience; the barriers to care they confront; the ways in which their knowledge, attitudes, and behaviors exacerbate the risk of their contracting serious illnesses; and the resources they have to deal with these problems.

These trends in asking tough questions of hard-to-locate respondents in order to gain information for the design of cost-effective public and private health programs to address the needs of these respondents will continue.

Techniques and Technologies

The topics to be addressed in health surveys present new and intensified challenges at each stage of the design and conduct of a study. Corresponding to these developments is the emergence of new technologies for assisting with these tasks.

Rapid growth in the number and diversity of journals and specialized publications dealing with health topics has made the job of identifying and evaluating the major research in any given area more challenging. Computerized text search programs have greatly facilitated access to published research, but knowledge of effective search techniques is required to carry out these searches efficiently. These databases encompass professional journals and related periodical literature, as well as increasingly expanded online access to books, government publications, and unpublished research in progress relevant to the topic of interest. For those health topics for which little information is available because of the newness of the topic or the corollary lag in the dissemination of research results, survey designers need to contact relevant public or private funding agencies and colleagues in the field who are known to have research in progress on the issue.

Training programs are needed to prepare both students and professionals for carrying out these searches and evaluating the credibility of sources that are identified. The credibility of Internet and unpublished research could be evaluated based on the authoritativeness and previous track record of the organization or individual to whom the work is credited (for example, National Center for Health Statistics reports are likely to be a more credible source than an unpublished manuscript posted by a university faculty member with little record of peer-reviewed publications or funding); the other research sources that the research draws on or references; as well as the standards for evaluating the possible sources of errors in research in general and surveys in particular discussed further later in this chapter and highlighted in each of the chapters that follow. (Also, see White, 1994, and Wortman, 1994, for a discussion of procedures and criteria for retrieving and evaluating scientific literature.)

In the interest of learning about health and health-related attitudes, knowledge, and behaviors, survey researchers are attempting to penetrate more deeply into the traditionally best-kept family and personal secrets. The application of principles of cognitive psychology to the design and evaluation of such questions has challenged many of the standardized approaches to asking questions. At a minimum, in the early stages of questionnaire development, survey designers should ask respondents what went through their minds when they were asked sensitive questions about themselves or other members of their family. Moreover, prominent survey methodologists have called for the development of theories of surveys. These theories would focus on the decisions that could be made at each stage of designing and carrying out a survey to maximize quality and minimize costs (Biemer & Lyberg, 2003; Dillman, 2000, 2002; Groves, 1987, 1989; Groves, Dillman, Eltinge, & Little, 2002; Groves, Singer, & Corning, 2000; Sudman, Bradburn, & Schwarz, 1996).

The technology that has had the largest influence on the techniques used in the design and conduct of health surveys is computerized information processing. These methods can be used to facilitate research on different survey techniques or methodologies (such as using different approaches to sampling respondents, phrasing questions, and training interviewers). The rapid turnaround of information made possible by computerized methods should expedite choices among design alternatives of this kind. More attention needs to be given to evaluating the overall quality of the information obtained using emerging computerized approaches, the impact on the interviewers and respondents of using computers to display the questions and enter respondents' answers, and the costs at each stage of the study. Computerized survey technologies are wonderful innovations. As with any other new invention, however, the most effective and efficient means of producing and using it needs to be explored and tested rather than simply assumed (Jones, 1999).

The topics and technologies evolving for health surveys present both challenges and opportunities in designing the samples for these studies. Health surveys have increasingly focused on rare or hard-to-locate populations. Innovative approaches are required to identify the universe or target population of interest, develop cost-effective methods for drawing the sample, and then find individuals to whom the questionnaire or interview should be administered. Survey designers must be aware of the methods that have been developed to identify and oversample rare populations and be prepared to invest time and resources to come up with the best sample design for their study.

Ethics

Asking people questions in surveys about aspects of their personal or professional lives always involves a consideration of the ethical issues posed by this process. Are the participants fully informed about the study, and do they voluntarily agree to participate? What benefits or harm may they experience if they participate? Will their right to remain anonymous and the confidentiality of the information they provide be maintained when the findings are reported? The evolution of the topics, techniques, and technologies just reviewed promises to heighten, rather than diminish, the importance of these ethical questions in the design and conduct of health surveys (Sudman, 1998).

The Privacy Rule enacted under the Health Insurance Portability and Accountability Act (HIPAA) of 1996 established minimum federal standards for protecting the privacy of individually identifiable health information. The Privacy Rule confers certain rights on individuals, including rights to access and amend their personal health information and to obtain a record of when and why this information has been shared with others for certain purposes. The Privacy Rule establishes conditions under which covered entities can provide researchers access to and use of personal health information when necessary to conduct research (National Institutes of Health, 2004; U.S. Department of Health and Human Services, Office for Civil Rights, 2005). The HIPAA legislation and related Privacy Rule requirements have imposed significant constraints on researchers in addressing issues of informed consent, the benefit versus harm to study participants, and rights of anonymity and confidentiality, as well as in obtaining Institutional Review Board (IRB) approval for the conduct of survey research. (An informative overview of the implications of these and related security and privacy issues for health surveys may be found in the series of papers presented in "Session 5: Security and Privacy," National Center for Health Statistics, 2004b.)

Informed Consent. The use of cold contact (unannounced) calls in random digit dialing telephone surveys permits very little advance information to be provided to the respondent about the nature of the study and the ways in which the information will be used. Survey designers are reluctant to spend much time giving respondents details on the survey for fear they will hang up. There is also little opportunity to elicit the formal written consent of respondents for what might be particularly sensitive topics. Respondents with what are perceived to be socially undesirable diseases and little means to pay for health care also may feel obligated to participate in a study if their providers ask them to do so, fearing that they will subsequently be refused treatment if they do not. From the providers' or researchers' perspectives, however, the increasingly complex and restrictive informed consent procedures may be viewed as seriously jeopardizing the ability to carry out reasonable scientific research protocols.

Benefit Versus Harm. Rational and ethical survey design attempts to ensure that the benefits outweigh the costs of participating. Asking people sensitive questions about threatening or difficult topics may call forth memories or emotions that are hard for them to handle. Most survey designers do not explicitly consider such costs to the respondents.

Providing monetary incentives does increase people's willingness to participate in surveys. However, more research is needed to examine the effect of such incentives on the quality of the information provided. Do respondents feel more obligated, for example, to give answers they think the interviewer wants to hear? Offering large incentives may also be viewed as raising questions about whether this is unduly coercive for certain respondents, such as poor or uninsured patients.

Rights of Anonymity and Confidentiality. Finally, an important issue in the design and conduct of surveys is guaranteeing the anonymity of survey respondents and the confidentiality of the information they provide. This issue is made more salient with the possibility of computerized linkages between sources, such as databases that link telephone numbers to household addresses or between survey data and medical records or billing information from providers. These issues have taken on even greater salience in the context of the HIPAA legislation, which sharply restricted the use of patient identifiers and introduced more stringent informed clearance for permitting access to medical record and related health plan data (National Institutes of Health, 2004; U.S. Department of Health and Human Services, Office for Civil Rights, 2005).

The United States has become an increasingly litigious society, as evidenced by the growing number of malpractice suits brought against health care providers. Survey designers can thus expect to confront more detailed and cumbersome review procedures for evaluating how the rights of study participants will be protected in carrying out the survey.

This environment compels that researchers, IRBs, and participating providers and funders devise means for constructive problem solving to protect the rights of study participants and ensure the feasibility of conducting sound research. *Reactive methodology* attempts to understand the dynamics that come into play and how best to resolve potential conflicts between those involved in the conduct and approval of the research (Sieber, 2004). "Reactive" refers to reactions to the proposed research by the potential study subjects, their community, the researchers, and other external forces such as HIPAA and related IRB procedures. It most essentially acknowledges that although regulations may dictate specific constraints on those who seek to conduct research, it is the relationships between and among the players that ultimately dictate whether the research can be conducted both responsibly and feasibly.

Defining Features of Surveys

Several key dimensions define the survey approach: (1) a research topic or problem of interest has been clearly delineated, (2) information on the issue is gathered by asking individuals questions, (3) the data collection process itself is systematic and well defined, (4) the purpose of the study is to generate group-level summary statistics, and (5) the results are generalizable to the groups represented by the individuals included in the study (American Statistical Association, Section on Survey Research Methods, 1998a, 1998b).

A number of these features are not unique to surveys, but taken together they tend to distinguish this data-gathering method from such other approaches as using existing record data, conducting participant or nonparticipant observational studies, or carrying out case studies of one or a limited number of programs, institutions, or related units. Researchers should not necessarily assume that surveys are always the best approach to use in gathering data. That decision depends on what best enables investigators to address the research questions of interest to them. Furthermore, survey developers are increasingly making use of qualitative research methods such as focus groups, in-depth unstructured interviews, or ethnographies to guide the development and interpretation of more structured surveys (Sale, Lohfeld, & Brazil, 2002; Sudman et al., 1996). The similarities and differences among these methods and surveys are reviewed in the following discussion.

Existing Record Sources

Health care investigators might decide that existing record data, such as the medical records available in hospitals or physicians' offices, claims data from private or public third-party insurers, or vital statistics records on births and causes of deaths, are the most useful and relevant sources for the types of information they need to gather for their study. Some of these sources may contain thousands of records that could be easily manipulated with high-powered personal computers. With these record sources, it will not be necessary to ask people questions directly to get the information. This is particularly true for factual data on concrete events that are fully and completely documented in existing sources. Data in such sources may, however, be inaccurate or incomplete, depending on the data quality standards governing gathering, entering, and verifying the information. If the investigator wishes to obtain more subjective, attitudinal data from individuals or to explore the probable accuracy or completeness of the information in the record sources, then designing a survey to ask people questions about the topic is required (Stewart & Kamins, 1993).

Participant or Nonparticipant Observation

In a second important method of data collection that differs from the survey approach, the investigator directly observes rather than asks individuals questions about particular situations or events. These observations may be relatively unstructured ones in which the researchers become, in effect, direct participants in the events. For example, this approach is used by medical anthropologists who live and work with members of a cultural subgroup (such as minority drug users or prostitutes) in order to establish the trust and rapport required to gain an understanding of certain health practices within that group (Jorgensen, 1989).

Structured observational methods require that the investigator have clearly delineated guidelines that indicate what to look for while observing the behaviors of interest. For example, researchers might want to record systematically patterns of interaction among family members during counseling sessions dealing with the addictive behavior of one of them. To do this, they could call on the procedures that social psychologists have developed for systematically inventorying and classifying such interactions. These approaches are also used in coding interviewers' and respondents' behaviors for the purpose of identifying problem questions during the instrument development phase of the study or to improve interviewer performance.

The principal way in which observational methods differ from surveys is that individuals are not asked questions directly to obtain needed information. In addition, the purpose of such research may be exploratory, that is, the investigator may want to get a better idea of what relationships or behaviors should be examined before going on to develop a comprehensive, formalized approach to gathering data on the topic. The investigator is usually not so interested in generating aggregate summary statistics that can be generalized to a larger target population when these methods are used. Instead, the focus is on the microcosm of activity being observed in the particular situation and what the investigator can learn from it.

Case Studies

Case studies of particular institutions or agencies (such as hospitals, managed care organizations, or neighborhood clinics) ask key informants questions about the organization, observe aspects of what is going on in the agency, or examine extant administrative or other record sources. The main difference between case studies and surveys is that in case studies, the investigators tend to focus on *a few elements to illustrate the type of unit* they are interested in learning about, whereas in a survey, they gather information *on a number of elements intended to represent a universe of units of that type.* Case studies take on more of the features of survey-based approaches to the extent that individuals are asked questions about themselves or their institutions; that a systematic, well-defined approach is used in deciding what questions to ask; and that the institutions or informants are selected with consideration given to the groups they represent (Yin, 2003).

If the investigators determine that a survey is the preferred method to elicit the information they need, they then have to decide whether they will try to do the study themselves, contract with a survey firm to carry it out, or make use of data that have already been gathered on the topic in other surveys.

Reasons for Studying Health Surveys

The reasons for studying health surveys are varied, but defining principles of survey design should guide the development, implementation, and assessment of all surveys.

To Design Good Surveys with Small Budgets

Most designers of health surveys do not have large grants or substantial institutional resources to support the conduct of large-scale studies. Students generally have a shoestring budget to carry out required thesis research. Academic researchers often use students in their classes or draw on limited faculty research funds to carry out surveys locally in their institutions or communities. State and community agency budgets are generally tight, and the boards of hospitals and health care organizations may encourage staff interested in conducting surveys to make use of institutional resources such as telephone, mail, or computer services to keep survey costs down. And doing good surveys does not always require large budgets. Either a Cadillac or a Ford will get you where you want to go; the same basic principles of sound engineering design apply to both. Survey developers should be aware of the fundamental principles behind the good design of even small surveys. It may be a matter of what you can afford. However, it is important to remember that the costs of poor survey design are also high.

To Learn About and from Well-Designed, Large-Scale Surveys with Large Budgets

Hundreds of millions of dollars have been spent in designing and executing large-scale national health surveys. The decennial census and Census Bureau–sponsored Current Population Surveys are useful sources of selected indicators of the health of the U.S. population. The National Center for Health Statistics routinely conducts surveys of the health of the U.S. population and the providers of health care. The Agency for Healthcare Research and Quality (formerly the Agency for Health Care Policy and Research) and the National Center for Health Statistics have conducted a number of large-scale special surveys on the health practices of the U.S. population and their levels and patterns of expenditures for medical care. In addition, a variety of methodological studies have been conducted in conjunction with these and other large-scale health surveys to identify sources of errors in this type of study and the decisions that should be made to reduce or eliminate them (Cohen, 2003; Mokdad, Stroup, Giles, & Behavioral Risk Factor Surveillance Team, 2003). The results of such studies are routinely published in the proceedings of conferences held by the American Statistical Association and the U.S. Bureau of the Census, as well as other governmental agencies (see Resource D).

Individuals interested in health surveys should be aware of these large-scale studies because they are a rich source of data on the nation's health and health care system. They also provide a gold mine of questions for inclusion in related studies, the answers to which can then be compared with national data. Finally, they have a great deal to teach us about how to do good surveys since resources are provided in the budgets of these surveys to assess the quality of the research itself.

To Be Aware of What to Look for in Conducting Secondary Analyses of Existing Health Survey Data Sets

Many researchers do not have the time or resources to carry out their own surveys. Extensive archives of national and local health survey data sets, such as the Inter-University Consortium for Political and Social Research at the University of Michigan, have been developed (see Resource D). Students, researchers, and program administrators and planners are being encouraged to make greater use of these secondary data sources, that is, data they were not involved in collecting (Kiecolt & Nathan, 1985; Moriarty et al., 1999; Shepard et al., 1999; Stewart & Kamins, 1993). These analyses can involve efforts to use existing data sets—state or national data collected for other purposes—to address a particular research question, such as the influence of the types of food children consume on obesity, or to make estimates for specific local areas or populations, such as the percentage of the population without insurance coverage. Small area estimation procedures have been developed to generate these latter estimates (Malec, 1995; Pfeffermann, 2002; Rao, 2003).

Users of secondary data sources should raise a number of questions, however, in considering the relevance of these data for their own research. How were people chosen for inclusion in the study? Were efforts made to evaluate the accuracy of the data obtained? How did researchers deal with people who refused to participate in the study or to answer certain questions? Are there particular features of how the sample was drawn that should be taken into account in analyzing the data? Awareness of these and other issues is essential to being an informed user of secondary health survey data sources.

To Know How to Evaluate and Choose Firms to Conduct Health Surveys

Health survey research is big business. Nonprofit, university-based survey organizations as well as for-profit commercial firms compete to obtain contracts with government agencies, academic researchers, and provider institutions for conducting national, state, and local health surveys. Some university-based or -affiliated survey research organizations that have conducted health surveys on a variety of topics include NORC (National Opinion Research Center, University of Chicago), Survey Research Center (University of California, Berkeley), Survey Research Center (University of Michigan), Survey Research Laboratory (University of Illinois), and the Wisconsin Survey Research Laboratory (University of Wisconsin). Other nonprofit firms that have been engaged in conducting large-scale health surveys include the Research Triangle Institute (University of North Carolina) and the RAND Corporation (Santa Monica, California). A number of commercial, for-profit firms have also carried out a range of health surveys under contract with public and private sponsoring agencies, including Abt Associates (Cambridge, Massachusetts), Gallup (Princeton, New Jersey), Louis Harris and Associates (New York), Mathematica Policy Research (Princeton, New Jersey), and Westat (Rockville, Maryland). The Web sites of these and other survey research entities could be consulted for descriptions of ongoing or completed studies and, in some cases, copies of survey questionnaires, summaries of study findings, and methodological reports.

These organizations emphasize different methods of data collection—in-person interviews, computer-assisted telephone interviews, or computer-assisted personal interviews—and different basic sample designs, and they use different types of data editing and data cleaning procedures. Researchers and agency and organizational representatives considering contracting with such organizations need to know their experience in doing health surveys and evaluate their capabilities for carrying out the proposed study.

To Become a Better-Informed Consumer of Health Survey Results

Opinion polls that summarize the American public's attitudes toward issues, such as whether children with HIV/AIDS should be admitted to public schools, often report that estimates vary plus or minus 3 percent for the sample as a whole or as much as plus or minus 7 percent for certain subgroups (African Americans, Hispanics) because only a small sample of the American public was interviewed to make these estimates. How does one use this information to decide whether a difference of 10 percent reported between African Americans and whites in support of the issue is "real" then? The administrator of a managed care organization is interested in the results of a survey of plan members' satisfaction with services in which only 50 percent of the members returned the questionnaire. Should she be concerned about whether the survey accurately represents all enrollees' attitudes toward the plan? Students and faculty conduct literature reviews of studies relevant to concepts of interest prior to formulating their own research proposals. If a study reports that an indicator of patient functional ability had a reliability coefficient of .80 when administered at two different times in the course of a week to a group of elderly patients, does that mean it is a fairly good measure? These are examples of the types of questions that could occur to consumers of health survey findings. This book identifies the criteria that can be applied in seeking to answer these and other questions about the quality of health survey data.

Framework for Classifying Topics in Health Surveys

Health surveys can cover a variety of topics, such as the ecology (distribution) and etiology (causes) of disease, the response to illness or maintenance of health on the part of the patient or the public, and the personnel and organizations in the health care professions (see Resource E). Health status is the explicit or implicit focus of health surveys, as defined here—studies that ask questions about factors that directly or indirectly influence, measure, or are affected by people's health. It is important to point out that health surveys may address more than one topic. A study may focus on one area of interest (out-of-pocket expenditures for care) but also include a range of related issues (health status, use of services) to examine their relationships to the major study variable. As will be discussed later, a survey may be principally concerned with describing a particular situation or with analyzing relationships between variables to explain why the situation is the way it is. The blocks outlined in Figure 1.1 reflect aspects that influence, measure, or are influenced by a person's health, and the arrows between them indicate relationships commonly hypothesized to exist between those elements. Health surveys can be used to examine the broader political, cultural, social, economic, and physical environment of a community, as well as the characteristics of the people who live there and the health care system that has evolved to serve them.

Characteristics of the Environment

Consideration of the predictors, indicators, and outcomes of health begins with the larger environment in which individuals live and work. Political, cultural, and social beliefs about health and medical care; the organization and status of the nation's or community's economy; and the nature of the physical environment itself

FIGURE 1.1. FRAMEWORK FOR
CLASSIFYING TOPICS IN HEALTH SURVEYS.

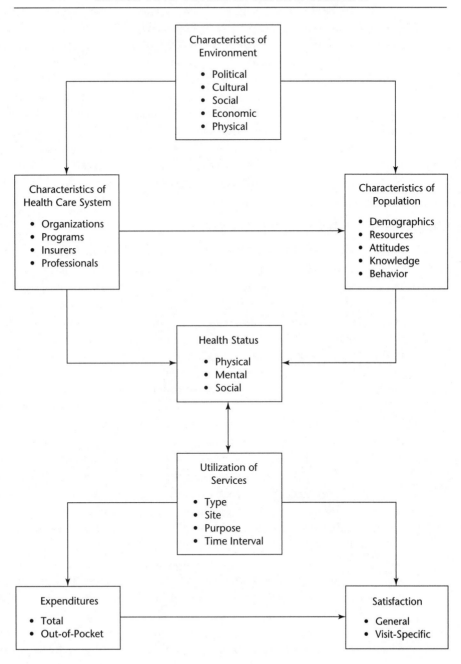

define both the limits and possibilities for health and health care of the individuals residing in a particular community.

Anthropologists and social scientists, for example, conduct cross-national or cross-cultural comparative surveys of how different groups define or respond to illness or the types of medical providers they consider appropriate for different symptoms. National, state, and local polls measure public opinion on issues, such as pending state health care reform legislation, and on more specific questions, such as whether universal health insurance should be provided, indigent undocumented residents should be entitled to Medicaid benefits, or persons with infectious diseases should be quarantined. Environmental and occupational safety and health scientists gather data on the waste disposal practices of major corporations and the extent to which residents report symptoms associated with radiation or chemical waste hazards identified in their neighborhoods or places of work.

Characteristics of the Health Care System

Surveys can be conducted of such health care organizations as hospitals, MCOs, community mental health centers, or hospices to learn about their basic structure or operations or their performance in terms of certain indicators—for example, the cost of delivering services. Many innovative health care programs have emerged in recent years, such as pain management clinics, programs for adult children of alcoholics, and employee work site programs, to deal with the special health care needs of selected groups. Surveys have been conducted of the client populations of these programs to determine whom they serve and what participants have gained from them. Managed care providers and health plans are developing and disseminating "report cards" on their performance, including the results of patient surveys of satisfaction and quality, to provide a more informed basis for consumers in choosing among competing options (Agency for Healthcare Research and Quality, n.d.-b; National Committee for Quality Assurance, n.d.).

Insurers are becoming an increasing focus of health care surveys because of concerns with the accelerating costs of medical care. Large-scale surveys of health care consumers often send questionnaires to insurers named by respondents to obtain detailed charge or cost data that individuals themselves may not be aware of when third parties pay their medical bills directly.

Health care professionals—physicians, dentists, nurses, allied health workers, and those in emerging health professions (such as complementary and alternative medicine specialties)—are a frequent focus of health care surveys. Surveys of health professionals have yielded information about the people who choose to go into the profession and why, the nature of the professional socialization experience and students' responses to it, factors that enter into the choice of specialty or practice location, the actual content and norms of care in professional practice, and the level of professional job or career satisfaction.

Characteristics of the Population

Surveys of the population at risk in a community have been widely used in needs assessment and strategic planning or marketing studies for new health care facilities or programs. Demographics, such as the age, sex, ethnic, and racial composition of a community, indicate the potential need and demand for certain medical services, such as prenatal care, preventive immunizations, hypertension screening, or elderly day care. Income levels and the type and extent of insurance coverage in a community reflect the resources available to individuals for purchasing medical care when they need it.

Responses to questionnaires about an individual's health and health care attitudes and knowledge may signal which groups are at particular risk of contracting certain illnesses (such as HIV/AIDS or cervical cancer) because of beliefs that demonstrate their ignorance of the disease or its causes or their unwillingness to seek appropriate screening or treatment services for it. There is increasing evidence that people who engage in certain personal health practices or behaviors, such as excessive smoking or alcohol consumption, and not others, such as exercising or eating breakfast regularly, experience higher morbidity (disease) and mortality (death) rates. With the promulgation by the U.S. Department of Health and Human Services of national objectives for promoting health and preventing disease, there has been a corresponding increase in national and local surveys that collect information on individual lifestyles and preventive self-care behaviors (National Center for Health Statistics, 2004g).

Health Status. A tremendous amount of effort has gone into clarifying and defining what is meant by the term *health* and in trying to develop valid and reliable indicators of the concept. The World Health Organization (WHO) offered a comprehensive definition of health as a "state of complete physical, mental, and social well-being and not merely the absence of disease or infirmity" (World Health Organization, 1948, p. 1). There is a growing interest in defining the goal of health policy to be improving the health of populations through broader medical and nonmedical public health and policy interventions. Measures of the health of populations reflect the health of individuals throughout the life course and take into account both premature mortality and measures of health-related quality of life (World Health Organization, 2002).

To determine health status, surveys can be based on individuals' own reports of their health or on clinical judgments or exams conducted by health professionals.

Furthermore, reports by individuals can reflect simply their subjective perceptions of how healthy they are (Is their health excellent, good, fair, or poor?) or describe the impact that being ill had on their ability to function in their daily lives (Did they have to take time off from work because of illness?). Differing conclusions about health can thus result depending on the dimension examined and the specific indicators chosen to measure it. A concern on the part of policymakers, consumers, insurers, and providers with measuring the outcomes of medical care has provided an added impetus to clarifying and refining both the predictors and indicators of health status (McDowell & Newell, 1996; Patrick & Erickson, 1993).

Utilization of Services. The environment in which individuals find themselves, the health care system available to serve them, their own characteristics and resources, and their state of health and well-being all influence whether they seek medical care and with what frequency. Surveys of health care utilization could ask questions to determine the type of service used (hospital, physician, dentist), the site or location at which the services are received (inpatient ward, emergency room, doctor's office, public health clinic), the purpose of the visit (preventive, illness related, or long-term custodial care), and the time interval of use (whether services were received, the volume of services received, or the continuity or pattern of visits during a given time period) (Aday & Awe, 1997). Presumably the use of health services also ultimately leads to improved health. This concept of health as both a predictor and an outcome of utilization is reflected in Figure 1.1 in the double-headed arrow between "health status" and "utilization of services." The growing focus on measuring the outcomes of medical care presents special challenges to survey researchers and others in developing or choosing the appropriate measures of health status and in designing studies that can accurately attribute observed outcomes to provider decision making. As when choosing health status measures in surveys, survey researchers should consider the particular dimensions they want to tap in their study and how precedents from other studies or methodological research on various ways of collecting health care utilization data inform those choices.

Expenditures. The cost of medical care has become a particular concern among consumers, policymakers, and health care providers. A number of large-scale national surveys and program demonstrations have examined patterns of expenditures for health care services for the U.S. population as a whole and for individuals in different types of health insurance plans (see Resource E).

Surveys are particularly useful for obtaining information on out-of-pocket expenditures for medical care and the private or public third-party payers, if any, that covered the bulk of the medical bills. As already mentioned, it is often necessary to go to insurers or providers directly to obtain information on the total charges for services that individuals received. It may require even more effort and creativity on the part of the researcher to estimate the actual "costs" of the care, which may differ from the "charges" for it because of markups to cover other services or patients for whom no payment was received.

Satisfaction. The experience people have when they go for medical care and how much they have to pay for it out of pocket have been found to be important influences on their satisfaction with medical care in general or with a particular visit to a health provider. Because of an increased emphasis on patient-centered care, many hospitals and provider settings have assigned greater weight to developing and implementing surveys of patient satisfaction with the services received (Rao, Weinberger, & Kroenke, 2000; Wensing & Elwyn, 2002; Wensing & Grol, 2000). A number of questions and attitude scales for measuring patient satisfaction with medical care have been developed and used in health surveys. (Specific examples are discussed in Chapter Eleven.) Designers of health surveys incorporating patient satisfaction measures should learn about these and other ways of asking satisfaction questions, how well they have worked in other studies, their relevance for the particular survey being considered, and how to modify them to increase their relevance or applicability to the population to be studied.

Examples of Health Surveys

It is not possible in the context of this book to provide a comprehensive inventory of the health surveys that have been conducted in the United States and other countries. However, Resource D offers a summary of sources of information on health surveys, and Resource E provides selected examples of major surveys that have been conducted internationally, nationally, and at the state and local levels. For each survey, a profile of the topics addressed, the research design, the population or sample included, and the method of data collection used are provided. Health survey researchers should be aware of the analyses that these studies have yielded on the topics of interest to them as well as the questions or methods used in those studies that they might employ in designing their own surveys.

In addition to numerous other examples, three surveys in particular will be used to illustrate many of the aspects of survey and questionnaire design that are in the chapters that follow. The UNICEF Multiple Indicator Cluster Survey (MICS) was intended to measure and monitor World Summit for Children indicators of child survival and development in participating countries and to compare the indicators within countries and across countries at mid-decade (1995) and end of decade (2000). A subsequent round of surveys (2005) was initiated to monitor World Fit for the Millennium Development Goals and related international health initiatives (UNICEF, n.d.). The California Health Interview Survey (CHIS) provides local-level estimates on a variety of public health topics, such as health status, health care access, and insurance coverage, for most counties in California as well as statewide estimates for California's overall population and its larger racial/ethnic groups, as well as for several smaller ethnic groups (UCLA Center for Health Policy Research, 2005). The CHIS was conducted in 2001, 2003, and 2005. The National Dental Malpractice Survey (NDMS) described dental malpractice insurance experience in a representative sample of U.S. dentists in 1991 and analyzed the practice characteristics that were predictive of dental malpractice insurance experience among U.S. dentists (Washington State University, Social and Economic Sciences Research Center, 1993). Sources for obtaining information on the questionnaires and the methodology for these studies are provided in Resources A, B, and C, respectively.

These three studies were chosen principally because they provide examples of the range of design alternatives that are available in doing health surveys. First, each involved different methods of data collection. The UNICEF MICS was conducted through personal interviews with family members in households selected for the study, the CHIS survey collected data through telephone interviews, and the dentist study sent a mail questionnaire to eligible providers. The UNICEF MICS is national and international in scope; the CHIS survey was a general population survey of people with telephones statewide, drawing sample from all counties; and the NDMS was based on a national list sample of dentists. The basic research designs for the studies were also different. (The different types of research designs that can be chosen in developing health surveys are discussed in Chapter Two.) The sample designs for the studies differed as well, with the UNICEF MICS relying on an area probability method of sampling, the CHIS primarily on random digit dialing, and the dentist survey on a list sample (these three designs are discussed in more detail in Chapter Six). The UNICEF MICS interview gathered information on the household in general, mothers, children under age five, and children ages five to fifteen, whereas the CHIS selected one adult respondent and, if present in the household, one child (under age twelve) and one adolescent (ages twelve to seventeen).

The survey questionnaires for the respective studies also reflect an array of health topics and different categories of questions relating to demographic characteristics, health behaviors, attitudes, knowledge, and need measured in a variety of ways. These three studies thus illustrate the range of choices that a researcher has in designing a survey.

Steps in Designing and Conducting a Survey

Good survey design is basically a matter of good planning. Exhibit 1.1 presents a picture of the survey research process experienced by investigators who fail to think about the steps involved in doing a study before they begin.

The principal steps in designing and conducting surveys and the chapters of this book in which they are discussed are displayed in Figure 1.2. A number of feedback loops appear in Figure 1.2 to reflect the fact that designing surveys is a dynamic, iterative, and interactive process. Many decisions have to be made in tandem; the advent of computerized systems that can be used to carry out many or all phases of the survey has made this even more true.

Previous experience and personal or professional interests can lead researchers to want more information about a particular issue. For academically oriented researchers, the problem could be stated in terms of study hypotheses about what they expect to find given their theoretical understanding of the topic. For business-oriented investigators, the problem could be stated in terms of precise questions that need to be answered to inform a firm's marketing, strategic planning, program development, or institutional evaluation decision-making activities.

The specification of the problem should be guided by what others have learned and written about it already. Reviewing the literature on related research, acquiring copies of questionnaires or descriptions of procedures used in studies on comparable topics, and consulting with experts knowledgeable in the field or associated with one's own institution can be extremely valuable in clarifying the focus of the survey.

The statement of the problem that emerges from this process should then serve as the reference point for all the steps that follow. This statement is the most visible marker on the landscape to guide the rest of the steps in the journey. These steps include defining the variables to be measured in the study, planning how the data will be used (or analyzed), choosing the methods for collecting the data, drawing the sample, formulating the questions and questionnaire to be used in the survey, collecting the data, preparing and analyzing them, and, finally, writing the research report.

A total survey design approach to planning surveys considers the impact of decisions at each of these steps on the overall quality and cost of the study (Biemer & Lyberg, 2003; Dillman, 2000; Groves, 1989). It also involves consideration of the fact that these steps are iterative and interdependent—that is, decisions made at one point in the survey design process should anticipate the steps that follow, and revisions to the original design will be required if unanticipated circumstances are encountered in the course of the study.

EXHIBIT 1.1. A TYPICAL SURVEY RESEARCH PROJECT.

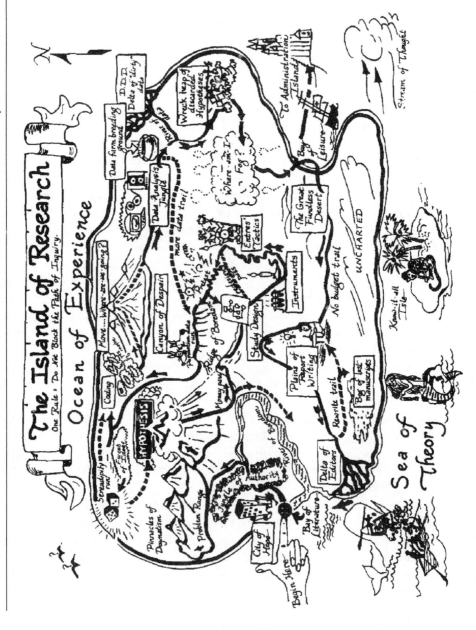

Note: Permission to reprint this figure granted by Ernest Harburg.

FIGURE 1.2. STEPS IN DESIGNING AND CONDUCTING A SURVEY.

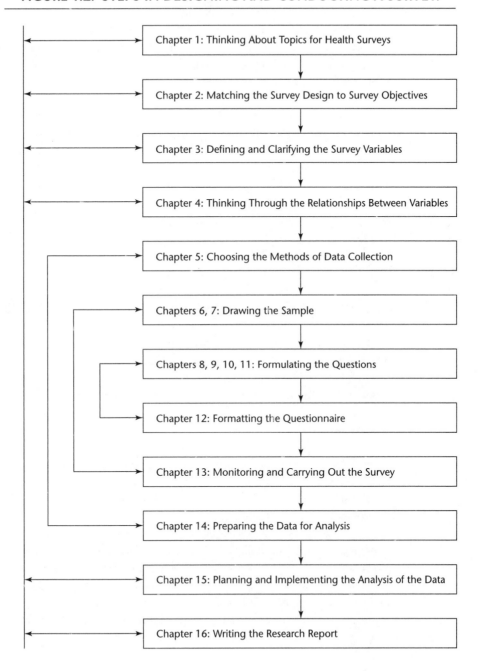

The method chosen for preparing the data for analysis can affect how the investigator decides to collect the data (see Figure 1.2). For example, if the researcher wants to build in checks on the accuracy of the data at the time they are being collected or otherwise expedite subsequent coding and data-processing procedures, it would be well to use a computer-assisted data collection approach. The quality of the training of the field staff and the specification of the data collection procedures will affect how well the sample design for the study is executed. Decisions about the ultimate format of the questionnaire and the way in which it will be administered to respondents will influence the questions that can be asked and how. Furthermore, the final form of the research report and the analyses that are carried out with the data should be planned at the beginning—not at the end—of the study, and they should be based on careful formulation of the research questions and an analysis plan for the project.

Framework for Minimizing Errors and Maximizing Quality in Surveys

A total survey error framework to guide decision making at each stage of the survey design process to help ensure accuracy and consistency of survey results will be used in presenting the steps for carrying out health surveys in the chapters that follow (see Table 1.1.) This framework is intended to provide a set of general principles, as well as specific guidelines, to facilitate survey developers' thinking critically about the implications of their decisions for the quality and usefulness of the data to which they and others have committed time and resources gathering.

A study carried out in the late 1970s by a special committee appointed by the Subsection on Survey Research Methods of the American Statistical Association, with support from the National Science Foundation, found—perhaps not surprisingly—that most surveys could be improved. Fifteen of twenty-six federal surveys and seven of ten nonfederal surveys studied had one or more major study design problems (Bailar & Lanphier, 1978).

In 1979 Andersen and his colleagues at the University of Chicago used a total survey error framework for identifying all the possible sources of bias and variable errors associated with both the sampling and nonsampling steps in designing health surveys. They then applied this framework to measure directly the magnitude of certain of these errors in a 1970 national survey of health care utilization and expenditures. The authors found that the type and magnitude of errors varied for different types of health and health care variables (Andersen, Kasper, Frankel, & Associates, 1979).

TABLE 1.1. TYPES OF SURVEY ERRORS.

A. No Bias, Low Variable Error

```
                    x
                    x
                    x
                    x
              x     x     x
              x     x     x
        x     x     x     x     x
        x     x     x     x     x
        x     x     x     x     x
        x     x     x     x     x
```

B. High (–) Bias, Low Variable Error

```
        x
        x
        x
        x
   x    x    x
   x    x    x
x  x    x    x    x
x  x    x    x    x
x  x    x    x    x
x  x    x    x    x
```

C. No Bias, High Variable Error

```
                 x    x
            x    x    x    x
        x   x    x    x    x    x
    x   x   x    x    x    x    x    x
x   x   x   x    x    x    x    x    x    x
```

D. High (–) Bias, High Variable Error

```
              x    x
         x    x    x    x
      x  x    x    x    x    x
   x  x  x    x    x    x    x    x
x  x  x  x    x    x    x    x    x    x
```

– Bias $\overline{X}$ + Bias

(True Value)

Presentations at a series of conferences on health survey research methods and procedures sponsored by the Agency for Healthcare Research and Quality (formerly the Agency for Health Care Policy and Research), National Center for Health Statistics, and other public and private sources have argued for the utility of a total survey design and related total survey error framework in enhancing the quality and reducing the costs of health surveys (National Center for Health Services Research, 1977, 1978, 1981, 1984, 1989; National Center for Health Statistics, 1996, 2001, 2004b). Robert Groves (1989), Don Dillman (2000), Paul Biemer, Lars Lyberg (Biemer, Groves, Lyberg, Mathiowetz, & Sudman, 1991; Biemer & Lyberg, 2003), and others (Lessler & Kalsbeek, 1992; Schwarz & Sudman, 1996; Sudman et al., 1996; Tanur, 1992; Weisberg, 2003) have made significant theoretical and empirical contributions to identifying and addressing the major types and costs of errors associated with the sampling and nonsampling aspects of designing both health and other surveys. The total survey error framework has led to the practical application of the related principles of Continuous Quality Improvement (CQI) and Total Quality Management (TQM) in designing systems to enhance the quality of survey data collection and processing (Biemer & Caspar, 1994; Biemer & Lyberg, 2003; Collins & Sykes, 1999; Lyberg et al., 1997; White & Hauan, 2002).

The field has evolved from focusing on constructing estimates of the total magnitude of error to designing and monitoring the study to ensure that standards of quality are maintained throughout the survey design and implementation process. Quantitative benchmarks of the quality of specific survey procedures become sentinel indicators of whether adjustments are needed to ensure a high-quality survey process and product. There is also a greater emphasis on the end users of survey data and results and whether the data and findings are applicable and interpretable on the part of the ultimate audience for the research.

The errors frequently made in designing and conducting surveys can be classified as either systematic ("bias") or random ("variable") errors (see Table 1.1). A bias involves a fixed departure of a statistic (such as a mean or proportion) across samples (or replications) in a particular (positive or negative) direction from the underlying actual (or true) population value for the estimate. Thus, the sample values are consistently higher or lower than the real value. Variable errors involve varying departures of the statistic (sometimes in a positive and sometimes in a negative direction) from the true population value. This means that the sample values vary or are spread out around the true value across samples (Andersen et al., 1979; Biemer & Lyberg, 2003; Groves, 1987, 1989). The combined or total error may be expressed as the mean square error (MSE), or the sum of the variable error (variance) and bias squared:

$$MSE = VARIANCE + BIAS^2$$

The further the estimate for the sample (such as a mean) is from the true population value—whether higher (+) or lower (−)—and the wider the spread (or variation) in the values obtained for a given sample, the greater the total survey error is. Though rarely measured fully and directly in a survey, the reference point provided by the concept of these two types of errors considered separately and in combination is useful for identifying and mitigating their occurrence or magnitude through thoughtful survey design. These two types of total survey error are portrayed graphically in Table 1.1, discussed in the following paragraphs, and elaborated in Chapter Sixteen (Table 16.2):

A. *No bias, low variable error.* When survey procedures yield estimates that basically cluster around the true value, as with example A in Table 1.1, they are said to be both unbiased and consistent. These are surveys in which the questions are valid and reliable. No substantial noncoverage or nonresponse problems were encountered in designing and executing the sample. That is, everyone who should have been eligible for the study had an opportunity to be included in the sample, a high proportion of those who were selected responded, and the size of the sample was large enough to minimize the standard (sampling) errors of the estimates derived from it.

B. *High bias, low variable error.* If procedures yield consistently inaccurate estimates (as with example B in the table), then the degree of bias is very high. One could, for example, design a question to ask about average weekly alcohol consumption that would yield fairly similar results if asked of the same respondents six months apart but that would still underestimate the rates of use for alcoholics. The refusal of heavy drinkers to participate in the survey could also create problems in this kind of study. The resulting nonresponse bias would contribute to the underestimation of alcohol use in the target population.

C. *No bias, high variable error.* Some measures or procedures may yield different results on different occasions or in different survey situations without any consistent pattern in one direction (higher or lower than the true value), as with example C in the table. These results could occur when questions with low reliability (stability) are used to measure the concept of interest (X) or when the sample size is too small to provide very precise estimates.

D. *High bias, high variable error.* If, in contrast, the researcher gets different answers each time the question is asked and these answers are consistently different (higher or lower, for example) from the right answer to the question, then the resulting estimate has a high degree of bias *and* variable error. Survey results are just the opposite of those described in example A. They are neither consistent nor accurate (as in example D in the table).

The total survey error summarized here and depicted in Table 1.1 will guide the presentation of both specific and general principles to apply in the aspects of designing a survey addressed in the chapters that follow.

No survey is ever error free. However, this book is intended to increase aware-ness of standards to use in identifying the type and magnitude of the problems that can arise in designing and conducting surveys and the alternatives available to minimize them.

Supplementary Sources

For a history and general overview of academic, governmental, and market-oriented polling and survey research, see Bulmer, Bales, and Sklar (1991) and Hyman (1991). Consult Resources D and E for additional sources and examples of health surveys. For an overview of survey design in general, see Abramson and Abramson (1999), Alreck and Settle (2004), Fowler (2002), and *The Survey Kit* (Fink, 2003). The approach to total survey error is discussed more fully in Chapters Eight and Sixteen.

CHAPTER TWO

MATCHING THE SURVEY DESIGN TO SURVEY OBJECTIVES

Chapter Highlights

1. Study designs for health surveys differ principally in terms of the number of groups explicitly included in the study—based on the criteria for including them—and the number of points in time and reference periods for collecting the data.
2. The first step in choosing the appropriate design for a survey is to formulate the research question to be addressed in the study based on who and what the focus of the survey will be, when and where it will be conducted, and (if applicable) what the researcher expects to find and why.
3. Study objectives help clarify what the researcher needs to do to answer the research question. Study hypotheses are statements of the answers the researcher expects to find based on previous research or experience.

This chapter provides guidance for designing surveys to address different types of research questions. In particular, it presents the types of designs that can be used to address various questions (Table 2.1), shows how to state the questions themselves (Tables 2.2 and 2.3), and discusses related study objectives and hypotheses (Figure 2.1).

The discussion that follows draws on contributions from the disciplines of epidemiology and sociology. Epidemiology is the study of the distribution and causes of disease and related medical conditions in populations. It addresses research questions such as, "Who gets sick in a community and why?" Since chronic, rather than infectious, diseases are now the leading cause of death in many countries, the discipline has turned to examining the total environment of an individual and the multitude of factors that can affect whether he or she develops a particular disease rather than focusing on a single causal agent of the condition.

Emerging paradigms within the field encourage exploring the causes of disease at a variety of levels (family, neighborhood, community) and within the historical context of societies *and* the life course of individuals. Corresponding to these developments, population-based health surveys are used by epidemiologists to explore the person's environment as a whole (community, neighborhood, family, and work) and the variety of both distal factors (income, education, social support) and proximal factors (diet, stress, smoking behavior) that could give rise to a greater risk of illness—that is, those that are more upstream versus downstream, respectively, in the sequence of exposures or events leading to the onset of illness. Qualitative ethnographic methods are also being increasingly used as a complement to such surveys to gain a fuller understanding of the role of culture and context in influencing these fundamental determinants of health, and in designing more culturally relevant surveys (Link & Phelan, 1995; Schwartz, Susser, & Susser, 1999; Susser & Susser, 1996a, 1996b).

Geographic information systems (GIS) provide another useful complement to surveys by facilitating the linking of socioeconomic and environmental characteristics to the geographical areas (such as census tracts, cities, or counties) in which survey respondents live (Krieger, Chen, Waterman, Rehkopf, & Subramanian, 2003; Ricketts, 2002).

Sociologists have also made major contributions to developing and refining the use of the survey method for gathering information from individuals representative of some population of interest (Babbie, 2004). They have, for example, developed broad conceptual frameworks to explain health care behavior that can be used to guide the development of study hypotheses and the selection of questions to include in the survey. Often, however, there is not an adequate translation of concepts and methods from either epidemiology or sociology in designing health surveys. This chapter draws on contributions from both disciplines to provide guidance for what different types of health survey designs can accomplish.

Types of Study Designs

Epidemiologists usually identify two major types of epidemiological study designs: *experimental* and *observational* (Hulley et al., 2001; Rothman, 2002). (See Table 2.1.) The two are distinguished principally with respect to whether the treatment or intervention (or major factor of interest in the study) is under the control of the investigator. In experimental studies, the investigator introduces a factor or intervenes in the environment of the study subjects (such as introducing a mass immunization program for preschool children in a certain community) to see what impact the intervention has on the study subjects (incidence of measles) compared with a group of subjects (in another community) that did not have the intervention.

In observational studies, the investigators do not directly intervene but instead develop methods for describing events that occur naturally without their direct intervention (identifying which children have already been immunized and which have not) and the effect that this has on study subjects (incidence of measles for both groups).

TABLE 2.1. TYPES OF STUDY DESIGNS.

| | *Characteristics* | | | |
| | *Groups* | | *Time Periods* | |
Types of Study Design	**Number of Groups**	**Criteria for Selection of Groups**	**Number of Periods of Data Collection**	**Reference Periods for Data Collection**
Observational Cross-sectional (one-group)	1	Population of interest	1	Present (and recall of past)
Group-comparison (Case-control)	2 or more	Population subgroups with and without characteristic of interest	1	Present and recall of past
Longitudinal (prospective)	1 or 2 or more	Population or subgroups that are and are not likely to develop characteristic of interest	2 or more	Present and future
Experimental "True" experiment	2 or more	Randomly determined subgroups of population	2 or more	Present and future

Furthermore, observational studies can be either descriptive or analytical in emphasis, depending on the types of research questions they address. *Descriptive surveys* provide a profile of the characteristics of a population or group of interest (proportion with measles). *Analytical studies* ask why the group has the characteristics (measles) it does (by examining the prior immunization status of study objects, for example). These studies entail testing statistical hypotheses regarding the likely association between variables or differences between groups. In general, the methods that have been increasingly used by epidemiologists are much more analytical than descriptive in design (Schwartz et al., 1999). There are three major types of observational study designs: *cross-sectional, group-comparison,* and *longitudinal.* The distinguishing features of these three designs, as well as of the experimental study design, are summarized in Table 2.1. The designs differ principally in two ways: (1) the number of groups explicitly included in the study and the criteria for choosing them and (2) the number of points in time and reference periods for gathering the data.

Cross-sectional designs generally focus on a single group representative of some population of interest. Data are gathered at a single point in time. The reference period for the characteristics that study subjects are asked to report may, however, be either for that point in time or for some reasonable period of time that they can recall in the past.

Group-comparison designs explicitly focus on two or more groups chosen because one has a characteristic of interest and the other does not. Data are collected at one point in time, as is the case with the cross-sectional design. Similarly, the reference period for asking study subjects questions may be either the present or some period of time in the past. Analytical group-comparison designs (termed *case-control* or *retrospective* designs in epidemiological studies) make an explicit effort to look back in time at the factors that may have given rise to one group having the characteristic (a particular disease, for example) and the other not having it.

Longitudinal designs focus on a population or subgroup, some members of which will be exposed to or experience certain events over time while others will not. Data are collected at more than one point in time, and the reference period is prospective rather than retrospective—that is, the investigator looks to the future, rather than the past, in describing and explaining the occurrence of the characteristic of interest.

In contrast to observational studies, experimental designs involve directly testing whether a treatment or a program that is thought to produce certain outcomes actually does produce them by assigning the treatment to one group but not another and then comparing the changes that take place in the two groups over time. Experimental designs thus include elements of cross-sectional, group-comparison, and longitudinal research designs.

Most observational studies combine elements of these respective designs as well. For example, a researcher might be interested in collecting data on high school seniors at the beginning of their senior year regarding their smoking practices; compare white, black, Hispanic, and Asian students regarding their smoking behavior; and then collect data at the end of their senior year to see if the practices had changed in general and across the different groups. The following discussion presents examples of each of the major types of observational and experimental designs to illuminate the distinctive features of each. Descriptive and analytical examples of each observational study design are also provided.

Observational Designs

The three principal types of observational designs are cross-sectional, group-comparison, and longitudinal designs.

Cross-Sectional Designs. A researcher may decide to do a one-time survey to profile a population or group of interest; this would be a descriptive cross-sectional survey design. It provides a slice of life at a particular point in time. For example, epidemiological prevalence studies estimate the prevailing rates of illness or related conditions in a population at a designated point in time (Hulley et al., 2001; Last, Spasoff, Harris, & Thuriaux, 2001; Rothman, 2002). Thus, a public health department might conduct a house-to-house survey in a neighborhood with high concentrations of Hispanics to estimate the proportion of preschool children who have not been immunized. Such a study would provide an assessment of the need for this service in the community at that time.

Analytical cross-sectional surveys search for explanations by examining the statistical association (or correlation) of variables gathered in a one-time survey. This type of survey addresses questions such as, "Are homosexual males who say they practice 'safe sex' less likely to have AIDS or HIV antibodies in their blood than are sexually active homosexual males who do not use these methods?" Analytical designs assume that the investigator has a specific statistical hypothesis in mind to test.

Many epidemiologists, as well as social scientists, do not draw sharp distinctions between descriptive and analytical cross-sectional surveys. Most investigators are interested in looking at the relationships of certain characteristics of the study subjects (such as their age, sex, race, and so on) to others (presence or absence of a disease) when doing cross-sectional surveys.

Designers of cross-sectional surveys should determine whether they simply want a snapshot of the population they will be surveying or if there are relationships between factors they will ultimately want to examine once the data are collected in order to be sure to ask questions about those factors in their survey. Even if the investigator simply wants to profile the population, thought should be given to what characteristics it is important to profile and why—*before* undertaking the study.

Group-Comparison Designs. In descriptive group-comparison designs, different groups are compared at approximately the same point in time. For example, a hospital administrator might be interested in the attitudes of physicians, nurses, and nonclinical staff toward a new patient safety monitoring system in the hospital. A survey could be administered to each of the groups and the results compared.

Analytical group-comparison designs are what epidemiologists call *case-control* or *retrospective* studies. In these studies, the past history of groups with and without a disease is retraced and compared to address the question of why the one group contracted it and the other did not. They are called *case-control* studies because the cases (that have the disease) are compared with the control group (that does not). With retrospective designs, the groups being compared are identified after the fact: it is known that one group has the illness (or condition) and the other does not. This is in contrast to prospective designs, which wait and see if the illness develops over time and for whom or to cross-sectional studies that take a look at who has the illness now and who does not and explore why statistically. However, epidemiologists do not generally distinguish between cross-sectional and between-group retrospective designs since both could focus on the recall of factors in the past that help explain a current characteristic of the groups of interest.

Longitudinal Designs. Surveys may also be conducted at different points in time to estimate how things change longitudinally, or over time. These longitudinal survey designs differ primarily in terms of whether the sample or populations surveyed are the same or different at the successive time periods (Binder, 1998; Ruspini, 2000; Trivellato, 1999).

Trend studies may be viewed as a series of cross-sectional surveys. They basically involve different samples of comparable populations over time. The National Center for Health Statistics, for example, conducts the National Health Interview Survey of the U.S. population annually. The size and composition of this population change each year, as does the particular sample chosen for the survey itself. Nevertheless, the survey provides a rich source of data over time on the health and health care of the American people (National Center for Health Statistics, 2005g).

Panel studies attempt to study the same sample of people at different times. The Medicare Current Beneficiary Survey, sponsored by the Centers for Medicare and Medicaid Services, is an example of a panel survey design. Respondents are interviewed three times each year over a four-year period. This panel design is intended to capture changes in health status, use, and coverage over time as well as to facilitate the quality and completeness of the complex utilization and expenditure data gathered in that study based on a shorter recall period (Centers for Medicare and Medicaid Services, 2004).

Longitudinal designs are used in epidemiological studies of disease incidence, that is, the rate of new occurrences (or incidents) of the disease over time (Hulley et al., 2001; Last et al., 2001; Rothman, 2002). Analytical longitudinal surveys refer to what epidemiologists term *prospective* or *cohort* studies. These involve studies of samples of populations over time to see whether people who are exposed at differing rates to factors (such as engaging in "unsafe" homosexual acts) thought likely to affect the occurrence of a disease (such as HIV/AIDS) do indeed ultimately contract the illness at correspondingly different rates. This type of design is termed *prospective* because it looks to the future "prospects" of the person's developing the illness, given the chances he takes over time in engaging in high-risk behavior.

Epidemiological cohort studies include the Framingham Study in Massachusetts, the Alameda County Study in California, and the Medical Research Council National Survey of Health and Development in Great Britain (also known as the British 1946 birth cohort study), among others, in which cohorts of members of selected individuals or communities are followed over decades and data gathered on health risks and related disease incidence (Inter-University Consortium for Political and Social Research, n.d.; Framingham.com, 1995; Imperial College London, 2004). Studies of this kind provide a better opportunity than one-time cross-sectional studies to examine whether certain behaviors do in fact lead to (or cause) the disease.

Experimental Designs

The most powerful type of design to evaluate what factors cause an illness or lead to certain outcomes is experiments in which the researcher directly controls who receives a certain type of treatment. Surveys can be used to collect both baseline (pretreatment) and follow-up (posttreatment) data on those who received the treatment (experimental group) and those who did not (control group). "True" experiments generally assume that individuals in the experimental and control groups are equivalent, so that the only reason they might differ on the outcomes of interest is the program or intervention itself. Randomly assigning a subject to either the experimental or control group is the means generally used to establish equivalence between the two groups. However, numerous ethical issues arise in implementing these kinds of studies. As a result, many social experiments or program evaluations are actually quasi-experiments in which some aspect of a true experiment has to be modified or dropped because of ethical or other real-world constraints

(Bickman, 2000; Campbell & Russo, 1999; Grembowski, 2001; Shadish, Cook, & Campbell, 2002).

Randomized trials have been a key component of clinical and pharmaceutical research to evaluate the efficacy of alternative therapeutic regimens and are being increasingly applied in health services research on the cost, quality, and effectiveness of medical care (Donenberg, Lyons, & Howard, 1999). Epidemiologists have conducted community or place-randomized trials in which entire communities are exposed to certain public health interventions, such as a water fluoridation program, prevention trials, or health education campaign, and indicators of health outcomes are compared over time or with communities that did not have such programs (Boruch et al., 2004; Stone, Pearson, Fortmann, & McKinlay, 1997; Victora, Habicht, & Bryce, 2004). The RAND Health Insurance Experiment (described in Resource E) is an example of a large-scale social experiment to evaluate the impact of varying the type and extent of insurance coverage on people's health, as well as on their utilization of and expenditures for health care. Surveys were a major part of that study.

Much can go wrong in the data collection process with surveys that take on special importance in social survey-based experiments or quasi-experimental program evaluations. In those studies, it is particularly important "to keep the noise down" so that one can detect whether the signals that the program worked are loud and clear. A variety of factors in the design of surveys administered at different points in time (such as minor revisions in question wording) or changes in the health care environment as a whole (improved medical diagnostic procedures, for example) that are not taken into account in designing longitudinal surveys can also directly affect interpretations of data collected to reflect changes in the nation's health over time (Murray, Moskowitz, & Dent, 1996; Stone et al., 1997).

This discussion of alternative designs for health surveys is intended to provide a framework to refine and clarify what a particular study might accomplish and at what level of effort and complexity.

Stating the Research Question for Different Study Designs

What are you interested in finding out? *Whom* do you want to study? *Where* are these people or organizations located? *When* do you want to do the survey? What do you expect to learn and *why?* These are the questions survey designers should ask themselves as guides to formulating the major research question or statement of the problem to be addressed by the study (see Table 2.2).

What investigators will be studying should be guided by the health topics they are interested in and what they would like to learn about them. A survey researcher

TABLE 2.2. STATING THE RESEARCH QUESTION FOR DIFFERENT STUDY DESIGNS.

Elements of Research Question	Descriptive			Analytical			
	Cross-Sectional	Group-Comparison	Longitudinal	Cross-Sectional	Case-Control	Prospective	Experimental
What?	What is the *prevalence* of cigarette smokers	Do the characteristics of those who are cigarette smokers and those who are not *differ*	What is the *incidence* of cigarette smokers	Are cigarette smokers *more likely* than nonsmokers	Are cigarette smokers *more likely* than nonsmokers	Is the *incidence* of cigarette smokers *greater*	Is the *incidence* of cigarette smokers *less*
Who?	among seniors	among seniors	among seniors	among seniors	among seniors	among seniors	among seniors
Where?	of a large urban high school	of a large urban high school	of a large urban high school	of a large urban high school	of a large urban high school	of a large urban high school	of a large urban high school
When?	in the last month of school?	in the last month of school?	between the first and the last month of school?	in the last month of school	in the last month of school	between the first and the last month of school	between the first and the last month of school
Why?	—	—	—	to have friends who smoke?	to have friends who have a history of smoking?	for those whose friends start to smoke?	for those randomly assigned to a teen peer antismoking program?

might, for example, be interested in the topic of smoking. Is he or she interested in people's attitudes or knowledge about smoking, their actual smoking behavior, or all of these aspects of the issue? Furthermore, is the researcher interested in studying smoking in general or one particular type of smoking, such as cigarette smoking? Perhaps the investigator is concerned with smoking as an aspect of some broader concept, such as health habits or self-care behavior. The researcher should then have an idea of how a study of smoking fits into learning about these more general concepts of interest. In either case, the investigator should clearly and unambiguously state *what* he or she is interested in studying and have in mind specific questions that could be asked of real-world respondents to get at those issues. In determining what the focus of their study will be, researchers should be guided not only by their own interests but also by the previous research that has been conducted on the topic.

A review of the example provided in Table 2.2 suggests that the focus of a study may be different for different survey designs. Descriptive studies focus on the characteristics of interest for a group at a particular point in time (cross-sectional design) or over time (longitudinal design) or on the differences that exist between certain groups on the characteristics of interest (group-comparison design). Analytical designs speculate on the relationship of the characteristics of interest (cigarette smoking behavior, for example) with some other factors (friends' smoking behavior). Experimental designs directly evaluate the impact of a program or intervention (antismoking seminars) on some outcome of interest (incidence of first-time smokers) in the experiment.

The principal distinguishing features of descriptive and analytical designs may be summarized as follows:

Descriptive	*Analytical*
Estimates	Explains
Is more exploratory	Is more explanatory
Profiles characteristics of group	Analyzes why group has characteristics
Focuses on *what?*	Focuses on *why?*
Assumes no statistical hypothesis	Assumes a statistical hypothesis
Does not require comparisons (between groups or over time)	Requires comparisons (between groups or over time)

At the same time that the investigator decides what the primary focus of the study will be, he or she should consider *who* will be the focus of the survey. The choice should be a function of conceptual, cost, and convenience considerations. Conceptually, whom does it make the most sense to study, given the investigator's interests? For example, is there a concern with learning about smoking behavior in the general U.S. population, among pregnant women, among nurses or other health professionals, among patients in the oncology ward of a particular hospital, or among high school students? All are possibilities; the choice depends on the researcher's interests and the constraints imposed by the varying costs of the study with different groups.

Deciding who will be the focus of the study is critical for determining the ultimate sampling plan for the survey. A researcher, for example, might be interested in learning about high school students' smoking behaviors and the impact that peer pressure has on their propensity to smoke (Table 2.2), but because of time and resource constraints, the study will have to be limited to a single high school in a city rather than include all the high school students in the community or a sample of students throughout the state.

A related issue is *where* the study will take place. This decision too is subject to time and resource constraints. There are also such issues as whether clearance can be obtained for conducting the survey in certain institutional settings or with selected population groups.

When the data will be collected is a function of what and whom the investigator is interested in studying and the research design chosen for the study, as well as practical problems related to gathering data at different times of the year. The *what* and the *who* may dictate the best time for data collection. It may make the most sense, for example, to gather information on students during the regular school year or on mothers of newborns just before discharge from the hospital or on recent health plan enrollees immediately following a company's open enrollment period.

As indicated in the example in Table 2.2, longitudinal and prospective as well as true experimental designs assume that data are collected at more than one point in time. The researcher will simultaneously need to consider whether there are seasonal differences that could show up on certain questions (incidence of upper respiratory illnesses, for example) depending on when the data are collected or if there might be problems with reaching prospective respondents at certain times of the year (such as during the Christmas holidays). Analytical and experimental designs attempt to explore *why* groups have certain characteristics in contrast to descriptive designs, which simply focus on *what* these characteristics are. The former types of designs assume that the researchers have some statistical hypotheses in mind about what they expect to find and why. Here is where previous experience and an acquaintance with existing research can be particularly helpful in shaping the research question and the particular issues to be pursued in any given study.

Stating the Study Objectives and Hypotheses for Different Study Designs

The research question is the major question that the study designer wants to try to answer. The specification of the study objectives and hypotheses are the first steps toward formulating an approach to answering this question. *Study objectives* reflect what the researcher wants to do to try to answer the question. *Study hypotheses* are statements of the answers the researcher expects to find and why, based on previous research or experience. Figure 2.1 provides templates for formulating the study objectives and hypotheses for different types of survey designs. "X" and "Y" refer to different variables. Groups being compared are designated as "A" and "B." Arrows (→) imply a relationship between variables. A plus sign means a positive relationship is hypothesized between the variables, that is, as one attribute of a study subject (fat consumption) increases, another attribute (cholesterol level) increases as well. A negative sign means a negative (or inverse relationship), that is, as a given characteristic (minutes of daily exercise) increases, another (body weight) declines. A zero implies that there is no statistically significant relationship between the variables.

Study Objectives

Study objectives may be stated in a form parallel to that of the expression *to do* to reflect the actions that the researcher will undertake to carry out the study. As suggested in the figure, the principal objectives will differ depending on whether the study is primarily descriptive, analytical, or experimental in focus. Again, the objective of descriptive studies is *to estimate,* of analytical studies *to test hypotheses,* and of experimental studies *to evaluate the impact of* certain factors of interest to the investigator. Whether the focus of the study is on a certain group at a particular point in time, over time, between different groups, or some combination of these will depend on the specific research question chosen by the investigator.

It is possible to address more than one research question in a study. An investigator may, for example, be interested in describing the characteristics or behaviors of certain groups (such as women who begin prenatal care after the first trimester of their pregnancy), in determining whether there are changes in their behavior over time (do they come in regularly for prenatal care, once seen?), and in discovering how they differ from other groups (such as women who begin prenatal care earlier). However, the precise question or set of questions the investigator wants to answer and the corresponding design or combination of designs and accompanying study objectives must be specified before the survey begins. In

FIGURE 2.1. STATING THE STUDY OBJECTIVES AND HYPOTHESES FOR DIFFERENT STUDY DESIGNS.

		Hypotheses	
Study Designs	*Objectives*	*Why?*	*What?*
Descriptive	To estimate. . .		
Cross-sectional	the characteristics (X, Y) of population.	—	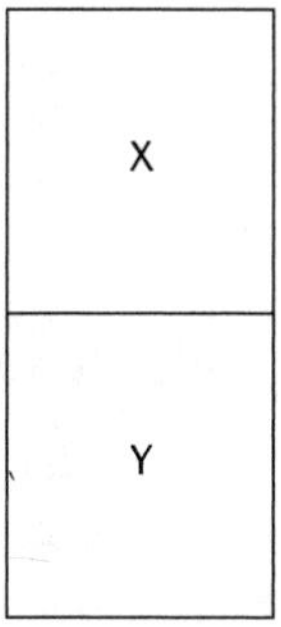 X
Group-comparison	whether the characteristics (X, Y) of subgroups A and B are different.	—	
Longitudinal	whether the characteristics (X, Y) of population or subgroups A and B change over time.	—	Y

Predictor. . .is related to. . .outcome.

Analytical	*To test hypotheses regarding whether. . .*	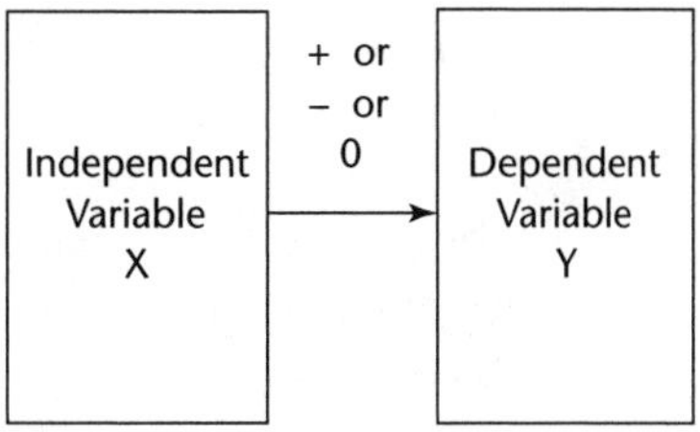 Independent Variable X →	+ or − or 0 → Dependent Variable Y
Cross-sectional	the characteristics Y of population are related to characteristics X.		
Case-control	differences in the characteristics Y of subgroups A and B are related to differences in characteristics X.		
Prospective	changes in the characteristics Y of population or subgroups A and B are related to changes or differences in characteristics X.		

Pretest. . .intervention. . .posttest.

Experimental	*To evaluate the impact of program (or treatment) X on Y for Group A that had it compared to Group B that did not.*	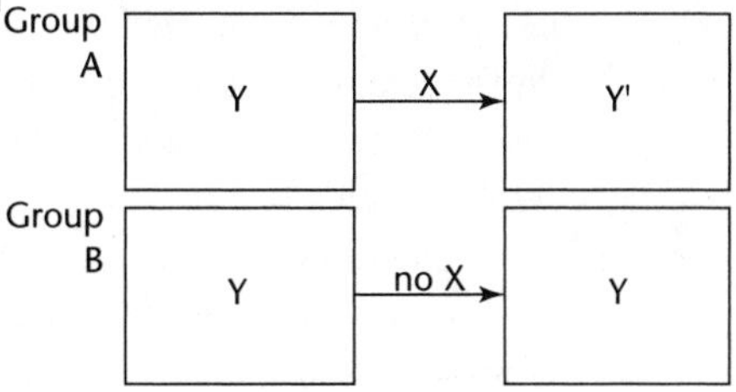 Group A: Y —X→ Y'	
		Group B: Y —no X→ Y	

addition, an investigator should not try to build too many objectives into a single study because the focus and nature of the study may become overly complex or ambiguous.

A clear statement of the study's objectives is essential to shaping the analyses that will be carried out to answer the major research question. Different data analysis plans and statistical methods are dictated by different survey designs. The three objectives—to estimate, test hypotheses, and evaluate the impact of—require different types of data analysis procedures. Having a clear idea of the study design and accompanying study objectives needed to address the major research question will greatly facilitate the specification of the analyses most appropriate to that design.

Study Hypotheses

Study hypotheses are statements about what the researcher expects to find in advance of carrying out the study and why. They are used in the physical and social sciences to express propositions about why certain phenomena occur. A theory represents an integrated set of explanations for these occurrences—explanations based on logical reasoning, previous research, or some combination of the two. Hypotheses, which are assumptions or statements of fact that flow from these theories, must be measured and tested in the real world. If the hypotheses are supported (or, more appropriately, not rejected), this provides evidence that the theory may be a good one for explaining how the world works. Theories provide the ideas and hypotheses the empirical tests of these ideas; in other words, they guide real-world observations of whether the theory's predictions do or do not actually occur.

Theories or frameworks predicting health and health care behavior can be tested in health surveys by empirically examining hypotheses that are based on those theories (Dilorio, Dudley, Soet, Watkins, & Maibach, 2000; Finney & Iannotti, 2001). Quite often, however, health surveys are applied rather than theoretical in focus. That is, they apply the theoretical perspectives to generate the questions that should be included in a study—to shed light on a health or health care problem and the best ways of dealing with that problem—rather than use the results to evaluate whether the theory itself is a good one. It was noted earlier that the science of epidemiology is concerned with studying the distribution and causes of disease in a community. Most often the data gathered in epidemiological surveys are used to design interventions to prevent or halt the spread of illness in a given community. In these applied surveys, theories about the spread of certain diseases can guide the selection of questions to be included in the study. But the survey results can also be examined to see whether they tend to support those theories per se, that is, do the findings agree with what the theory predicted?

In either case, researchers should begin with a review of the theoretical perspectives and previous research in an area before undertaking a study. They will then better understand what questions have and have not been answered already about the health topic that interests them, how their research can add to the current body of knowledge on the topic, and what the theories in the field suggest about the questions that should be included in studying it. They will also gain insights into ways in which their own research can serve to test the accuracy of prevailing theories in the field.

As stated earlier, hypotheses generally state what the investigator expects to find and why. In some instances, however, theories or previous research on a topic of interest will be limited. The researchers will then have to conduct exploratory studies to gather information on the issue or to generate hypotheses, using their own or others' practical experience in the area.

Traditionally, hypotheses refer to statements about *why* certain characteristics or behaviors are likely to be observed. These causal hypotheses are what guide the conduct of analytical or experimental survey designs. (See the analytical and experimental study designs in Figure 2.1.) In these cases, the hypotheses go beyond simple descriptions of certain characteristics to statements about differences on selected characteristics (high school seniors' smoking practices) between groups (seniors whose friends tend to smoke [Group A] compared to those whose friends mostly do not smoke [Group B]).

The phenomena for which explanations or causes are being sought (smoking practices) are termed *dependent variables (Y)*, while factors suggested as the explanations or causes of these phenomena (friends' smoking practices) are termed *independent variables (X)*. The hypothesis states that some relationship exists between these (independent and dependent) variables. If the hypothesis suggests that as one variable changes, the other changes in the same direction, the variables are positively (+) associated. If they change in opposite directions, they are inversely or negatively (–) associated. A hypothesis may also theoretically state that there is no (0) relationship between the variables or no differences (in smoking practices) between groups.

The hypothesis of no difference is a null form of the hypothesis also used in statistical tests of relationships between variables, to be discussed further in Chapters Four and Fifteen. A research or alternative hypothesis states that there is a difference or association between the variables.

The research hypothesis underlying the analytical study designs in Table 2.2 is, "The prevalence (or incidence) of smoking (dependent variable) will be higher (+ relationship) among high school seniors who have friends who smoke (or start to smoke) (independent variable)." The null hypothesis is that there is no association or no difference in the smoking practices of seniors whose friends smoke and those who do not.

Analytical surveys focus on whether there are empirically observed relationships between certain characteristics of interest. Theories, previous research, or the investigators' own experiences can help suggest which should be considered the dependent and which the independent variable in the hypothesized or observed relationship. However, for the independent variable to be considered a "cause" of the dependent variable, (1) there has to be some theoretical, conceptual, or practical basis for the hypothesized relationship; (2) the variables have to be statistically associated (that is, as one changes, so does the other); (3) the occurrence of the independent variable has to precede the occurrence of the dependent variable in time; and (4) other explanations for what might "cause" the dependent variable have to be ruled out.

In the real world, however, and especially in the health and social sciences, there are very often a variety of explanations for some phenomenon of interest. In that case, the major study hypothesis will have to be elaborated (more variables will have to be considered) to test adequately whether the hypothesized predictor (independent) variable is the "cause" of the outcome (dependent) variable of interest. Most important, the researcher must think through the variables of interest before undertaking the study in order to reduce the chance that a critical variable for stating or elaborating the study objectives or hypotheses will be omitted.

In experimental study designs, the underlying hypothesis is that the experimental group (group A) that receives the intervention or program (X) is more likely to have an outcome (Y) than the control group (group B) that does not receive the intervention (no X). Data are collected over time for both groups before and after X is administered to group A, to establish the temporal priority of X, and the groups are made as equivalent as possible through randomization to rule out any other possible explanations for differences observed between the groups except for X.

Special Considerations for Special Populations

The underlying objectives and associated design for addressing them have direct implications regarding whom to include in the study. Both the complexity and costs of capturing the target population for a survey are increased if the groups of interest are rare, hard to locate, highly mobile, non-English speakers, or otherwise different from modal demographic or social-cultural groupings. These implications will be addressed more fully in Chapter Six, in discussing the design of the sampling plan for the survey. It is, however, none too soon to anticipate these parameters in the initial formulation of the study design on which it is based.

Selected Examples

The study objectives and related study designs and research questions for the surveys in Resources A, B, and C are summarized in Table 2.3.

The UNICEF Multiple Indicator Cluster Survey (MICS) and the California Health Interview Survey (CHIS) represent descriptive longitudinal surveys (UCLA Center for Health Policy Research, 2005; UNICEF, n.d.). They provide trend data over time—for 1995, 2000, and 2005 in the instance of the MICS, and biennially beginning in 2001 for the CHIS. They are, however, not longitudinal *panel* designs, in that different respondents are sampled at each of the time periods. The MICS is based on national surveys of participating countries and the CHIS is designed to provide estimates at the state and local level, as well as for racial/ethnic subgroups, in the state of California. Both studies have a group-comparison dimension as well in that they were designed to permit comparisons of estimates across countries (MICS) or between areas and subgroups within a state (CHIS).

The National Dental Malpractice Survey (NDMS) is also a cross-sectional survey of a national sample of U.S. dentists conducted at a single point in time: 1991. It has both descriptive and analytical objectives in that it was intended (1) to estimate dental malpractice insurance experience among U.S. dentists, as well as (2) to test hypotheses regarding the practice characteristics that are predictive of their dental malpractice insurance experience. The NDMS was grounded in theoretical and empirical research regarding the likely factors accounting for dental malpractice insurance experience (Conrad, Milgrom, Whitney, O'Hara, & Fiset, 1998; Conrad et al., 1995; Milgrom et al. 1994; Milgrom, Whitney, Conrad, Fiset, & O'Hara, 1995).

Guidelines for Minimizing Survey Errors and Maximizing Survey Quality

Two major types of systematic errors are of primary concern in formulating analytical and experimental designs: *internal validity* and *external validity* (Bickman, 2000; Campbell & Russo, 1999; Grembowski, 2001; Rossi, Lipsey, & Freeman, 2004; Shadish, Cook, & Campbell, 2002) (see Table 2.4). Internal validity refers to whether the design adequately and accurately addresses the study's hypotheses, particularly with respect to demonstrating a causal relationship between the independent and dependent variables. External validity deals with how widely or universally the findings are likely to apply to related populations or subgroups. These types of validity can be affected by both the variable and systematic errors that

TABLE 2.3. SELECTED HEALTH SURVEY EXAMPLES—
STUDY OBJECTIVES, STUDY DESIGNS, AND RESEARCH QUESTIONS.

Design Dimensions	UNICEF Multiple Indicator Cluster Surveys (MICS)	California Health Interview Survey (CHIS)	National Dental Malpractice Survey (NDMS)
Study objectives	1. To estimate and monitor World Summit for Children and related World Fit for the Millennium Development Goals (MDGs) indicators of child survival and development for children and mothers in participating countries.	1. To provide statewide estimates for the population of the state of California overall and local-level estimates for most counties in the state of California on a variety of public health topics such as health status, health care access, insurance coverage.	1. To estimate dental malpractice insurance experience in a representative sample of U.S. dentists in 1991.
	2. To compare the indicators over time, as well as across countries.	2. To compare estimates across local areas and between larger racial/ ethnic groups, and selected smaller ethnic groups.	2. To test hypotheses regarding the practice characteristics that are predictive of dental malpractice insurance experience.
Study designs	Descriptive longitudinal, comparative national surveys conducted in 1995, 2000, and 2005 in participating countries	Descriptive longitudinal, comparative state and local surveys conducted on a biennial basis, beginning in 2001, in the state of California	Analytical cross-sectional national survey of U.S. dentists, conducted in 1991
Research questions			
What?	World Summit for Children and MDG indicators of child survival and development	Health status, chronic conditions, health behaviors, health care access, insurance coverage, and so forth	Malpractice insurance experience and practice characteristics
Who?	Children and mothers	State and county populations	Dentists
Where?	Participating countries	State of California	United States
When?	1995, 2000, 2005	2001, 2003, 2005	1991
Why?	—	—	To test hypotheses regarding the practice characteristics that are predictive of dental malpractice insurance experience.

TABLE 2.4. SURVEY ERRORS: SOURCES AND SOLUTIONS— MATCHING THE SURVEY DESIGN TO SURVEY OBJECTIVES.

	Systematic Errors		*Variable Errors*
	Poor Internal Validity	**Poor External Validity**	**Design Specification Ambiguity**
Solutions to Errors	Use randomization, matching, or statistical controls to rule out other factors that may account for relationships between variables.	Clearly specify where, with whom, and when the survey will be done in stating the study objectives, and design the sample frame and survey sampling procedures accordingly.	Clearly specify the study objectives and related concepts to be measured in the survey, particularly in relationship to the underlying study design and data analysis plan for the study.

plague a given design. Variable errors can, for example, result from design specification ambiguity, in which the statement of the study objectives and related concepts to be measured in the survey are not clearly and unambiguously articulated, particularly in relationship to the underlying study design and data analysis plan for the study.

Internal Validity

Analytical cross-sectional designs have the least control over two major conditions in determining whether a hypothesized relationship between two variables (X, Y) is causal: the temporal priority of the independent variable in relationship to the dependent variable and the ability to rule out other explanations. In these types of designs, procedures for statistically controlling for the influence of other factors are employed. (These types of procedures are more fully discussed in Chapters Four and Fifteen.) Case-control designs try to rule out competing explanations about whether some factor X caused one group to have a condition Y and another group not to have that condition by matching the groups as nearly as possible on everything else that could "cause" Y. Prospective designs attempt to establish more clearly whether one factor (X) does indeed precede the other (Y) in time. The true experimental design, which entails randomization of individuals to an experimental or control group, provides the most direct test of whether a certain outcome Y is "caused" by X. (See the experimental study design in Figure 2.1.) However, much applied public health and health services research is based on quasi-experimental designs that do not entail the full randomization of individuals to experimental and control conditions. These types of designs present more threats to the internal validity of the study. (For a discussion of these threats for different designs, see Bickman, 2000; Campbell & Russo, 1999; Grembowski, 2001; Rossi et al., 2004; and Shadish et al., 2002.)

External Validity

The major limitations with respect to the external validity of a design are directly linked to its spatial and temporal dimensions, that is, where and with whom, in addition to when, the study is done. The results of cross-sectional surveys, as well as those based on other designs, are generalizable only to those groups and time periods that were eligible to be represented in the study. Group-comparison designs place a special premium on who is included in the study and longitudinal designs on when it is conducted. A defining strength of experimental designs from the point of their internal validity (random assignment of participants to the experimental and control conditions) may, in contrast, introduce problems in terms of their external validity or generalizability (because of the artificiality of the experimental situation or who is willing to participate in such experiments). To minimize issues of external validity, the researcher should clearly specify where, with whom, and when the survey will be done in stating the study objectives and design the survey sampling procedures accordingly. (The procedures for designing samples to maximize the external validity of survey findings are discussed in Chapters Six and Seven.)

Design Specification Ambiguity

The different types of study designs may be viewed as maps that are available to chart the spatial and temporal dimensions of the study—or where, with whom, and when the survey will be done. The research questions reflect the destination, or what the investigator is interested in discovering. The specific itinerary is mapped out in the study objectives based on the guidance provided by an appropriately chosen research design. The hypotheses represent the points of interest the traveler (or researcher) expects to find once the undertaking is completed. The analysis plan provides a specific idea of how the data that are gathered are to be used. The study objectives provide the road map for formulating the analysis plan and related methods of analyzing and reporting the results of the study. (Specific guidance for the formulation of an analysis plan in relationship to the study objectives is provided in Chapters Four and Fifteen.)

If survey researchers fail to articulate clearly the research questions, study design and objectives, and their interrelationship, they may not accomplish what they set out to do and may spend resources in gathering data that will ultimately be disappointingly irrelevant or imprecise.

Supplementary Sources

Sources to consult on alternative research designs for surveys from the point of view of different disciplines include the following: epidemiology (Abramson & Abramson, 1999), sociology and the social sciences (de Vaus, 2002), and program evaluation (Grembowski, 2001; Rossi, Lipsey, & Freeman, 2004).

CHAPTER THREE

DEFINING AND CLARIFYING THE SURVEY VARIABLES

Chapter Highlights

1. The researcher should start with a clear idea of the concept that he or she wants to measure to guide the choice of questions to ask about that concept.
2. The phrasing of the questions chosen to operationalize the concept of interest should reflect the level of measurement—nominal, ordinal, interval, or ratio—appropriate for the types of analysis that the researcher wants to carry out using those questions.
3. The reliability of survey questions can be evaluated in terms of the stability of responses to the same questions over time (test-retest reliability) and their equivalence between data gatherers or observers (inter-rater reliability). They can also be evaluated in terms of the consistency of different questions related to the same underlying concept (internal consistency reliability).
4. The validity or accuracy of survey measures can be evaluated in terms of how well they sample the content of the concept of interest (content validity) and how well they predict (predictive validity) or agree with (concurrent validity) some criterion. Their validity is also based on the extent to which empirically

observed relationships between measures of the concepts agree
with what theories hypothesize about the relationships between
the concepts (construct validity), that is, whether they are
correlated (convergent validity) or not (discriminant validity).
5. Survey items that relate to the same topic can be summarized
into typologies, indexes, or scales (such as Likert or other scales),
depending on the underlying concept and level of measurement
desired.

Once they start looking at questionnaires used in other studies, researchers
can identify literally dozens of questions they may wish to include in their
survey. This chapter presents criteria to apply in deciding the types of questions
it would be appropriate to take from existing sources and evaluating the soundness of items that researchers develop themselves. Researchers should have a clear
idea of (1) the precise concept they want to capture in asking the question; (2) how
the question should be asked and how variables should be created from it to yield
the type and amount of information required for analyzing the data in certain
ways (Table 3.1); and (3) the methods and criteria to use in evaluating the reliability and validity of the question (Figures 3.1 and 3.2 and Tables 3.2 and 3.3).

The reliability of information obtained on a topic by asking a question about
it in a survey refers to the extent of *random variation* in the answers to the question
as a function of (1) when it is asked, (2) who asked it, and (3) that it is simply one
of a number of questions that could have been asked to obtain the information.

The validity of a survey question about a concept of interest (such as health)
refers to the extent to which there is a *systematic departure* in the answers given to
the question from (1) the meaning of the concept itself, (2) answers to comparable questions about the same concept, and (3) hypothesized relationships with other
concepts.

In the measurement of attitudes toward health issues or practices, a variety
of questions are often asked to capture a respondent's opinion. Procedures have
been developed to collapse responses to numerous items of this kind into single
summary scores (or scales) that reflect how respondents feel about an issue. The
procedures used to develop such scales and integrate the answers from several
different survey questions into one variable (or scale score) as well as the procedures
for critically evaluating the potential sources of errors in these procedures are presented in this chapter (Figure 3.3 and Table 3.4). An understanding of these data
summary or reduction devices can facilitate the development of empirical definitions of complex concepts that are both concise and meaningful, reduce the overall number of variables required to carry out the analyses of these concepts, and
acquaint the researcher with criteria to use for determining whether the summary

devices that other researchers have developed are valid and reliable—and therefore worth using in his or her own studies.

The criteria and procedures for developing a multidimensional approach to measuring health status in connection with the Medical Outcomes Study (MOS), a major health services research study that compared health outcomes for patients in managed care organizations (MCOs), multispecialty groups, and solo practices in three cities (Boston, Chicago, and Los Angeles) and has been widely adapted and applied internationally, will be used to illustrate reliability and validity analyses and associated scale construction procedures (Gandek & Ware, 1998; McHorney, Ware, Lu, & Sherbourne, 1994; McHorney, Ware, & Raczek, 1993; Stewart & Ware, 1992; Ware & Gandek, 1998a, 1998b; Ware & Sherbourne, 1992).

Translating Concepts into Operational Definitions

Researchers often begin with a variety of concepts they would like to measure in a health survey. For example, they may be interested in finding out about levels of alcohol consumption or drug use of survey respondents and how these levels affect people's reported well-being as well as if the findings are different for people at different income levels, for men and women, for employed and unemployed persons, for individuals who are married and those who are not, and so on. The precise selection of topics and the relationships to be examined between them are dictated by the study's principal research question and associated study objectives and hypotheses.

The actual questions to be asked or the procedures to be used to gather information about the major concepts of interest in a study are called the *operational definitions* of the concepts. They specify the concrete operations that will be carried out to obtain answers to the overall research questions posed by the investigator. Other surveys that have dealt with comparable issues should be the starting point for the selection of the questions to be asked. In the absence of previous questions on a topic, the researcher will have to draft new questions based on an understanding of the concept of interest and the principles of good question design (detailed in Chapters Eight to Eleven). The answers to these survey questions will then be coded into the variables that will ultimately be used in analyzing the data.

It is imperative that the precise questions asked in the survey and the resulting variable definitions adequately and accurately capture the concepts that the investigator has in mind. Formal methods for testing the correspondence between these empirical measures and the original theoretical or hypothetical concepts will be presented later when various approaches to evaluating the validity of survey variables are discussed. In general, however, researchers should consider exactly what they want to capture in operationalizing the concept (such as "obesity") and how they expect to use the data gathered on that concept (for example, to construct an objective composite index of the relationship between the respondent's height and weight) in deciding how best to phrase a survey question about it.

The process for translating ideas or concepts into questions to be asked of study subjects in a survey is illustrated in Table 3.1.

Applying Different Levels of Measurement to Define Study Variables

The form and meaning of the variables constructed from answers to survey questions have important implications for the types of analyses that can be carried out with the data. As will be discussed in more detail in Chapter Fifteen, certain statistical techniques assume that the study variables are measured in certain ways. Table 3.1 summarizes examples of ways in which study concepts would be operationalized differently depending on the type or level of measurement used in gathering the data. The respective measurement procedures—nominal, ordinal, and interval or ratio—provide increasingly more quantitative detail about the study variable.

In general, constructing variables involves assigning numbers or other codes to represent some qualitative or quantitative aspect of the underlying concept being measured. The codes assigned should, however, be mutually exclusive in that a value should represent only one answer (not several). They should also be exhaustive, that is, the codes should encompass the range of possible answers to that question. For example, the use of only two income categories, such as $0–$25,000 and $25,000–$50,000, would reflect groupings that are neither exhaustive (some people may earn more than $50,000) nor mutually exclusive (persons with incomes of $25,000 could place themselves in either category).

Nominal Variables

Nominal variables reflect the names, nomenclature, or labels that can be used to classify respondents into one group or another, such as male or female; African American, white, or Hispanic/Latino; and employed, unemployed, or not in the labor force. Numerical values assigned to the categories of a nominal scale are simply codes used to differentiate the resulting categories of individuals.

Nominal scales do not permit the following types of quantitative statements to be made about study respondents: "The first respondent is higher than the second on this indicator," or "The difference between respondents on the measure is

TABLE 3.1. APPLYING DIFFERENT LEVELS
OF MEASUREMENT TO DEFINE STUDY VARIABLES.

Definitions and Selected Examples	*Levels of Measurement*		
	Nominal	**Ordinal**	**Interval or Ratio**
Conceptual Definition (concept or issue of interest) . . . family income from wages or salaries. . . . obesity.	*Classification* of study subjects by . . .	*Ranking* of study subjects according to . . .	*Quantifying* or comparing *levels* reported by study subjects on . . .
Operational Definition (questions asked to obtain information on concept or issue)	Did anyone in your family have income from wages or salaries in the past twelve months?	Which of the following categories (SHOW CARD) best describes your family's total income from wages and salaries in the past twelve months?	What was your family's total income from wages and salaries during the past twelve months?
	Do you consider yourself overweight, underweight, or just about right?	Would you say you are very overweight, somewhat overweight, or only a little overweight?	About how tall are you without shoes? *and* About how much do you weigh without shoes?
Variable Definition (variable constructed from questions to be used in the analysis of the data)	*Family Wages and Salaries* 1 = had wages or salaries 2 = did not have wages or salaries	*Family Wages and Salaries* 1 = income category 1 2 = income category 2 k = income category k	*Family Wages and Salaries* = $ _____ /year
	Obesity 1 = overweight 2 = underweight 3 = about right	*Obesity* 1 = very overweight 2 = somewhat overweight 3 = only a little overweight	*Obesity* *Construct* index of obesity, based on body mass index (BMI), calculated as weight divided by height, squared.

X units." These more quantitative applications are possible only with the other (ordinal, interval, or ratio) measurement procedures.

Data for the concepts in Table 3.1—family income from wages and salaries and obesity—could be summarized in quantitative terms depending on how the question is asked. The examples given of a nominal level of measurement for these concepts reflect questions primarily intended to classify a respondent into one group or another: (1) whether someone in the family had income from wages or salaries or not, and (2) whether the person considers himself or herself to be overweight, underweight, or just right. To obtain more detailed quantitative information on these concepts, different questions (such as those listed under the other levels of measurement in Table 3.1) would have to be asked.

Ordinal Variables

Ordinal variables are a step up on the measurement scale in that they permit some ranking or ordering of survey respondents on the study variable. Ordinal measures assume an underlying continuum along which respondents can be ranked on the characteristic of interest—from high to low, excellent to poor, and so on. In Table 3.1, for example, people who say they are overweight are asked to indicate the extent to which they think they are overweight—very, somewhat, or only a little. However, ordinal scales make no assumptions about the precise distances between the points along this continuum (that is, how much more obese a man who says he is "very" overweight is compared with another who says he is "only a little" overweight).

The Medical Outcomes Study developed a number of ordinal-level questions related to dimensions of physical, mental, and social role functioning and well-being. Among these, for example, was a question asking if the respondent's health limited his or her activities during a typical day (such as lifting or carrying groceries or climbing several flights of stairs) a lot, a little, or not at all (Stewart & Ware, 1992; Ware & Gandek, 1998b; Ware & Sherbourne, 1992).

Interval or Ratio Variables

Interval and ratio levels of measurement assume that the underlying quantitative continuum on which the study variable is based has intervals of equal length or distance, much as the inches of a ruler do. The main difference between interval scales and ratio scales is that the latter have an absolute zero point—meaning that the total absence of the attribute can be calibrated—while the former do not. Because of the anchor provided by this zero point, the ratio scale allows statements to be made about the ratio between these distances, that is, whether one score is X times higher or lower than another, as well as about the magnitude of these distances.

Examples of interval scales are measures of intelligence and temperature. Theoretically, there is never a total absence of these attributes, and therefore no real zero point on the scales that measure them. On certain variables used in health surveys, such as measures of a person's height or weight or scores on interval-level attitude scales, a substantively meaningful zero point either does not exist or is hard to define. Scales used in measuring other variables in health surveys—such as number of physician visits, nights spent in the hospital, number of cigarettes smoked per day, or days of limited activity due to illness during the year—do have meaningful zero points. Interval-level measures are treated like ratio measures for most types of analysis procedures in the social sciences. Interval and ratio measures can be collapsed to create nominal variables (saw a doctor or not) or ordinal variables (0, 1–2, 3–4, 5 or more visits).

In summary, survey researchers should think through how much and what kind of qualitative and quantitative information they want to capture in asking a question about some concept of interest in their study. Knowing whether the resultant survey variable represents a nominal, ordinal, or interval or ratio level of measurement will help in deciding which way of asking the question is best given the objectives of the study.

Evaluating the Reliability of Study Variables

The reliability of a survey measure refers to the *stability* and *equivalence* (or reproducibility) of measures of the same concept over time or across methods of gathering the data. The stability of a measure refers to the consistency of the answers people give to the same question when they are asked it at different points in time, assuming no real changes have occurred that should cause them to answer differently. In contrast, the equivalence of different data-gathering methods refers to the consistency of the answers when different data gatherers use the same questionnaire or instrument or when different but presumably equivalent (or parallel) instruments are used to measure the same individuals at the same point in time (American Psychological Association, 1999; DeVellis, 2003; Nunnally & Bernstein, 1994).

Questions with low reliability are ones in which respondents' answers vary widely as a function of when the questions are asked, who asks them, and the fact that the particular questions chosen from a set of items seem to be asking the same thing but are not.

The consistency of answers to the same questions over time may vary as a function of transient personal factors, such as a respondent's mental or physical state at the different time periods, situational factors (whether other people are present at the interview), variations in the ways interviewers actually phrase the questions at the different time periods, and real changes that may have taken place between these periods.

Variations in the consistency of responses to what are thought to be equivalent ways of asking a question could be the result if different observers or interviewers elicit or record the data differently or if apparently equivalent items do not actually tap the same underlying concept.

Estimates derived from survey data always reflect something of the true value of the estimate as well as random errors that result from the unreliability of the measure itself. Good survey design seeks to anticipate the sources of these variations and, to the maximum extent possible, control and minimize them in the development and administration of the study questionnaire.

The estimates of reliability to be examined reflect the extent to which (1) the same question yields consistent results at different points in time, (2) different people collecting or recording data on the same questions tend to get comparable answers, and (3) different questions that are assumed to tap the same underlying concept are correlated. These are termed *test-retest, inter-rater,* and *internal consistency reliability,* respectively (DeVellis, 2003).

Figure 3.1 summarizes the various procedures for evaluating the reliability of survey variables. Correlation coefficients are the statistics used most often in developing *quantitative measures* of reliability (these statistics are discussed in more detail in Chapter Fifteen). Quantitative measures can also be readily computed using standard social science and biomedical computer software (for example, SAS, SPSS, STATA). In general, correlation coefficients reflect the degree to which the measures "correspond" or "co-relate." That is, if one tends to be high or low, to what extent is the other high or low as well? Correlation coefficients normally range from -1.00 to $+1.00$. The most reliable measures are ones for which the reliability (correlation) coefficient is closest to $+1.00$.

The precise coefficient (or formula) to use in estimating the reliability of an indicator differs for different approaches to measuring reliability (DeVellis, 2003; Nunnally & Bernstein, 1994). The following sections discuss the appropriate coefficient to use with particular approaches and the criteria that can be applied to evaluate the reliability of a given question based on the resulting value of the coefficient.

Test-Retest Reliability

The test-retest reliability coefficient reflects the degree of correspondence between answers to the same questions asked of the same respondents at different points in time. A survey designer might, for example, try out some questions on a test

FIGURE 3.1.   EVALUATING THE RELIABILITY OF STUDY VARIABLES.

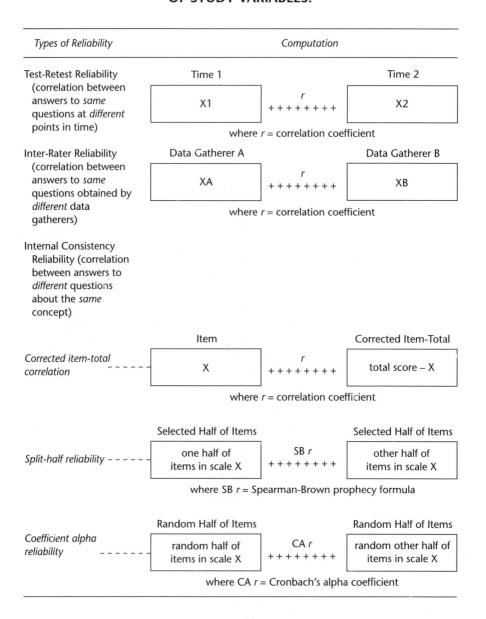

Types of Reliability	Computation

Test-Retest Reliability (correlation between answers to *same* questions at *different* points in time)

Time 1 — X1 — *r* +++++++ — Time 2 — X2
where *r* = correlation coefficient

Inter-Rater Reliability (correlation between answers to *same* questions obtained by *different* data gatherers)

Data Gatherer A — XA — *r* +++++++ — Data Gatherer B — XB
where *r* = correlation coefficient

Internal Consistency Reliability (correlation between answers to *different* questions about the *same* concept)

Corrected item-total correlation

Item — X — *r* +++++++ — Corrected Item-Total — total score – X
where *r* = correlation coefficient

Split-half reliability

Selected Half of Items — one half of items in scale X — SB *r* +++++++ — Selected Half of Items — other half of items in scale X
where SB *r* = Spearman-Brown prophecy formula

Coefficient alpha reliability

Random Half of Items — random half of items in scale X — CA *r* +++++++ — Random Half of Items — random other half of items in scale X
where CA *r* = Cronbach's alpha coefficient

sample of respondents and then go back a month later to see if they give the same answers to the questions asked earlier, such as how many drinks of alcoholic beverages they have on average each week. There could be real changes in the behavior or situation about which the questions are asked to account for a less-than-perfect correspondence between the data gathered at different times. Changes that occur at random between the respective time periods could also give rise to any differences observed. The researcher needs to consider these possibilities in selecting the questions to include in a test-retest reliability analysis, deciding how long to wait before going back, and ultimately interpreting the coefficient obtained between the two time periods. On average, a maximum of two to four weeks is a reasonable period of time between the initial and follow-up administration of the questionnaire to minimize the possibility of real or random changes occurring.

In the original Medical Outcomes Study (MOS) to develop the thirty-six-item short form (SF-36) health status scale, data were gathered on the same person for selected questions four months apart. Because real changes in health could occur over this period, the correlation between answers at the two time periods was deemed to represent the "lower-bound estimate of reliability," that is, it was likely to represent the lowest reliability coefficient for a given question, especially compared to its likely performance in terms of internal consistency reliability (Stewart & Ware, 1992, p. 83).

It would be desirable to have a much shorter period of time between the first and second measurements (perhaps two to four weeks), particularly if there is a possibility that real changes might take place in the underlying construct of interest (emotional well-being) within a short period of time. In the evaluation of a twelve-item version of the SF-36 (the SF-12), a two-week test-retest interval was employed. The test-retest reliability coefficient (or correlation) was somewhat higher for the physical health component of the scale (.89) compared to the mental health component (.76), suggesting somewhat more instability, but still an acceptable level of reliability, for the mental health subscale (Ware, Kosinski, & Keller, 1996).

Test-retest reliability can be computed using correlation coefficients such as the Pearson correlation coefficient for interval-level data, the Spearman rank-order coefficient for ordinal-level variables, or nominal-based measures of association for categorical data to examine the stability of the answers a respondent gave to the same question (or item) at two different points in time (Table 3.2).

The closer the values of the test-retest correlation coefficients are to +1.00, the more stable or consistent the indicator can be said to be at different points in time. In general, minimum test-retest reliabilities of .70 are satisfactory for studies focusing on group-level differences. Higher coefficients (.90 or above) are preferred when the emphasis is on changes in individuals over time, especially if

TABLE 3.2. METHODS OF COMPUTING RELIABILITY.

Types of Reliability	Data Records		Correlation Coefficients
	Cases	Data/Answer	
Test-retest		*Item Over Time*	
	Respondent	*Time 1* *Time 2*	*Interval:* Pearson r
	1	X11 X12	*Ordinal:* Spearman rho
	2	X21 X22	*Nominal:* Chi-square-based
	3	X31 X32	
	4	X41 X42	
	5	X51 X52	
Inter-rater		*Item Across Data Gatherers*	where two data gatherers = A,B
	Respondent	*A* *B*	*Interval:* Pearson r
	1	X1A X1B	*Ordinal:* Spearman rho
	2	X2A X2B	*Nominal:* Kappa
	3	X3A X3B	
	4	X4A X4B	where three+ data gatherers = A,B,C, etc.
	5	X5A X5B	*Mixed:* Intra-class correlation (eta)
Internal consistency	*Respondent*	*Item 1* *Item 2*	
	1	X11 X12	*Interval* Corrected item total r
	2	X21 X22	*or Ordinal:* Spearman-Brown
	3	X31 X32	Cronbach's alpha
	4	X41 X42	*Dichotomy:* Kuder-Richardson
	5	X51 X52	

Formula: Cronbach's alpha $= kr/[1+(k-1)r]$

where,
k = number of items in the scale
r = average correlation between items

Example: Cronbach's alpha $= 10(.32)/[1+(10-1)*.32]$
$= 3.20/[1+(9)*.32]$
$= 3.20/3.88$
$= .825$

where,
k = 10
$r = [.185+.451+.048+\ldots+.233=14.557]/45=.32$

Correlation Matrix (numbers in cells=correlation between items)

	1	2	3	4	5	6	7	8	9	10
1	–	.185	.451	.399	.413	.263	.394	.352	.361	.204
2	–	–	.048	.209	.248	.246	.230	.050	.277	.270
3	–	–	–	.350	.399	.209	.381	.427	.276	.332
4	–	–	–	–	.369	.415	.469	.280	.358	.221
5	–	–	–	–	–	.338	.446	.457	.317	.425
6	–	–	–	–	–	–	.474	.214	.502	.189
7	–	–	–	–	–	–	–	.315	.577	.311
8	–	–	–	–	–	–	–	–	.299	.374
9	–	–	–	–	–	–	–	–	–	.233
10	–	–	–	–	–	–	–	–	–	–

Source: Table 3, "Correlation Matrix of Self-Esteem Items." Carmines, E. G., & Zeller, R. A., *Reliability & Validity Assessment,* p. 64, copyright © 1979 by Sage Publications, Inc. Reprinted by permission of Sage Publications, Inc.

the measure is to be used to make clinical judgments regarding treatment or outcomes on a case-by-case basis.

The computation of correlation coefficients is affected by the variability that exists between study subjects, that is, the variation in how the questions are answered by different respondents. Analysis of variance (ANOVA) procedures permit this variation between respondents to be calculated. Procedures for adjusting the correlation coefficients through the application of ANOVA procedures that remove this variation *between* subjects would provide more precise estimates of the variation *within* subjects, that is, the stability in the answers to the same question that the same respondents give at two different times—which is the focus of test-retest reliability (Bland & Altman, 1995). In addition, using procedures that assume related samples, such as the paired *t*-test, to compare a respondent's answers at the two time periods would more accurately take into account that the first and second measurements are not independent, as well as more directly compare the actual answers at the two points in time. (See also Chapter Fifteen.)

Inter-Rater Reliability

Inter-rater reliability examines the equivalence of the information obtained by different data gatherers or raters on the same (or comparable) groups of respondents.

We have seen, in the examples of possible sources of variation in survey questions, that different interviewers may ask the same survey questions differently. Survey designers may also engage raters or observers to record and observe behaviors rather than ask questions directly. For example, observers might report on study subjects' level of functioning on physical tasks or patterns of interaction with family members. Inter-rater reliability correlation coefficients reflect the level of agreement between interviewers or observers in recording this information. In general, a correlation of the answers between or among raters of .80 or higher is desirable.

As indicated in Table 3.2, a Pearson, Spearman rank order, or kappa coefficient can be used to measure the strength of agreement between *two* data gatherers (A and B) for interval, ordinal, or nominal-level variables. An intraclass correlation coefficient measures the agreement among all the data gatherers in the study: A, B, C, and so on (Nunnally & Bernstein, 1994). The intraclass correlation coefficient may be preferable to the Pearson correlation coefficient in evaluating inter-rater reliability between two raters for continuous variables because the Pearson correlation describes the extent to which the scores covary but not the extent to which the scores from the different raters are actually the same (Ebel, 1951).

The inter-rater reliability between survey interviewers is rarely computed. Different interviewers do not usually go back to ask respondents the same questions, and groups of respondents interviewed by different interviewers are not always comparable. Especially in personal interview surveys, interviewers may be assigned to different areas of a city or region that differ a great deal compositionally. Survey designers should, however, consider what might give rise to random variation in interviewers' performance before starting the study and standardize the training and field procedures to reduce these sources of variation as much as possible.

Internal Consistency Reliability

Whereas test-retest and inter-rater reliability analysis can be used to evaluate individual items or summary scales, internal consistency reliability analysis is used primarily in constructing and evaluating summary scales. The sources of variability examined with this type of reliability analysis include the inconsistency or nonequivalence of different questions intended to measure the same concept. If the questions are not really equivalent, then different conclusions about the concept will result, depending on which questions are used in constructing the summary scale to measure it. The main procedures for estimating the internal consistency or intercorrelation among a number of different questions that are supposed to reflect the same concept are the *corrected item-total correlation* and *split-half* and *alpha reliability coefficients*. The procedures were originally developed in connection with multiple-item summary scores or scales of people's attitudes toward a particular topic. People's attitudes (toward persons with HIV/AIDS or banning smoking in public places, for example) are often complex and multidimensional and therefore difficult to tap with a single survey question.

As will be seen later in this chapter, the process of developing attitude scales begins with the identification of a large number of questions that seem to capture some aspect of how a respondent feels about an issue. The corrected item-total correlation, split-half, and internal consistency reliability procedures are used to estimate the extent to which these items tap the same basic attitude (toward persons with HIV/AIDS, for example, rather than toward homosexuals, who are one of several risk groups for the disease; or toward policies about banning smoking in the workplace rather than toward the practice of smoking in general). There could, of course, be a variety of dimensions that characterize the attitudes that individuals hold on certain topics. Attitude scaling and the reliability analyses required to construct those scales help identify what those dimensions are and which survey items best tap those dimensions.

A useful indicator for initially assessing whether all the items that are intended to measure a given concept do and therefore warrant being combined into a single scale is the correlation of the item with the sum of all the other items in the scale. This is sometimes referred to as the *corrected item-total correlation* since the item is not included in computing the total scale score. Doing this serves to remove the bias associated with correlating an item with itself. A correlation of .40 or higher was used as a cutoff for identifying candidate items in constructing a thirty-six-item health status questionnaire in the MOS. This was deemed to be a substantively meaningful and robust level of association between variables. All the items except one exceeded this criterion (McHorney et al., 1994).

Split-half reliability reflects the correspondence between answers to two subsets of questions when an original set of questions about a topic (such as patient satisfaction with various aspects of medical care) is split in half, and a correlation coefficient is computed between scores from the two halves. The correlation coefficient used to compute the correspondence between the scores for these two subsets of items is the Spearman-Brown prophecy formula (DeVellis, 2003; Nunnally & Bernstein, 1994). The reliability estimate based on this formula will be higher (1) the more questions asked about the topic and (2) the higher the correlation between the scores for the respective halves of the entire set of questions.

The process for computing *coefficient alpha reliability* is similar to that for the split-half approach except that it is based on all possible ways of splitting and comparing sets of questions used to tap a particular concept. Cronbach's alpha or coefficient alpha is the correlation coefficient used to estimate the degree of equivalence between answers to sets of questions constructed in this fashion. The Kuder-Richardson formula is a special case of the alpha coefficient that is used when the response categories for the questions are dichotomous rather than multilevel. In other words, they require a *yes* or *no* rather than a *strongly agree, agree, uncertain, disagree,* or *strongly disagree* response to a statement that reflects an attitude toward some topic (DeVellis, 2003; Nunnally & Bernstein, 1994).

The coefficient alpha (and associated Kuder-Richardson) formula is used more often than the split-half formula in most internal consistency analyses of multiple-item scales because it enables the correlations between scores on all possible halves of the items to be computed. The coefficient alpha will be higher (1) the more questions asked about the topic and (2) the higher the average correlation between the scores for all possible combinations of the entire set of questions.

In most applied studies, the lowest acceptable level of internal consistency reliability is .70 for group-level and .90 or higher for individual-level analysis (Nunnally & Bernstein, 1994). Values any lower than this mean that some items in the summary scale do not tap the attitude in the same way as the others. When a researcher evaluates scales that others have constructed, an alpha of less than .70 should be a red flag that the items used in the scale to tap a particular concept are not entirely consistent in what they reflect about the person's attitudes toward the issue. These internal consistency coefficients are then helpful in deciding whether different questions are yielding similar answers.

A formula based on the number of questions (or items) in a scale and the average correlation among the items, as well as an example of the computation of Cronbach's alpha using this formula, is provided in Table 3.2. The values in the correlation matrix reflect the correlations among items in a ten-item scale of self-esteem reported by Carmines and Zeller (1979, p. 64). The average correlation is a mean (.32) of all (forty-five) unduplicated correlations in the correlation matrix (which range from .048 to .577). The coefficient alpha resulting (.825) reflects an acceptable level of reliability. If the alpha for the scale as a whole increases when an item is removed, this suggests its correlation with the other items is low and should perhaps be deleted. If the alpha remains unchanged or decreases, it should be retained.

Internal consistency reliability coefficients were computed for eight summary scales used to tap various dimensions of health status in the MOS (McHorney et al., 1994). These coefficients ranged from a low of .78 to .93, well above the overall standards for reliability. However, the MOS investigators pointed out that if the principal analyses involve comparisons between groups (such as patients in different delivery settings), the minimum reliability standard could perhaps be somewhat lower (.50 to .70). But if the focus is on individuals (whether a particular patient experiences an improvement in health over time), then a more rigorous standard may be required (.90 to .95) to ensure that sound decisions are made regarding the individuals' care.

Evaluating the Validity of Study Variables

The validity of survey questions refers to the degree to which there are systematic differences between the information obtained in response to the questions relative to (1) the full meaning of the concept they were intended to express, (2) related questions about the same concept, and (3) theories or hypotheses about their relationships to other concepts. Such differences generally reflect assessments of content validity, criterion validity, and construct validity, respectively. Figure 3.2 summarizes these three approaches to estimating the validity of survey measures, and Table 3.3 highlights the principal methods used to evaluate each (American Psychological Association, 1999; Nunnally & Bernstein, 1994).

Content Validity

Content validity relies on judgments about whether the questions chosen are representative of the concepts they are intended to reflect. More precisely, it refers to how good a sample the empirical measures are of the theoretical domain they are

FIGURE 3.2. EVALUATING THE VALIDITY OF STUDY VARIABLES.

	Computation	
Types of Validity	Measure	"True Value"
Content Validity (extent to which measures adequately represent concept)	Variables	Concept

Content Validity (extent to which measures adequately represent concept)

Variables

x1
x2
x3
x4

$=$
$= = = = = = = =$

Concept

X1
X2
X3
X4

Criterion Validity (extent to which measure predicts or agrees with criterion indicator of concept)
—Predictive
—Concurrent

Variable

x1

r
$+ + + + + + + +$

Criterion

x1'

where r = correlation coefficient

Variable (x1)   Criterion (x1')

+   −

	a = true +	b = false +
+		
−	c = false −	d = true −

Sensitivity = $a \div (a + c)$ Specificity = $d \div (b + d)$

Construct Validity (extent to which relationships between measures agree with relationships predicted by theories or hypotheses)
—Convergent
—Discriminant

Observed Relationships

+
x1 + + + + x1'
0
x1 + + + + x2
0
x1 + + + + x3
+
x1 + + + + x4

$=$
$= = = = = = = =$

Theoretical Relationships

+
X1 + + + + X1'
0
X1 + + + + X2
0
X1 + + + + X3
+
X1 + + + + X4

TABLE 3.3. METHODS OF COMPUTING VALIDITY.

Methods	Types of Validity		
	Content	Criterion	Construct
Literature review	X		
Expert judgment	X		
Sensitivity-specificity analysis		X	
Correlation coefficients		X	X
Known-groups validity			X
Factor analysis			X
Multitrait multimethod			X

presumed to represent. It is therefore important that there be some clear idea of the domain or universe of meaning implied in the concept being evaluated. One way to ensure that a series of questions has a fair amount of content validity is to begin with questions and variables on the same topic that have been used in other studies. The researcher could also ask expert consultants in the area whether, in their judgment, the questions being asked adequately represent the concept. This approach could be formalized by asking the experts to rate specific items in terms of whether they are not relevant, somewhat relevant, quite relevant, or very relevant to the study concept and empirically assessing the evaluator's level of endorsement of the respective items (Wynd, Schmidt, & Schaefer, 2003).

Investigators in the MOS were interested in validating empirical measures of the dimensions of physical, mental, and social functioning and well-being, as well as general health perceptions and satisfaction. The content validity analyses in that study involved thorough reviews of the literature on the concepts and measures within each dimension. The content of the items being considered for inclusion in the study was then compared with the universe of items distilled from this literature review to evaluate whether at least one item was included to represent each of the major dimensions of health and certain concepts within each dimension (such as depression and anxiety within the mental health dimension) and whether a sufficient number of items were included to represent each dimension and concept adequately (Stewart & Ware, 1992; Ware & Gandek, 1998b).

Criterion Validity

Criterion validity refers to the extent to which the survey measure predicts or agrees with some criterion of the "true" value (or "gold standard") for the measure. The two major types of criterion-based validity are *predictive* and *concurrent validity*, depending on whether the criterion is one that can be predicted by or currently corresponds with the survey estimate.

Both types of criterion validity are generally quantified through correlation coefficients between the survey measure and the (future or concurrent) criterion source value. The higher the correlation, the greater the validity of the survey measure is said to be. The predictive validity of a survey-based measure of functional status, for example, could be based on the correlation of this measure with the ability of the respondent to carry out certain physical tasks in the future. This form of validity analysis is often used in designing tests to choose good candidates for certain programs (such as health promotion programs) based on the correlation of scores (of probable adherence) on screening tests with participants' later performance in the program (actual adherence to prescribed health promotion regimens). Tests of predictive validity may be particularly applicable to measures to be employed in longitudinal studies or experimental or quasi-experimental designs that are used to reflect changes in respondents' behavior, attitudes, or knowledge over time. Concurrent validity, in contrast, reflects the correspondence between the survey measure and a criterion measure obtained at essentially the same point in time. For example, concurrent validity could be evaluated by correlating patient reports of the types of conditions for which they had seen their physicians during a year with the physicians' medical records for the same time period.

Another approach to quantifying both predictive and concurrent criterion validity is to use sensitivity and specificity analyses. The diagram in Figure 3.2 shows the outcomes that could result, for example, when patient and physician data are compared by means of this approach. The proportion represented by the number of times that the patient reports a condition that also appears in the physician records $[a/(a + c)]$ reflects the sensitivity of the survey question to picking up the condition in the survey when it is known, from the physician records, to have occurred. The extent to which patients do *not* report conditions that do *not* appear on the medical record $[d/(b + d)]$ reflects the "specificity" or accuracy of the aim of the measure in not netting something it should not. When a respondent reports an extra condition that is not found in the physician's record, it is said to be a "false-positive" response. If, in contrast, the respondent fails to report a condition that is found in the medical record, it is said to be a "false-negative" survey response. The higher the sensitivity and specificity of the survey measure, and correspondingly, the lower the false-positive and false-negative rates of the indicator when compared with the criterion source, the greater is its criterion validity. Highly unreliable survey measures are likely to have low sensitivity and specificity as well (Hennekens & Buring, 1987).

Examples of concurrent validity analyses conducted in the MOS included examining the correlation between a survey-based measure of depression and a gold standard measure derived from the Diagnostic Interview Schedule of the *Diagnostic and Statistical Manual of Mental Disorders* (American Psychiatric Association, 2000), as well as the correlation of a short-form measure of physical functioning with a validated longer form measure of the same concept. The predictive validity of a perceived health measure gathered at the time of enrollment in the study was assessed by examining its association with the use of health services in the following year (Stewart & Ware, 1992).

Construct Validity

Evaluations of the construct validity of a survey variable assume that there are well-developed theories or hypotheses about the relationships of that variable to others being measured in the study. Construct validity examines whether and how many of the relationships predicted by these theories or hypotheses are empirically borne out when the data are analyzed. The more often these hypothetical relationships are confirmed, the greater the construct validity of the survey variables is assumed to be. Construct validity tests whether a hypothesized association between the survey measure and a measure of the same concept (convergent validity) or a different concept (discriminant validity) is confirmed.

Construct validity analysis is appropriate when the concept being measured is more abstract and/or for which there is not an equivalent empirically verifiable criterion available against which to compare the survey question, such as attitudes toward physicians. In contrast, criterion (particularly concurrent) validity principally examines the strength of the association of the survey question (regarding physician visits, for example) with what is deemed to be an equivalent, accurate, objective measure of the same concept (say, physician visits recorded in the patient's medical record).

Correlational analyses can be used to quantify construct validity as well. For example, in the MOS, it was hypothesized that different indicators of physical health (such as physical functioning, mobility, and pain) would be correlated (as in the example of the positive correlation between x1 and x1' in Figure 3.2). Measures of physical health (x1) would not, however, be highly correlated with measures of mental or social health (x2 or x3, respectively). Furthermore, measures of general health status and vitality (x4) would be correlated with the measures of physical health (x1) as well as with the mental and social health indicators. The construct validity analyses in that study did in fact confirm these hypothesized relationships for the health status variables (Gandek & Ware, 1998; McHorney et al., 1993).

The more that different measures meant to measure the same concept (such as physical health) agree (that is, have convergence) and the more that they differ from those intended to tap other concepts (such as mental or social health), the greater the convergent and discriminant validity of the indicators, respectively, is said to be. Other approaches to examining convergent and discriminant construct validity, in addition to correlational analyses, include known-groups comparisons, factor analysis, and the multitrait multimethod approach (Table 3.3) (Streiner & Norman, 2003).

Known-groups validity analysis is based on comparing a given health survey measure of physical or cognitive functioning, for example, between groups with known clinically diagnosed (physical or mental) status. The hypothesis would be that the survey measures would clearly differ between the groups on those measures that were most reflective of the underlying clinical differences between them. The MOS compared four patient groups—those with (1) minor chronic medical conditions, (2) serious chronic medical conditions, (3) psychiatric conditions only, or (4) serious medical and psychiatric conditions—on both physical and mental health status measures. The results confirmed hypotheses regarding expected differences between the groups on the respective types of health status measures (McHorney et al., 1993).

Factor analysis basically uses the correlation matrix between variables as the basis for examining whether subsets of the variables are related in such a way (or form a factor) so as to suggest that they are measuring the same underlying concept. Factor loadings are used to express the correlation between each item and a given factor (DeVellis, 2003; Nunnally & Bernstein, 1994).

The MOS conducted extensive factor analyses of the variety of scales developed to measure physical or mental health status or overall health status and vitality. A strong correlation (or factor loading) was defined to be greater than or equal to .70, moderate to substantial as .30 to .70, and weak as less than .30. The results strongly confirmed that the hypothesized associations among the respective dimensions of health status at a strong, moderate, or weak level were correlated as expected (McHorney et al., 1993).

Psychologists have developed the multitrait multimethod approach to formally test the construct validity of measures of complex concepts. A matrix is constructed that displays the correlations between two or more health concepts (physical and cognitive functioning), for example, measured by two or more methods (health survey and clinical exam). With this approach, a measure is hypothesized to be more highly correlated with other measures of the same concept (physical or cognitive functioning) across methods (survey or clinical exam) than with a different concept measured using the same method. The matrix also provides a look at the underlying internal consistency reliability of the items intended to measure the same construct (DeVellis, 2003; Scherpenzeel & Saris, 1997). The multitrait multimethod approach was not used in evaluating the MOS-36 survey measures because the information used to measure the health status constructs was gathered through essentially the same data collection method (respondent self-reports) (Stewart & Ware, 1992).

It is important for the researcher to have a good idea of the soundness of the theory or hypotheses on which the predictions about the relationships between variables are based in order to make judgments about the construct validity of the measures.

Measures must be reliable to be valid. Conceptually, if there is a great deal of instability in answers to questions that are posed about monthly drug use to measure the presence and severity of drug abuse, for example, it would be very difficult to conclude that it has been measured accurately. Empirically the maximum observable correlation between two scales (used to measure the criterion or construct validity of one of them, for example) is defined by the theoretically maximum correlation multiplied (reduced) by the square root of the product of the respective scale's reliability coefficients (test-retest or coefficient alpha, for example). The maximum possible correlation between two scales with coefficient alphas of .60 and .80, even if the concepts they measure were theoretically perfectly correlated (1.00), would be only .69, that is, $1.00 * (\sqrt{.60 * .80})$ (Carmines & Zeller, 1979).

Constructing Typologies, Indexes, and Scales to Summarize Study Variables

As indicated in the previous discussion, many different questions may be asked in a survey to obtain information about a concept of interest. Using several questions rather than only one or two to tap concepts that are particularly complex or have a number of different dimensions (such as health status or preventive care behavior) can result in data that are more valid and reliable. For example, if the researcher wants to operationalize adequately the comprehensive World Health Organization definition of health, it will be necessary to ask questions about the physical, mental, and social well-being of the respondent. Sources and summary scales tapping a number of common social, psychological, and health status concepts are highlighted in Chapter Nine.

Figure 3.3 and Table 3.4 present different approaches for collapsing and summarizing a variety of questions about the same underlying concept into typologies, indexes, or scales that capture the overall meaning of a number of different measures of a concept. However, the choice of a method for summarizing the data is dependent on the level of measurement (nominal, ordinal, interval or ratio) of the variables to be included.

Typologies

An approach to combining one or more variables that are basically nominal scales might be a cross-classification of these variables to create a typology mirroring the concept of interest. Each cell of the cross-classification table results in identification of a type of respondent or study subject. For example, Shortell, Wickizer, and Wheeler (1984), in an analysis of the characteristics of community hospital–based group practices to improve the delivery of primary medical care in selected communities, created a typology of the groups based on whether their institutional and community environment was favorable or unfavorable to a group's development (X1) and the actual performance (high or low) of the group in meeting its goals (X2) (see Figure 3.3). The resulting classification of these two variables yielded a profile of different types of programs. Those programs that were started in a favorable environment and did well were called "hotshots" (Type 11). "Overachievers" were initiated in unfavorable environments but did well anyway (Type 21). In contrast, "underachievers" began in favorable settings but did not really achieve what they set out to accomplish (Type 12). "Underdogs" did not have favorable environments and did poorly (Type 22). Typologies are particularly helpful in descriptively profiling an underlying study concept of interest, such as the potential and realized success of participating organizations in the above example.

Indexes

Another approach to summarizing a number of survey questions about an issue is simply to add up the scores (or codes) of the variables related to the concept that the researcher wants to measure. The resulting total is a simple summary measure or index of the constituent items. This is a particularly useful approach for summing up the correct answers to questions that test the respondent's knowledge regarding a certain topic, such as the risk factors for HIV/AIDS or breast cancer.

Index scores do not, however, provide information on the patterns of the responses that were given. For example, do respondents seem to have more knowledge about certain diseases than others? Index construction per se does not assume a process for verifying that the individual items tap the same underlying concept: Do they reflect knowledge about these conditions or some underlying attitude toward the scientific practice of medicine? Furthermore, such summaries may make more sense for certain types of variables than others, depending on what the constituent numbers mean in terms of the respective levels of measurement. The sum of codes for types of the kind described earlier, for example, has no meaning in

FIGURE 3.3. CONSTRUCTING TYPOLOGIES AND INDEXES TO SUMMARIZE STUDY VARIABLES.

Typologies and Indexes	Level of Measurement	Scoring Methods		
		Methods		Scoring
Typology (cross-classification of answers to questions)	Nominal	Variable X2	Variable X1 1 2	Codes
		1	1 = Type 11 | 2 = Type 21	1 = Type 11 2 = Type 21
		2	3 = Type 12 | 4 = Type 22	3 = Type 12 4 = Type 22
Index (accumulation of scores assigned to answers to questions)	Ordinal	*Variable* X1 X2 X3 X4 X5	*Answers* 1 = yes 2 = no 1 = yes 1 = yes 1 = yes	*Scores* 1 0 1 1 1 — 4

itself. The process of constructing scales to summarize questions presumed to tap the same underlying concept attempts to address these issues.

Scales

The construction of scales follows this pattern: (1) a large number of items or questions thought to reflect a concept are identified (that is, an *item pool* is created), (2) items that are poorly worded or seemingly less clear-cut indicators of the concept are eliminated, and (3) some process for deciding whether the items fit into the structure for the variables that are assumed by a particular scale is chosen (that is, are they "scalable" according to that scale's requirements?). The major type of scale discussed here and presented in Table 3.4 is the Likert summative scale.

An implicit assumption in the construction of a summary scale is that the scale items are observable (empirical) expressions of an underlying, unobservable (latent) construct (attitude). Scale development methods such as internal consistency reliability and construct validity analyses serve to quantify the extent to which responses to the survey questions that are actually developed to measure this construct are correlated with or may be said to be "caused by" this underlying abstract

TABLE 3.4. CONSTRUCTING A LIKERT SCALE TO SUMMARIZE STUDY VARIABLES.

Scale	Level of Measurement	Method (Scaling and Scoring Method)						Scoring
		Variables	Response Categories					Scores
	Ordinal		Strongly Agree	Agree	Uncertain	Disagree	Strongly Disagree	
Likert scale (sum of scores assigned to answers to questions in scale)		X1	1	2	3	(4)	5	4
		X2	1	(2)	3	4	5	2
		X3	1	2	3	4	(5)	5
		X4	(1)	2	3	4	5	1
		X5	1	2	(3)	4	5	3
								15

but nonetheless real influence (DeVellis, 2003; Jöreskog, Cudeck, du Toit, & Sörbom, 2001; Nunnally & Bernstein, 1994).

As mentioned earlier, survey designers may want to use scales developed by other researchers. In that case, they should have some idea of how the respective scales are constructed, what they mean, whether the reliability and (when possible) the validity of the scales have been documented, and whether the findings for the populations included in those studies are relevant to the current population of interest. With the Likert scale, investigators can include items in the survey that they have developed on their own and that they think can be collapsed into these scales and then test the actual scalability of the data during analysis. Or, ideally, if the necessary time and resources are available at the front end of the study, the investigators can develop and test such scales on a set of subjects similar to those who will be in the survey and then incorporate only those items in the study questionnaire that turn out to be scalable.

The Likert approach to developing questions and summary scales is used with great frequency in surveys. It basically relies on an ordinal response scale in which the respondent indicates the level of his or her agreement with an attitudinal or other statement. This, of course, reflects a subjective rather than a factual response of the individual to an issue. Generally five categories—*strongly agree, agree, disagree, strongly disagree,* and *uncertain* (or *neutral*)—are used in such questions, although as few as three or as many as ten could be used.

Scores can be assigned to each of the responses to reflect the strength and direction of the attitude expressed in a particular statement. For example, a code of 1 could be used to indicate that respondents strongly agree with a statement regarding their satisfaction with an aspect of medical care and 5 when they strongly disagree. The scores associated with the answers that respondents provide to each question (indicated in parentheses in Table 3.4) would then be added up to produce a total summary score of the strength and direction of a respondent's attitude on the subject (with a higher score meaning a more positive attitude, for example). Likert-type scales are referred to as *summative scales* because the scores on the constituent question are summed or added up to arrive at the total scale score.

A good scale should have a mix of positive and negative statements (about satisfaction with aspects of medical care, for example). Let us assume that the following codes are used to reflect responses to such statements: 1 = strongly agree, 2 = agree, 3 = uncertain, 4 = disagree, and 5 = strongly disagree. A person who strongly disagrees (code of 5) with a negative statement ("I am sometimes ignored by the office staff in my doctor's office") or strongly agrees (code of 1) with a positive statement ("The office staff treats me with respect") would be deemed to have a positive attitude about their care (Weiss & Senf, 1990). When summing the answers to each question to create a summary score, if a higher score were intended to represent higher levels of satisfaction on this five-item scale, then a code of 1 assigned for strongly agreeing with a positive statement would need to be recoded to 5, for example. A formula for converting (reversing) the coding for this and other possible responses is as follows: $R = (H + L) - I$, where H is the highest possible value or response (5), L is the lowest possible value (1), and I is the actual response (or code) for a given item. For a five-item ordinal response scale that ranges from 1 to 5, the results would be: $(5 + 1) - 1 = 5$; $(5 + 1) - 2 = 4$; $(5 + 1) - 3 = 3$; $(5 + 1) - 4 = 2$; $(5 + 1) - 5 = 1$ (Spector, 1992, p. 22).

Other types of response gradients may be applied as well for the items to be used in developing Likert summary scales, depending on the nature of the question being asked. For example, in question 3 in the National Dental Malpractice Survey (Resource C), dentists were asked to indicate the extent to which different statements tended to be typical of "unsatisfactory patient encounters." The ordinal response gradient for this question ranged from 1 to 5, with a score of 1 indicating the characterization was very typical and 5 that it was "not at all typical" of such encounters. These items were used to develop a twenty-two-item summary scale characterizing "frustrating patient visits" (FPV), described more fully later in this chapter in the discussion of "Selected Examples" (Mellor & Milgrom, 1995).

The reliability indicators reviewed earlier can then be used to determine just how stable and consistent summary scores computed from the series of items are over time, across interviewers, and among the array of items on which the summary scores are based. The alpha coefficient can be used to assess the feasibility of combining a variety of attitudinal items into a Likert-type scale. As mentioned earlier, a minimum coefficient of .70 is required to document that items included are fairly consistent in how they tap the underlying concept.

More sophisticated procedures, such as factor analysis, can also be carried out to determine whether different factors or subdimensions of the same concept are being tapped by different subgroups of questions.

The MOS has made extensive use of many of the procedures outlined here in developing Likert-type summary scales of health status, including the MOS 36-Item Short-Form Health Survey (SF-36) and related forms of this scale (the SF-20 and SF-12, for example) (McHorney et al., 1993, 1994; QualityMetric Incorporated, n.d.; Stewart & Ware, 1992; Ware et al., 1996; Ware & Sherbourne, 1992).

Survey researchers need to consider whether they may be tapping a variety of subdimensions of a concept when creating summary scores based on different questions; they should also be aware of formalized procedures for testing whether they are in fact doing so.

Two other types of scaling that have been used in connection with health status index development in particular are item response theory (IRT) and utility scaling. Utility-scaling approaches to health status scale development are discussed in more detail in Chapter Nine.

The Likert summative scaling method is grounded in classical measurement theory (CMT). CMT assumes that scale items are essentially caused by an underlying, unobservable (latent) construct (such as satisfaction with health care or level of physical functioning) and that individual items selected to include in the scale are essentially equivalent (parallel) measures of this underlying concept. CMT also assumes that scores on the summary scales are the result of the respondent's true score as well as random error or variability and that the true score and error are essentially equivalent across items within a scale for a given respondent.

Item response theory also posits that items to be grouped together relate to a single latent (unobservable) variable. In contrast to classical measurement theory, however, IRT assumes that items are not necessarily equivalent, and, in fact, each individual item taps different degrees or levels of the underlying attribute (such as levels of physical functioning). CMT tends to create aggregate or summary scores from individual items, whereas IRT scores are based on estimates derived from modeling of the probability of choosing a given response category for a selected item (for example, need the help of other people in handling routine tasks none of the time, rarely, sometimes, often, or all of the time) in relationship to the overall level of the attribute (such as physical functioning). Guttman and Thurstone scoring procedures represented an earlier form of scale construction that permitted the creation of items and scale scores to reflect such gradients as well. These scaling approaches have, however, been largely supplanted by the IRT scale development procedures (Andrich, 1988; DeVellis, 2003; Hambleton, Swaminathan, & Rogers, 1991; Sijtsma & Molenaar, 2002).

Another unique and important contribution of IRT is its ability to disaggregate and quantify error within an item according to (1) the item's level of difficulty, (2) its capacity to discriminate among responses, and (3) its susceptibility to false positives. *Item difficulty* refers to the level of the attribute being measured that is associated with a transition, from "failing" to "passing" the item, that is, to what extent elderly respondents can pass a selected test of physical function implicit in a given item. *Item discrimination* is concerned with the degree to which a response can be unambiguously classified as a "pass" or "fail." Estimates of false-positive rates mirror the likelihood of respondents' guessing rather than knowing the answer to a given item with surety.

IRT is particularly useful in the development of summary scales that are hierarchical (items progress from easy to difficult along a hypothesized continuum, such as indicators of physical functioning), unidimensional (represent a single dominant concept), and reproducible (the order and meaning of the points along the scale, such as degree of difficulty, are not highly variable across different groups and over time). IRT assumes that each item has its own characteristic sensitivity to the underlying concept being measured that can be expressed as a logistic probability function (or the probability of answering the question in a certain way as a function of the magnitude of the underlying level of functioning). This approach can be particularly useful if one is interested in classifying scale items according to an underlying hierarchy (of task difficulty, for example) ranging from tasks that may be relatively easy (bathing and dressing) to relatively difficult (engaging in vigorous physical activity) to perform. An IRT analysis of the ten-item physical functioning scale (PF-10) from the MOS SF-36 confirmed that the items in this scale could be arrayed in this fashion (Haley, McHorney, & Ware, 1994; McHorney, Haley, & Ware, 1997).

Another important utility of IRT is its capacity to distinguish the extent to which the characteristics of items differ across groups. This application addresses differential item functioning (DIF), that is, the tendency of the item to perform differently in different groups (for example, across racial/ethnic or linguistic groups) that are actually equivalent in terms of the underlying attribute (such as physical functioning) being assessed. DIF analyses generate estimates of the level of item difficulty, discrimination, and false-positive rates across groups. They are therefore particularly helpful in developing and evaluating the cross-cultural equivalence of scales and are of particular benefit in cross-national and cross-cultural studies (Laroche, Kim, & Tomiuk, 1998).

IRT is increasingly being used in developing hierarchical scales, as well as an important adjunct to the development and evaluation of summative scales of health status and health impact (Conrad & Smith, 2004; Kosinski, Bjorner, Ware, Batenhorst, & Cady, 2003; McHorney & Cohen, 2000).

Critics of classical measurement theory argue that IRT more accurately and appropriately acknowledges that selected CMT assumptions—of equivalent true score and error across items for an individual, for example—are not necessarily met. The estimates derived from IRT analyses are, however, heavily dependent on the underlying model and measurement assumptions underlying the IRT analyses.

The principal driver for selecting and applying an approach to scale development should be grounded in the underlying concept the scale is intended to measure. If questions asked to measure an underlying concept (such as health status) are assumed to reflect a gradient (of physical functioning, for example), then IRT may be the place to begin in scale development. If the questions are assumed to be parallel or equivalent measures (of health or physical functioning), then Likert scaling would be appropriate. IRT could be then used as an adjunct procedure to verify that the assumptions underlying the Likert scale development procedures are accurate. Unified test theory is an emerging field of study that explores the methods for integrating classical measurement theory and item response theory (McDonald, 1999).

Special Considerations for Special Populations

Other important criteria, in addition to those reviewed here, for evaluating items and summary measures used in surveys are practical ones related to their responsiveness, interpretability, respondent and administrative burden, alternative forms of administration, and cultural and language adaptations. These are important criteria to consider in general, but they take on particular importance in studies of special populations. *Responsiveness* refers to the tool's ability to detect changes (in health status, for example) that are deemed relevant by individuals (persons with HIV/AIDS, for example) targeted for a particular intervention (a new drug). *Interpretability* means that the quantitative findings on the measure (scale scores) can be translated into qualitative meanings (health status) that can be understood by users or consumers (patients or providers). *Respondent and administrative burden* refers to the time and effort in administering the instrument, as well as responding to it. It would also be important to evaluate the comparability and reliability and validity of information obtained through *alternative modes of administration* (for example, self-report, interviewer administered, observer rating, or computer assisted). The evaluation of *cultural and language adaptations* is concerned with the assessment of conceptual and linguistic equivalence of other language versions of the instrument, as well as whether their psychometric properties (reliability and validity) are comparable for different language or cultural groups. It may also be important to evaluate the reading level of the survey instrument in relationship to the likely literacy levels of the target population (Scientific Advisory Committee of the Medical Outcomes Trust, 2002; Sullivan et al., 1995).

Generalizability theory uses analysis of variance to explore formally the extent to which the measurement process is similar across different measurement situations (data gatherers or mode of administration), referred to as facets. This procedure may be particularly useful to employ in evaluating the equivalence of items using different data collection modes or language versions of an instrument (DeVellis, 2003).

Selected Examples

The twelve-item short form of the Medical Outcomes Study Health Survey (MOS-12), which reproduces the Physical Component and Mental Component summary scales derived from the MOS-36, was incorporated into the 2001 California Heath Interview Survey (see questions AB1 through AB12, CHIS 2001).

The MOS-12 and MOS-36 have been widely used in providing overall measures of health status in a variety of population and patient surveys in the United States and other countries. The algorithms for computing the summary scores for the respective components of the scale, as well as findings for various referent populations, such as from national surveys or selected samples of patients, are available from the survey developers (QualityMetric Incorporated, n.d.).

Question 3 in the National Dental Malpractice Survey Questionnaire (Resource C) is illustrative of a series of questions that could be combined into a Likert summary scale. The latent construct being measured with this set of questions is dentists' characterizations of frustrating patient visits. Dentists are asked to reflect the extent to which a series of statements about likely attributes are very typical or not at all typical of such visits.

In a companion study to the NDMS, the questions were administered to 356 dentists in the Family Health Service Authority of Greater Manchester, England. A twenty-two-item summary scale of frustrating patient visits (FPV) was developed, based on the questions. Factor analyses confirmed five subscales or dimensions of such visits: unpleasant dentist feelings, lack of communication, patient noncompliance, patient control, and practice organization. Cronbach's alpha on the respective subscales ranged from 0.59 to 0.77. All five of the subscores were greater (meaning higher levels of frustration) for dentists who reported larger numbers of unsatisfactory visits and expressed greater dissatisfaction with dental practice in general. Three of the five subscale scores (unpleasant feelings, lack of communication, and practice organization) were significantly greater for dentists who had official malpractice complaints to insurers (Mellor & Milgrom, 1995). In general, then, the subdomains of the FPV scale were confirmed to have acceptable internal consistency reliability based on the Cronbach's alpha analysis and good discriminant construct validity, based on the factor analysis and comparisons between groups of dentists who were known to differ in important ways related to the scale.

A series of questions in the UNICEF Multiple Indicator Cluster survey (questions 3–12, HIV/AIDS Module, UNICEF MICS-2, Resource A) could be used to construct a Knowledge of HIV/AIDS Index:

3. Now I will read some questions about how people can protect themselves from the AIDS virus. These questions include some issues related to sexuality which some people might find difficult to answer. However, your answers are very important to help understand the needs of people in (*country name*). Again, this information is all completely private and anonymous. Please answer yes or no to each question. Can people protect themselves from getting infected with the AIDS virus by having one uninfected sex partner who also has no other partners?
4. Do you think a person can get infected with the AIDS virus through supernatural means?

5. Can people protect themselves from the AIDS virus by using a condom correctly every time they have sex?
6. Can a person get the AIDS virus from mosquito bites?
7. Can people protect themselves from getting infected with the AIDS virus by not having sex at all?
8. Is it possible for a healthy-looking person to have the AIDS virus?
9. Can the AIDS virus be transmitted from a mother to a child?
10. Can the AIDS virus be transmitted from a mother to a child during pregnancy?
11. Can the AIDS virus be transmitted from a mother to a child at delivery?
12. Can the AIDS virus be transmitted from a mother to a child through breast milk?

The answer categories provided for these questions are yes, no, or DK (for don't know). The answers to the series of questions could be assigned a score of 1 to mean a correct answer and a 0 to mean an incorrect answer. The scores could then be summed up to create an index ranging from 0 to 10, with a higher score on the index indicating more knowledge of HIV/AIDS. "Yes" responses to questions 3, 5, 7, 8, 10, 11, and 12 would be coded as correct answers (yes = 1). "No" responses to questions 4 and 6 would be coded as "correct" (no = 1). Any other answers to the respective questions would be deemed to be incorrect responses and assigned a code of 0.

Question 9, "Can the AIDS virus be transmitted from a mother to a child?" is, however, somewhat ambiguous. Given that it is placed before a series of questions regarding the virus being transmitted from a mother to child during pregnancy (question 10), during delivery (question 11), or through breast milk (question 12), the implication is that question 9 refers to transmission through mother-to-child contact more generally. In that case, the correct answer would be no. If the question is referring to more specific modes of mother-to-child transmission, addressed in detail in questions 10 to 12, then yes would be the correct response. The specificity of the referent for a given question and the order and context in which it appears should be carefully evaluated in formulating questions in general and in unambiguously scoring correct and incorrect answers to questions in constructing knowledge indexes in particular.

Guidelines for Minimizing Survey Errors and Maximizing Survey Quality

Reliability and validity analysis represent classic and important approaches to evaluating the magnitude of random and systematic error in survey data (see Table 3.5). A consideration of these norms may be applied at many stages of survey de-

TABLE 3.5. SURVEY ERRORS: SOURCES AND SOLUTIONS— DEFINING AND CLARIFYING THE SURVEY VARIABLES.

	Systematic Errors: Low or Poor Validity	Variable Errors: Low or Poor Reliability
Solutions to Errors	Monitor and evaluate systematic departures in the content of a survey question from the meaning of the concept itself (content validity), the accuracy of answers based on comparisons with another data source (criterion validity), or the strength of hypothesized relationships of the concept being measured with other measures or concepts (construct validity).	Monitor and evaluate random variation in answers to a survey question due to when it is asked (test-retest reliability), who asked it (inter-rater reliability), or as one of a number of questions asked to construct a summary scale (internal consistency reliability).

sign: in identifying the relevant principles to apply in wording certain types of questions (threatening, nonthreatening, attitudinal, and so on) in order to ensure the accuracy and stability of people's answers; evaluating the questions or scales developed in other studies; designing a pretest or pilot study to evaluate the reliability and validity of the instrument before going into the field; and constructing and validating summary scales based on the information gathered in the survey on a key study concept of interest.

High reliability and validity coefficients for a scale to measure a given concept do not in and of themselves ensure that the scale is either meaningful or relevant. Theoretical knowledge and practical wisdom are both useful in informing the development of questionnaire items and summary scales to measure a concept of interest. Limiting the dimensions of consumer satisfaction considered to the experiences of those who regularly use medical care may fail to surface the considerable dissatisfaction of those who do not. And asking questions that make sense to people who stroll the main street in, say, suburban Peoria may not necessarily play to those who live out their days on inner city streets.

This chapter suggested a number of criteria for survey designers to consider in deciding what questions to include in their studies and how to go about reducing an array of questions about the same topic into parsimonious and reliable summary indicators for analysis. Readers may want to return to this chapter as they think about how to analyze the data in their own studies. The alternatives are presented here, however, to encourage survey designers to think about these types of analyses early on so that they will know what kinds of items or summary scales to look for or create in designing their own studies as well as the criteria to use in evaluating them. In fact, it may be desirable to use well-developed scales that have undergone rigorous development and evaluation of the kind described here to measure key study constructs. The next chapter outlines the elements to consider when thinking through the analyses for the study—before asking the first question of a respondent.

Supplementary Sources

Explanations of the steps involved in constructing a summated rating (Likert) scale may be found in Spector (1992) and DeVellis (2003). See Hennekens and Buring (1987) for an example of sensitivity and specificity analysis. Andrich (1988), Hambleton, Swaminathan, and Rogers (1991), and Sijtsma and Molenaar (2002) provide a discussion of the fundamentals of Rasch models of measurement and item-response theory, and Haley, McHorney, and Ware (1994) and McHorney, Haley, and Ware (1997) usefully demonstrate the application of the IRT methodology to the evaluation and refinement of the MOS-36.

CHAPTER FOUR

THINKING THROUGH THE RELATIONSHIPS BETWEEN VARIABLES

Chapter Highlights

1. An informed approach to survey design identifies not only the specific variables that will be used to measure the study concepts but also the relationships between them, which are implied in the study's research objectives and hypotheses.

2. The basis for identifying relevant variables and their interrelationships may be a theory or conceptual framework, previous research, or practical experience.

3. The study objectives and type of design underlying them (cross-sectional versus longitudinal, for example) dictate the type of analyses that can be conducted.

4. To establish that an independent variable is a "cause" of the dependent variable, (1) there must be a statistical association or correlation among the variables; (2) a theoretical, conceptual, or practical basis for an hypothesized relationship must exist; (3) the occurrence of the independent variable must precede the occurrence of the dependent variable in time; and (4) other explanations for what might "cause" the dependent variable have to be ruled out.

Before developing the survey questionnaire and approaches to gathering the data, researchers must consider not only the major variables but also their interrelationships that will be examined and why. The study objectives and hypotheses and associated research design are the defining guides for specifying these relationships.

As pointed out in Chapter Two, a theory or conceptual framework, previous research, or practical experience may serve as the basis for delineating the objectives and hypotheses. The analytical thrust (descriptive, analytical, or experimental), as well as the temporal and spatial parameters (cross-sectional, group-comparison, or longitudinal) of the design, are meant to mirror and underlie the questions that the study will address (see again Tables 2.2 and 2.3 and Figure 2.1).

Testing Study Hypotheses

As mentioned in Chapter Two, longitudinal or experimental designs allow the investigator to detect more clearly the "cause" of an outcome of interest than do one-time cross-sectional surveys. In one-time surveys, the researcher relies on theoretical models of the causal chain of events that lead to certain outcomes and on statistical approaches to testing those models. The process of statistically controlling for other variables in such analyses is comparable to creating equivalence between groups through the random assignment of subjects to an experimental and control condition in a true experimental design. Then the only condition that varies between the two groups is the administration of the experimental stimulus, which is analogous to the operation of the "independent variable" in cross-sectional survey analyses. Correspondingly, the sampling design for the study must anticipate the number of cases required to carry out the resulting subgroup analyses.

Discovering the determinants of human behaviors or attitudes requires consideration of a range of complex, interrelated factors. Sociologists in particular have developed and refined approaches for sorting out the most important reasons that people behave the way they do. In the main, these approaches are based on procedures for elaborating study hypotheses (Hirschi & Selvin, 1996; Raftery, 2000; Rosenberg, 1968; Zeisel, 1985). The discussion that follows provides examples of how these approaches can be used to refine the hypotheses that guide the design and conduct of health surveys.

In a chemistry lab, students may be given two known compounds and one unknown and asked to identify the unknown compound on the basis of prior assumptions about the reactions that will occur when the chemicals are mixed. Testing study hypotheses is like sorting out the chemistry between two variables when another one is added to the equation. In addition to the main independent and dependent variables, the variables that could be included in a study are termed *test* or *control* variables. They help in examining whether one variable does indeed cause another or whether the relationship observed between the variables is "caused" by some other factor. It is important to identify these other variables in advance of doing a survey to ensure that data are available to examine adequately and accurately the variety of competing explanations for relationships observed between the main independent and dependent variables in a study.

As mentioned in Chapter Two, other conditions in addition to a statistical association or correlation must be satisfied for an independent variable to be considered a "cause" of the dependent variable: (1) there has to be some theoretical, conceptual, or practical basis for an hypothesized relationship; (2) the occurrence of the independent variable has to precede the occurrence of the dependent variable in time; and (3) other explanations for what might "cause" the dependent variable have to be ruled out.

Researchers should also decide whether they are principally interested in testing for the simple *existence of a relationship* (or association) between two variables or groups of interest or the *strength of the relationship* (or association) between the two variables, or both. An array of statistical procedures and associated tests of significance (such as chi-square, *t*-tests, and analysis of variance) can be used to test for the existence of a relationship between variables. Correlation coefficients appropriate to the level of measurement of the respective variables—most of which range between 0 and 1.0 or -1.0 to $+1.0$—can be used to measure the strength and direction of the relationship between variables (or groups). Specific statistical techniques for examining these relationships for different study designs and types of variables are reviewed in Chapter Fifteen.

The variables in the hypotheses used here to illustrate the approaches to analyzing health survey data are expressed in terms of dichotomous categorical variables. The same basic logic can be applied, however, to examining the relationships between study variables based on other (higher) levels of measurement.

The first step in developing and testing a hypothesis is to specify the relationship that one expects to find between the main independent and dependent variables of interest. For example, in Table 2.2, the analytical designs were guided by the hypothesis that friends' smoking behavior (independent variable) was predictive of high school seniors' propensity to smoke (dependent variable). The simplest type of statistical procedure for testing the relationship between nominal-level independent and dependent variables is to construct a data table that looks at a cross-classification of the dependent variable Y (whether the senior smokes or not) by the independent variable X (seniors with friends who smoke versus those whose friends do not smoke). (See the sample table in Figure 4.1.) If a large proportion

(say, 75 percent) of the seniors whose friends are smokers smoke and a smaller proportion (say, 30 percent) of those whose friends are not smokers smoke, then the
findings would seem to bear out the study hypothesis.

An approach that epidemiologists use in examining the relative importance
of exposure to different health risks (elevated cholesterol levels) in accounting for
whether a person has a disease (heart disease), using a case-control design, is the
odds ratio or relative risk (Kahn & Sempos, 1989). This ratio can be computed by

FIGURE 4.1. TESTING THE MAIN STUDY HYPOTHESIS.

Theoretical Model and Sample Table

Theoretical Model

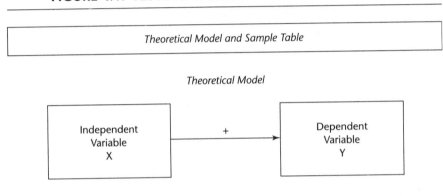

Sample Table

Student Smoking Status (Y)	Friends' Smoking Status (X)		Total
	Some or All	None	
Smoker	*a* 75% (75)	*b* 30% (30)	53% (105) *(a + b)*
Nonsmoker	*c* 25% (25)	*d* 70% (70)	48% (95) *(c + d)*
Total	100% *(a + c)* (100)	100% *(b + d)* (100)	100% (200) *(a + b + c + d)*

odds ratio (OR) $= \dfrac{a/b}{c/d} = \dfrac{ad}{bc} = \dfrac{75*70}{30*25} = \dfrac{5{,}250}{750} = 7.0$

chi-square = 40.6
p = .000

calculating the ratio of the odds (or likelihood) of exposure among the cases (with the disease) to that among the controls (without the disease) (an example of these computations is provided in Figure 4.1):

$$\text{odds ratio (OR)} = \frac{a/b}{c/d} = \frac{ad}{bc}$$

where, a = number of cases exposed (elevated cholesterol level), b = number of cases not exposed (normal cholesterol level), c = number of controls exposed (elevated cholesterol level), and d = number of controls not exposed (normal cholesterol level).

If the variables are not related, their respective odds would be identical (or nearly so) and the ratio of their odds (odds ratio, OR) equal to 1.00 (OR = 1.00). Odds ratios of greater than one indicate a positive covariation between variables (the presence of or the greater the magnitude of an attribute, the *more* likely the other attribute is to be present), while odds ratios less than one reflect a negative or inverse covariation (the presence of or the greater the magnitude of an attribute, the *less* likely the other attribute is to occur).

Odds ratios are most appropriately used with case-control designs to reflect the probability of having a disease or not as a function of having been exposed to selected risk factors. The examples presented in Figure 4.1 and the figures and tables that follow are based on a cross-sectional analytical design. Chi-square tests of differences are reported to document whether there is a statistically significant relationship between the independent and dependent variables (as defined in the respective examples). Odds ratios are reported as well to demonstrate the strength of the relationship between a given outcome (smoking or not) as a function of selected risk factors (parents' or friends' smoking), should this be an appropriate analytical strategy given the underlying study objectives and design. (See Chapter Fifteen for further discussion of guidelines for matching the analytical procedures to the study design.)

The strong association of students' smoking behavior with that of their friends is confirmed by the highly significant results for the chi-square test of differences between groups (p = .000, meaning de facto that it approximates .000) (Figure 4.1). The odds ratio (7.0) for the relationship of friends' smoking status (X) to whether a high school student smokes indicates that smokers are seven times more likely than nonsmokers to have friends who smoke. With cross-sectional studies, the time frame being referenced is embedded in the questions asked of the respondent, that is, whether it refers to current or past smoking practices, for example (see Table 2.1 in Chapter Two).

However, it is possible that other variables (for example, family history of elevated cholesterol or smoking) that might be related to the main (independent and dependent) variables (X and Y) in the study actually account for the relationship observed between these variables. The statistical procedures for examining the impact of these other variables attempt to consider *what if* the influence of these other variables were removed. Would the original relationship still exist? This process of removing the influence of these other variables involves not allowing them to vary (or "controlling" them, "adjusting" for them, "stratifying" on them, or holding them "constant") when looking at the original relationship.

The simplest way to control the operation of these other variables is to look at the original relationship between the independent and dependent variables in the study separately for groups of people who have the same value on the variable being controlled. In the cross-classification table of the relationship between friends' smoking behavior (X) and a student's propensity to smoke (Y), the impact of some variable Z could be controlled by looking at that table separately for different categories of Z—for example, students whose parents smoke versus students whose parents do not smoke, students who view smoking as a socially acceptable practice versus those who do not, or minority students versus white students. The variable Z takes on the same value, that is, it is "held constant" within each of the respective categories of Z. Statistical techniques used with higher-order levels of measurement accomplish the same thing through statistically "controlling for," or removing the effects of, these other variables.

As in the chemistry example given earlier, three results are possible when the impact of this third factor (Z) is controlled: (1) the original relationship between X and Y disappears, (2) the original relationship between X and Y persists or becomes stronger in one category of Z but not in the other, or (3) there is no change in the original relationship between X and Y. The first result represents an *explanation* or *interpretation* of why the relationship between X and Y seems to be affected so dramatically. The second provides a *specification* of the conditions under which the original relationship is most likely to hold. This is also referred to as "statistical interaction" or "effect modification," meaning that the original relationship between X and Y is different under different conditions defined by the control variable Z. The third outcome is essentially a *replication* of the original study results. These possible outcomes are displayed in Figures 4.2 through 4.5 and are discussed in the following paragraphs.

If the relationship disappears when the effects of Z are removed, it may mean one of two things: (1) X appeared to be linked to Y in the original relationship only because they were both tied to Z, or (2) Z really is an important link in the causal chain between X and Y. In either case, removing the influence of Z affects the relationship between X and Y.

The discussion that follows shows how these relationships can be tested empirically. Which aspect the investigator elects to emphasize depends on the theoretical perspective chosen to guide the collection and analysis of the survey data.

Explanation

One may be interested in further understanding the dynamics of the relationship of having friends who smoke to the likely adoption of smoking among teenagers as a basis for designing interventions to reduce this occurrence. Based on theory, previous research, or knowledge of the study population, investigators may wish to explore the influence of parents' smoking behavior as well as students' perceptions of the social acceptability of smoking as factors that determine or mediate the impact of peers' smoking practices.

If the investigator views the students' parents' smoking behavior as predictive of whether the students have friends who are smokers ($Z \rightarrow X$) and of whether they themselves are likely to take up smoking ($Z \rightarrow Y$), then the relationship between students' and their peers' smoking behaviors ($X \rightarrow Y$) would hypothetically be explained largely by these parental or family influences (Z), as shown in the theoretical model in Figure 4.2.

This model is called *explanatory* because the original relationship can be explained by some other "cause" (Z) for the apparent relationship observed between X and Y. As mentioned earlier, the strength of the causal argument must be grounded in the theoretical and temporal ordering of variables, in addition to the existence and strength of statistical associations between variables. The test variable in this type of model is an *extraneous* or *confounding* variable. It lies outside the direct causal chain between the independent and dependent variables. The original relationship between variables is, as a result, labeled "spurious" because although it looked as though there was a direct causal relationship between X and Y, the investigator's theory and findings indicate that something else was the real cause of both. Implicitly this extraneous or confounding influence is temporally and instrumentally prior to each of the other factors, that is, the fact that parents smoke is likely to influence the choice of friends who do so, as well as set up a predisposition for the student to take up smoking.

The sample tables in Figure 4.2 show how each of these relationships can be tested empirically. First, the relationship between parents' smoking behavior (Z) and friends' smoking status (X), $Z \rightarrow X$, is tested (Table a in Figure 4.2). The data show that the percentage with friends who smoke is much higher among those with parents who smoke than among those whose parents do not: 67 percent versus 19 percent. These findings establish that parents' and friends' smoking practices are related. Also, it is reasonable from both theoretical and temporal points

FIGURE 4.2. ELABORATING THE
MAIN STUDY HYPOTHESIS—EXPLANATION.

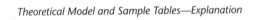

Theoretical Model and Sample Tables—Explanation

Theoretical Model

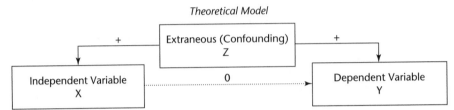

Sample Tables

Table a			Table b		
Friends' Smoking Status (X)	Parents' Smoking Status (Z)		Student Smoking Status (Y)	Parents' Smoking Status (Z)	
	One or Both	Neither		One or Both	Neither
Some or All	67% (87)	19% (13)	Smoker	69% (90)	21% (15)
None	33% (43)	81% (57)	Nonsmoker	31% (40)	79% (55)
Total	100% (130)	100% (70)	**Total**	100% (130)	100% (70)

Table c Z = One or both parents			Table d Z = Neither parent		
Student Smoking Status (Y)	Friends' Smoking Status (X)		Student Smoking Status (Y)	Friends' Smoking Status (X)	
	Some or All	None		Some or All	None
Smoker	69% (60)	70% (30)	Smoker	23% (3)	21% (12)
Nonsmoker	31% (27)	30% (13)	Nonsmoker	77% (10)	79% (45)
Total	100% (87)	100% (43)	**Total**	100% (13)	100% (57)
$OR = \dfrac{60 \times 13}{30 \times 27} = \dfrac{780}{810} = .96$ chi-square = .01 p = .926			$OR = \dfrac{3 \times 45}{12 \times 10} = \dfrac{135}{120} = 1.1$ chi-square = .03 p = .872		

of view that if their parents smoke, students are more likely to be comfortable with friends who smoke.

Next, the relationship between the parents' and students' behavior ($Z \rightarrow Y$) is examined (Table b in Figure 4.2). These data show that 69 percent of the students whose parents smoke also smoke compared with only 21 percent of those whose parents are nonsmokers. Parents' smoking practices then influence what their children do.

The final set of tables in Figure 4.2 examines the original relationship hypothesized between their peers' (X) and the students' own behavior (Y), controlling for parental influences (Z), which was found to be related to both, based on the cross-sectional analytical design. The data in Tables c and d in Figure 4.2 show that regardless of what their friends do, the majority (around 70 percent) of the students with parents who smoke also smoke. Among those whose parents do not smoke, the majority (almost 80 percent) do not smoke no matter whether their friends are smokers.

The odds ratios for the original relationship displayed in those tables controlling for parents' behavior (Tables c and d) are close to 1.0, and the chi-square tests of difference are not significant, indicating that the relationship between peer and student practices can be largely explained by whether the students' parents smoke. These results bear out the important influence that parental role modeling has on student behavior.

Interpretation

If the investigator hypothesizes that peers' smoking practices directly influence students' perceptions of the social acceptability of smoking ($X \rightarrow Z$) and that this in turn predicts whether the student is likely to take up smoking ($Z \rightarrow Y$), then a different temporal and causal ordering of variables is suggested. The underlying hypothesis here is that peer influences play an important role in reinforcing whether smoking is okay, which leads to a greater chance of teenagers' taking up the practice.

This model reflects an "interpretation" of the direct causal linkages between variables that lead to the outcome of interest: $X \rightarrow Z \rightarrow Y$ (Figure 4.3). The control variable that is thought on the basis of the investigator's theory to facilitate an interpretation of why and how X leads to Y is called an *intervening* or *mediating* variable. It theoretically intervenes in or mediates the causal linkage between X and Y.

The investigator may want to go back even further in the causal chain to trace the importance of other determinants of this outcome. For example, there might

FIGURE 4.3. ELABORATING THE
MAIN STUDY HYPOTHESIS—INTERPRETATION.

Theoretical Model and Sample Tables—Interpretation

Theoretical Model

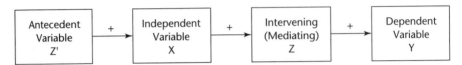

Sample Tables

Table a			Table b		
Attitude Toward Smoking (Z)	Friends' Smoking Status (X)		Student Smoking Status (Y)	Attitude Toward Smoking (Z)	
	Some or All	None		Socially Acceptable	Socially Unacceptable
Socially Acceptable	67% (87)	19% (13)	Smoker	69% (90)	21% (15)
Socially Unacceptable	33% (43)	81% (57)	Nonsmoker	31% (40)	79% (55)
Total	100% (130)	100% (70)	**Total**	100% (130)	100% (70)

Table c — Z = Socially Acceptable			Table d — Z = Socially Unacceptable		
Student Smoking Status (Y)	Friends' Smoking Status (X)		Student Smoking Status (Y)	Friends' Smoking Status (X)	
	Some or All	None		Some or All	None
Smoker	69% (60)	70% (30)	Smoker	23% (3)	21% (12)
Nonsmoker	31% (27)	30% (13)	Nonsmoker	77% (10)	79% (45)
Total	100% (87)	100% (43)	**Total**	100% (13)	100% (57)

$OR = \dfrac{60 \times 13}{30 \times 27} = \dfrac{780}{810} = .96$ chi-square = .01 p = .926

$OR = \dfrac{3 \times 45}{12 \times 10} = \dfrac{135}{120} = 1.1$ chi-square = .03 p = .872

be an interest in the impact of some variable (Z') antecedent to X (such as race or ethnicity) as a determinant of X (having friends who smoke).

In the example in Figure 4.3, students with friends who smoke are much more likely to believe it is an acceptable practice than those who do not have friends who are smokers: 67 percent versus 19 percent (Table a in Figure 4.3). Those who think it is a socially acceptable practice are also more likely to be smokers: 69 percent versus 21 percent (Table b in Figure 4.3). When controlling for students' perceptions of the social acceptability of smoking (Tables c and d in Figure 4.3), the original relationship between peers' and students' behavior disappears, as reflected in the odds ratios of around 1.00 and accompanying statistically non-significant chi-square results. Regardless of what their friends do, the majority (around 70 percent) of the students who believe smoking is socially acceptable smoke. Among those who do not, however, the majority (almost 80 percent) do not smoke, no matter whether their friends are smokers. In this case, the key link in the causal chain is student attitudes toward the social acceptability of this practice (Z).

Although parental and peer influences are considered separately in the examples provided here, the analyst may want to consider the impact of both in understanding the propensity to become a smoker. Multivariate procedures that permit a number of different factors to be considered as predictive or determinant of a given outcome of interest (such as multiple regression, logistic regression, path analysis, or LISREL, discussed in Chapter Fifteen) could be used for this purpose. The same basic logic applies. The investigator, guided by theory, previous research, or practice, must think through the study variables and their hypothesized interrelationships before formulating the survey questionnaire to make sure that the objectives that he or she sets out to accomplish can be achieved.

Interaction or Effect Modification

Another possible outcome when the original relationship between X and Y is looked at for different categories of Z or Z' is that the same relationship remains or grows stronger for some categories of the control variable but not for others. This finding further specifies under what conditions or for whom the hypothesized relationship is likely to exist (Figure 4.4). It may, for example, be important to look at the relationship between peer and student smoking practices for different racial or ethnic groups of students (Z'). Among Hispanic students, the percentage of those who smoke is high among those whose friends are smokers compared with those whose friends do not smoke: 86 percent versus 35 percent. But among African American students, the percentage who are nonsmokers is high (almost 80 percent) regardless of whether they have friends who smoke. The odds ratios and chi-square tests of significance for the impact of peer behavior on smoking confirm that it is a major influence among Hispanic students (OR = 12.0, p = .000) but not consequential for African American students (OR = 1.1, p = .872). (This phenomenon of finding that different relationships exist between the independent and dependent variables for different values of a third variable is said to reflect *effect modification* or *statistical interaction* between variables—X and Z' in this case.)

Replication

If the same relationship is found between the original variables when the control variable is considered in the analysis, then the original relationship—in this case, between peer and student behavior—is replicated (Figure 4.5). The odds ratios for this relationship, controlling for other factors, are essentially the same (around 7.0, p = .000) as observed originally (Figure 4.1). The control variable (parental influence, attitudes toward smoking, or race and ethnicity, depending on the model of interest) does not appear to have an effect on the original relationship. The hypothesis that peer behavior directly influences students' smoking practices is not rejected. The investigator will need to explore other possible explanations for this result if he or she is interested in pursuing that question.

Not every study is necessarily guided by formal causal hypotheses between study variables. However, even descriptive studies examine the relationships of certain attributes of the study population (such as their age, sex, and race) to others (such as whether they saw a physician within the year). The researcher should consider what these variables will be so that questions that should be asked are not omitted and questions that will never be used are not included.

Setting Up Mock Tables for the Analysis

One of the most important steps in developing a proposal for the conduct of a survey is to formulate a plan for analyzing the data to address the specific study objectives. A component of the analysis plan is outlining the tables that will be used to report the data to address each objective. These tables are called "mock" tables because they help the researcher to mock up the specific setup they will be used for summarizing and displaying the data once they are gathered and analyzed. Basic tables for displaying the data to address selected types of objectives and related study designs are provided in Exhibit 4.1. Researchers should also consult published articles or other resources in their field to glean ideas for how they might want to set up tables to best display the data to address their specific objectives (Nicol &

FIGURE 4.4. ELABORATING THE
MAIN STUDY HYPOTHESIS—INTERACTION.

> *Theoretical Model and Sample Tables—Interaction*

Theoretical Model

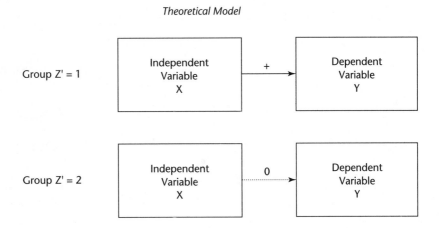

Sample Tables

	Table a Z' = Hispanic			Table b Z' = African American	
Student Smoking Status (Y)	Friends' Smoking Status (X)		Student Smoking Status (Y)	Friends' Smoking Status (X)	
	Some or All	None		Some or All	None
Smoker	86% (75)	35% (15)	Smoker	23% (3)	21% (12)
Nonsmoker	14% (12)	65% (28)	Nonsmoker	77% (10)	79% (45)
Total	100% (87)	100% (43)	**Total**	100% (13)	100% (57)

$$OR = \frac{75 \times 28}{15 \times 12} = \frac{2100}{180} = 12.0 \quad \text{chi-square} = 35.6 \quad p = .000$$

$$OR = \frac{3 \times 45}{12 \times 10} = \frac{135}{120} = 1.1 \quad \text{chi-square} = .03 \quad p = .872$$

FIGURE 4.5. ELABORATING THE
MAIN STUDY HYPOTHESIS—REPLICATION.

Theoretical Model and Sample Tables—Replication

Theoretical Model

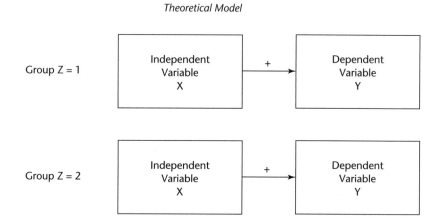

Sample Tables

	Table a Z = 1				Table b Z = 2		
Student Smoking Status (Y)	Friends' Smoking Status (X)			Student Smoking Status (Y)	Friends' Smoking Status (X)		
	Some or All	None			Some or All	None	
Smoker	75% (49)	31% (20)		Smoker	74% (26)	29% (10)	
Nonsmoker	25% (16)	69% (45)		Nonsmoker	26% (9)	71% (25)	
Total	100% (65)	100% (65)		**Total**	100% (35)	100% (35)	

$$OR = \frac{49 \times 45}{20 \times 16} = \frac{2205}{320} = 6.9 \quad \text{chi-square} = 26.0 \\ p = .000$$

$$OR = \frac{26 \times 25}{10 \times 9} = \frac{650}{90} = 7.2 \quad \text{chi-square} = 14.6 \\ p = .000$$

EXHIBIT 4.1. SETTING UP MOCK TABLES FOR THE ANALYSIS.

Purpose of Analysis	Examples of Mock Tables

To describe the sample

Table a. Characteristics of High School Students.

Characteristics	Percent (Frequencies)			
	White	African American	Hispanic	Total
Student Smoking Status Smoker Nonsmoker				
Parents' Smoking Status One or both parents Neither parent				
Friends' Smoking Status None smoke Some smoke All smoke				
Attitude Toward Smoking Socially acceptable Socially unacceptable Not sure				

To test for relationship between variables (test a hypothesis)

Table b. Student Smoking Status by Friends' Smoking Status.

Student Smoking Status	Friends' Smoking Status	
	Some or All	None
Smoker Nonsmoker		
Total	100%	100%

To explain relationships between variables (elaborate a hypothesis)

Table c. Student Smoking Status by Friends' and Parents' Smoking Status.

	Parents' Smoking Status			
	One or both parents		Neither parent	
Student Smoking Status	Friends' Smoking Status			
	Some or All	None	Some or All	None
Smoker Nonsmoker				
Total	100%	100%	100%	100%

Pexman, 2003). The procedures for developing the analysis plan and related mock tables are more fully elaborated in Chapter Fifteen.

The first step in carrying out the analysis of any data set, regardless of the type of study design, is to analyze the sample itself according to the major study variables of interest. In a descriptive cross-sectional study design, a key study objective might be to estimate the characteristics (X, Y) of a population (see Figure 2.1 in Chapter Two). In mock Table a in Exhibit 4.1, the number (frequencies) and percentage of people in each category of the major analysis variables can be displayed. One can then see what percentage (and how many) of the sample were smokers, what percentage (and how many) had parents or friends who smoked, and what percentage (and how many) thought smoking was socially acceptable. Univariate summary statistics for describing the distribution of the sample on the variables (such as a mean, median, and standard deviation) are reviewed in Chapter Fifteen. If certain subgroup breakdowns (by race, for example) are important for carrying out the analysis plan for the study, then special efforts may be required in the design of the sampling plan for the study (described in Chapter Seven) to obtain a sufficient number of individuals in the respective subgroups (white, African American, and Hispanic).

In addition to providing a profile of the members of the sample, the frequencies alert the researcher to (1) whether there is a large proportion of missing values for a particular variable, (2) whether there are too few cases of a certain kind to conduct meaningful analyses for a given group, and (3) whether there are outliers, that is, cases with extremely large or extremely small values on a variable compared with the rest of the cases. Based on this information, the researcher can make decisions regarding how best to handle these variables in the analyses. Imputing or estimating variables for those respondents for whom the information is missing, combining response categories, or deleting outliers may help to reduce bias and increase the precision of estimates. These procedures may, however, introduce other types of errors (see Chapter Fourteen). As with other types of research design decisions, the researcher has to be aware of possible trade-offs in survey errors at every stage of decision making and be explicit in addressing and reporting them.

Mock Table b in Exhibit 4.1 allows the researcher to look at a hypothesized relationship between the dependent and independent variables, paralleling the approach to hypothesis testing for cross-sectional or case-control designs outlined earlier. In cross-tabular analyses of the kind outlined here and in Figures 4.1 through 4.5 for cross-sectional analytical designs, the percentages should be computed within categories of the independent variable ("friends' smoking status"), that is, each column in Table b should sum to 100 percent. The percentages within the table would reflect the percentage of students who were smokers among those who had no friends who smoked versus those for whom either some or all of their friends smoked to address the question of whether friends were likely to influence the students to smoke. In contrast, in case-control designs, the percentages would be computed within categories of the outcome variable ("student smoking status"), that is, each row in Table b would sum to 100 percent. In that case, the data would reflect the percentage of students whose friends smoked among students who were smokers ("cases") versus those who were not ("controls") to address the question of whether smokers were more likely to have been exposed to friends who smoke.

It is not imperative that categories be combined or collapsed (as is done here for those for whom *some or all* of their friends smoke). The decision to do so should be based on both substantive and methodological considerations. Are the groups enough alike to warrant combining? Is the number of cases for one of the categories too small to be analyzed separately?

In Exhibit 4.1, mock Table c shows how a third (control) variable could be introduced into the analysis to see if the relationship observed between friends' smoking status and student smoking status is a function of parents' smoking practices. In this example, the relationship examined in mock Table b is examined separately for whether one or both versus neither parent smoke. This is analogous to the process of examining the relationship between X and Y for different categories of Z displayed in Figures 4.2 through 4.5. More than three variables can be considered in the analysis, but some multivariate statistical procedures are better able to handle analyses of a large number of variables than are others. (Specific types of univariate, bivariate, and multivariate analysis procedures are discussed in Chapter Fifteen.)

The number of tables used to report the study findings should be kept to a minimum, and each should be clearly related to the study objectives. Chapter Fifteen provides additional guidelines on how to construct mock tables to address different types of study objectives, and Chapter Sixteen offers suggestions regarding how to most clearly format and display data tables in the final report of the study.

Special Considerations for Special Populations

Issues that come into play in pursuing the types of analyses outlined in this chapter with special populations revolve around choosing subgroup breakdowns on interest (minorities versus whites *or* whites, African Americans, Hispanics, Asian Americans, Native Americans, or others) and designing the sample to permit a sufficient number of cases of each type to analyze these subgroups separately. Selected demographics (such as age, gender, and race or ethnicity) are frequently used as control variables in sociological and epidemiological analyses due to their assumed social or biologic relevance. These variables are most often cast either in the role of confounder (extraneous) variables, since they affect rather than are affected by other factors, or in the role of variables for which interaction effects are expected, that is, when the nature or magnitude of the hypothesized relationship between an independent (or predictor) and dependent (outcome) variable is assumed to be different for different groups (for example, males versus females, young adults versus the elderly, or African American versus Hispanic).

Selected Examples

A rich array of hypotheses may be tested and elaborated with the data from the three case studies in Resources A, B, and C. Theoretical models and previous epidemiological and behavioral surveys informed the selection and formulation of questions to include in those studies and, ultimately, the analyses of the resulting data. The California Health Interview Survey was grounded in the well-established Behavioral Model of Health Services Utilization and Access (Aday & Awe, 1997; Andersen, 1995). The UNICEF Multiple Indicator Cluster Survey was concerned with monitoring and comparing indicators and correlates of child development, health, and survival within and across countries (UNICEF, n.d.). The National Dental Malpractice Survey described trends in the dental malpractice liability system and analyzed policy and practice-related factors that helped to explain dentists' premiums and claims experience (Conrad et al., 1995). Examples of analyses conducted using these data sets are discussed in Chapter Fifteen.

Guidelines for Minimizing Survey Errors and Maximizing Survey Quality

To pick up a clear signal, background noise must be subdued. The same principle applies in ruling out sources of variation other than the main ones that are expected to give rise to a hypothesized outcome. Four main approaches can be undertaken to control for these other factors. Two of them can be implemented in the initial design of the study (randomization or matching of cases and controls, for example) and the other two during analyses of the data (stratified or multivariate analysis). The design-based alternatives were discussed in Chapter Two. This chapter presented the logic of stratifying (or conducting the analyses separately for different subgroups or categories of variables) as a basis for clarifying whether these variables are a source of noise. The use of multivariate analyses will be more fully discussed in Chapter Fifteen. (See Tables 2.4 and 15.5 for a review of relevant survey errors and the related means for addressing them.)

This chapter introduced the logic and techniques to use in thinking through a plan for collecting and analyzing the survey data. The reader should return to this chapter after giving more thought to the precise questions that will be included in a survey questionnaire. After the data are collected, the reader can use this chapter to review the steps that might be undertaken to analyze them.

Supplementary Sources

For the classic approach to stratified analysis from a sociological perspective, see Hirschi and Selvin (1996), Rosenberg (1968), and Zeisel (1985). From an epidemiological perspective, consult Abramson and Abramson (2001), Gordis (2004), and Rothman (2002).

CHAPTER FIVE

CHOOSING THE METHODS
OF DATA COLLECTION

Chapter Highlights

1. Nonresponse and noncoverage are bigger problems in telephone surveys and Internet surveys than in personal interview surveys; however, telephone surveys and Internet surveys can produce data of comparable quality to those of personal interviews at lower cost.
2. Mail questionnaires and Internet surveys may offer advantages when asking about sensitive or threatening topics, but constraints on the complexity and design of the survey questionnaire may be a problem.
3. Computer-assisted telephone interviews (CATI), computer-assisted personal interviews (CAPI), computer-assisted self-interviews (CASI), and Internet surveys are increasingly being used to collect health survey data.

This chapter provides an overview of methods for gathering data in health surveys and the relative advantages and disadvantages of each. The choice of data-gathering method has significant impacts on decisions made at every subsequent stage of a study: designing the sample, formulating the questions, formatting the questionnaire, carrying out the survey, and preparing the data for analysis.

The principal methods for gathering data in surveys are *personal interviews, telephone interviews,* and *self-administered questionnaires* (by mail, over the Internet, or in office, classroom, or other group-administered settings). Sometimes the methods are combined to capitalize on the advantages of each. In the discussion that follows, the advantages and disadvantages of the respective modes of data collection are compared to provide guidance in selecting the approach that might best fit the researcher's objectives and budget. The comparative advantages hypothesized for the computerized alternatives are also discussed. Finally, the chapter offers examples of how the respective data-gathering methods may be combined in a single study to enhance the unique advantages of each and to reduce the overall costs of the survey.

Criteria for Choosing the Data Collection Method

Researchers should ask themselves three general questions when deciding on the approach to use in gathering their data: Which method is most appropriate, given the study question and population of interest? Which method is most readily available? And how much money has been budgeted for carrying out the study?

The particular study question or population may suggest that a certain method of data collection must be used or is, at least, highly appropriate. For example, if the investigator is interested in finding out about the health care practices in a low-income Hispanic community, the majority of whose members do not speak or read English or have telephones, then an in-person interview in Spanish may be the only way to do the study. If a company's management is interested in enhancing the candor and confidentiality of responses to a survey that asks employees about health risks resulting from their own behaviors (such as excessive smoking or drinking) or perceived hazards in the workplace, then an anonymous mail questionnaire would be more appropriate than personal or telephone interviews. If a drug company wants to get a quick sense of the probable consumer response to alternative nationwide marketing strategies that it is considering for a new sinus headache remedy, telephone interviews are the best way to reach the right people in a timely and cost-effective way.

In some instances, certain modes of data gathering may not be available to researchers within their institutions or areas or may not be feasible within the proposed scope of their project. For example, projects carried out in large measure by a single student or researcher may necessitate the use of mail, Internet, or other self-administered questionnaires because there is no staff available to carry out personal or telephone interviews with prospective respondents. Again, computerized data collection strategies may seem preferable for a given study, but the firm or organization charged with doing the survey may not have that capability. Often the most fundamental determinant of what method is chosen is how much money is available to do the study and what the respective methods of gathering data will cost. As will be seen in this chapter's discussion, there are major disparities in the costs of different data-gathering methods.

The purpose of the study, the availability of a particular method, and its price tag are the overarching questions to have in mind when choosing among the methods.

Computerized Data Collection Methods

Before discussing the relative advantages of personal, telephone, and self-administered forms of data gathering in particular, a description of the computerized versions of each of these methods will be presented.

Computer-Assisted Telephone Interviewing (CATI)

CATI was the first widely applied computerized data-gathering technology. In the CATI system, the questionnaire is programmed and displayed on a terminal or microcomputer screen. The interviewers call respondents, ask the questions displayed on the screen, and then enter the respondents' answers into the computer using the computer keyboard. The earliest CATI systems were developed in the 1970s by Chilton Research Services of Radnor, Pennsylvania, to carry out large-scale market research surveys rapidly and cost-effectively for AT&T and other commercial clients, and by the University of California, Los Angeles, to conduct academic, social science-oriented surveys (Fink, 1983; Shanks, 1983).

The CATI technology accommodates a broad range of functions in the conduct of telephone surveys. These include selection of the sample by means of a random digit dialing (RDD) approach; the assignment, scheduling, and monitoring of interviews; building in specific probes or help menus that the interviewer can access during the interview; programming the logical sequence for a series of questions; and entering the allowable range of codes for certain items so that the interviewer can correct mistakes during the interview. Interviewers in centralized CATI systems can be linked (or networked) through a host computer that controls and monitors this array of functions.

Computer-Assisted Personal Interviewing (CAPI)

CAPI is essentially an adaptation of computer-assisted telephone interview technologies. The CAPI interview is programmed into a portable computer that the interviewer can carry to the respondent's home or other location to conduct the interview. CAPI technology has evolved with the development of smaller and smaller portable computers with sufficient storage to accommodate the complex program for the questionnaire, the data gathered from respondents, and the software needed to run the program.

Computer-Assisted Self-Interviewing (CASI)

The promises and approaches to *computer-assisted self-interviewing* (CASI) have blossomed with the advent of new and innovative information exchange technologies. Video-CASI and audio-CASI make use of the video and audio capabilities of small portable computers to present the questions on the computer screen (monitor) or over headphones connected to the computer to respondents, who then enter their answers on the computer keyboard or pad. This and related approaches offer particular promise for interviewing special populations (adolescents) about sensitive issues such as drug or alcohol use or sexual practices (Couper, Singer, & Tourangeau, 2003; O'Reilly, Hubbard, Lessler, Biemer, & Turner, 1994).

In some ways, *portable digital assistants (PDAs)* can be seen as a natural evolution in CASI technology in that a computer is used to collect data from the respondent. The primary difference between the previous generation of CASI and a PDA is that the latter is a handheld device, while the former can be administered using a desktop or laptop computer. Although the first PDA was developed in the 1970s, its popularity as a form of computing did not take hold until the advent of the Palm Pilot in the mid-1990s. PDAs are now used for many functions, including tracking student homework assignments (Fagerberg, Rekkedal, & Russell, 2002; Ray, McFadden, Patterson, & Wright, 2001), facilitating the training of medical interns (Criswell & Parchman, 2002; Smørdal & Gregory, 2003), monitoring patient care (Giammattei, 2003), and obtaining pharmaceutical updates (Cameron, 2002), in addition to facilitating survey research.

PDAs have been seen as more advantageous over paper-and-pencil surveys because of their portability and the ability to interface them with a database such as Microsoft Access (Giammattei, 2003). Their limitations include the difficulties associated with reading information on a small screen, including eye strain and visual disturbances (Kukulska-Hulme, 2002). O'Reilly (2001) reported that the use of PDAs led to the logging of more procedures by interns than using the standard approach. The study did not, however, document the accuracy of the reports. More research is needed to evaluate the validity of using PDAs in health surveys.

Like PDAs, the use of the *Internet* goes back several decades. Its viability as a means for conducting research increased with the expansion of the use of the Internet for commercial purposes. Internet-based surveys now include intercept surveys where a pop-up screen appears polling every *n*th visitor to a Web site; e-mail–based surveys where the respondent receives an e-mail invitation to participate in a survey by clicking a universal resource locator (URL) link, which opens a survey for them to complete online; or as an option that is provided to the respondent as an alternate way of completing a paper-and-pencil version of the survey. In this case, the respondent is instructed to go to a specific URL to complete the survey online. The common theme among these options is that they are all based on the use of an online form (or shell) for recording data into an online database (Couper, 2000; Gunn, 2002; Schaefer & Dillman, 1998; Solomon, 2001).

Internet surveys are seen as being convenient for the respondent and less expensive to administer than other approaches. They can save time in data editing because they can be designed to correct data entry errors while the data are being entered. They have an additional advantage over other methods in that they can be programmed to be dynamic, that is, the set of questions presented to the respondent can change based on the response to a previous question, as in the case of a response to a skip pattern in a questionnaire (Mertler, 2002; Pitkow & Kehoe, 1995; Scriven & Smith-Ferrier, 2003).

Computerized networks available through e-mail, the Internet, and related electronic highways offer promising channels, as well as new challenges, for the conduct of computer-assisted self-administered questionnaires and interviews. These methods may greatly facilitate and speed access to potential respondents, but they also pose a number of problems to be solved with respect to clearly delineating the target population, calculating noncoverage and nonresponse biases, and protecting the confidentiality of electronically transmitted responses (Wyatt, 2000).

Other CASI technologies include touchtone data entry to answer questions using the numeric keypad of a touchtone telephone; voice recognition entry, which entails a digitized voice functioning as an interviewer to read the questions, recognize the respondent's vocalizations, and echo them back for confirmation; FAX machines or the FAX capabilities of personal computers to transmit survey questions and return responses; and the accompanying processing of the information through computerized optical imaging or optical character recognition that translates the text into computer-readable form (Blyth & Piper, 1994; Dillman, 2000; Dillman & Miller, 1998; Janda, Janda, & Tedford, 2001; Tourangeau, Steiger, & Wilson, 2002; U.S. Department of Labor, Bureau of Labor Statistics, 2005; Walker, 1994).

Computer-assisted self-interviewing is a promising innovation that is likely to greatly expand the scope and possibilities of the older generations of data-gathering approaches. It will be used more and more as computers become more commonplace in homes and work environments.

Computerized data collection systems have been refined and expanded through the years, and many firms and organizations have developed software and associated hardware technologies for carrying out computer-assisted telephone interviews. CATI, CAPI, and CASI (including PDAs) have come to be widely applied in studies conducted by the U.S. Bureau of the Census; the National Center for Health Statistics, Substance Abuse and Mental Health Services Administration; the Centers for Medicare and Medicaid Services; the U.S. Department of Agriculture; and a variety of other federal agencies, academic institutions, and commercial and academic survey research organizations that carry out national, state, and local health or health-related surveys. Computerized data collection approaches, including possibly expanded use of the Internet, are likely to be defining of large-scale governmental and academic surveys in the future (see Resources D and E).

Comparison of Personal Interviews, Telephone Interviews, and Self-Administered Questionnaires

Table 5.1 provides a comparison of the advantages and disadvantages of personal interviews, telephone interviews, and self-administered questionnaires and computer-assisted adaptations of these at each stage in carrying out a survey. The comparison is based on a synthesis of critiques provided by other survey research methodologists as well as on current research on health surveys in particular (Dillman, 1978, 1991, 2000; Fowler, 2002; Groves, 1990; Groves & Kahn, 1979; Groves et al., 1988; Groves, Dillman, Eltinge & Little, 2002; National Center for Health Statistics, 2004b; Salant & Dillman, 1994).

The use of the plus and minus signs in Table 5.1 indicates whether there is an advantage or disadvantage of the approach, using the paper-and-pencil personal interview as the standard. A plus sign means that the approach tends to be equivalent or have advantages compared to the paper-and-pencil personal interview. A minus sign means that the approach tends to have disadvantages compared to the paper-and-pencil personal interview.

Drawing the Sample

Drawing a sample for a survey entails developing the sampling frame that will be used for selecting sample respondents to minimize noncoverage bias, procedures for calculating and evaluating the response rate and related nonresponse

TABLE 5.1. COMPARISON OF PAPER-AND-PENCIL AND COMPUTER-ASSISTED ADAPTATIONS OF PERSONAL INTERVIEWS, TELEPHONE INTERVIEWS, AND SELF-ADMINISTERED QUESTIONNAIRES.

Steps in Conducting Survey	Personal		Telephone		Self-Administered	
	Paper-and-Pencil	CAPI	Paper-and-Pencil	CATI	Paper-and-Pencil (Mail)	CASI
Drawing sample						
Coverage of the population	+	+	−	−	−	−
Response rates						
Calculation	+	+	−	−	−	−
Level (high/low)	+	+	−	−	−	−
Noncoverage and nonresponse bias	+	+	−	−	−	−
Accuracy in selecting respondent	+	+	−	−	−	−
Design effects	−	−	+	+	+	+
Formulating the questions						
General format						
Complex questions	+	+	−	+	−	−
Open-ended questions	+	+	−	+	−	−
Use of visual aids	+	+	−	−	−	+
Types of questions						
Nonthreatening	+	+	+	+	+	+
Threatening	−	−	+	+	+	+
Formatting the questionnaire						
Longer length	+	+	−	−	−	−
Control of sequence of response to questions	+	+	−	+	−	+
Carrying out the survey						
Supervision of interviewers	−	+	+	+	NA	NA
Length of data collection period	−	+	+	+	−	+
Preparing the data for analysis						
Need for editing/cleaning	+	+	−	+	−	+
Need for imputation of missing values	+	+	−	+	−	+
Speed of turnaround	−	+	+	+	−	+
Costs	−	+/−	+	+	+	+

Note: Plus and minus signs indicate whether there is an advantage or disadvantage of the approach, using the paper-and-pencil personal interview as the standard. NA = not applicable. A plus sign means that the approach tends to be equivalent or have advantages compared to the paper-and-pencil personal interview. A minus sign means that the approach tends to have disadvantages compared to the paper-and-pencil personal interview. See the text regarding the basis for the ratings assigned here. The evaluation of different aspects of drawing the sample is based on the assumption of the following types of designs: personal interviews—area probability sample; telephone interviews—random digit dialing; self-administered questionnaires—list sample. These assessments would be different for different designs. CASI includes notebook computer, PDA, and Internet computer-assisted self-interview technologies.

bias in the study, assuring the random selection of study respondents, and calculating and adjusting for design effects due to the complex nature of certain sample designs. (See Chapter Six for a fuller discussion of these issues.)

Coverage of the Population. A central issue in designing a sample for a survey is making sure that everyone the researcher is interested in studying has a chance of being included in the survey. In sampling terminology, this refers to the extent to which the sample design ensures coverage of the population of interest.

Methods for sampling households in communities and then selecting an individual or individuals within those selected households (area probability sampling) have been used most often in identifying respondents for personal interviews. This sampling methodology generally requires that field staff go out and list the addresses of all the eligible housing units (businesses or institutions would, for example, be excluded). The units in which the study will be conducted are then systematically selected from all the lists compiled by the field staff using methodologies designed by the study's sampling consultant. With this in-person approach to identifying eligible houses and then contacting them for the interview, the coverage of the study population is generally less of a problem than is the case with telephone surveys.

The National Health Interview Survey and many other national health and health care surveys have used these traditional in-person approaches to sample selection and subsequent data collection. Moreover, in-person field and sampling methods are essential for locating certain hard-to-reach populations that have become of increasing interest in health surveys, such as American Indians, Hispanics, and the homeless or drug-using populations that congregate in certain blocks or neighborhoods of a city (National Center for Health Statistics, 2004a, 2004b).

With the telephone interview approach, however, certain people will be left out of the study simply because the sample includes only people with telephones. Blumberg, Luke, and Cynamon (2004) used data from the 2003 National Health Interview Survey on trends in telephone coverage across time and between subgroups to estimate both landline and wireless telephone use in the United States. In 2003, 98.4 percent of adults had either a cell phone or a landline telephone. The noncoverage rate for U.S. adults as a whole was estimated to be 1.6 percent. Those who had no telephone service were more likely than those with telephones to live in the South; in one-person households; be renting their apartment or homes; disproportionately Hispanic or black; between the ages of twenty-five and forty-four; male; to have had less than a high school education; and not currently working.

The United Nations provided statistics on the proportion of households in 211 countries that have telephone coverage. Estimates varied considerably from

56 per 100 persons and 68 per 100 persons in Canada and Sweden, respectively, to 10 per 100 persons and 7 per 100 persons in Hungary and Mexico, respectively (United Nations Statistics Division, 2005).

As in the case of other approaches, there are challenges posed by using Internet surveys to collect data as well. The most notable problems are self-selection bias, sampling bias, and coverage bias (Pitkow & Kehoe, 1995; Saxon, Garratt, Gilroy, & Cairns, 2003; Solomon, 2001); concerns about privacy and confidentiality (Shannon, Johnson, Searcy, & Lott, 2002); and differential response rates across groups (Solomon, 2001).

Self-selection and sampling bias typically occurs in Internet surveys as a result of using nonprobabilistic sampling methods such as the posting of flyers on Web sites or bulletin boards to recruit survey respondents. This method of sampling respondents tends to lead to self-selection bias since respondents are often individuals who "volunteered" to participate after reading a flyer or announcement. Coverage bias occurs because samples are typically restricted to those who have access to computer technology. It may also occur because multiple submissions of a survey are possible when computers are used. The reliance on nonprobabilistic methods to recruit participants also poses additional concerns regarding privacy and confidentiality. Some respondents might see these solicitations as junk mail or spam and may feel that their e-mail address was obtained as a result of an invasion of privacy (Saxon, Garratt, Gilroy, & Cairns, 2003; Scriven & Smith-Ferrier, 2003; Shannon et al., 2002).

In light of these concerns, researchers have provided recommendations that are believed to improve the design and implementation of Internet-based surveys. Placing computers in private settings (for example, homes) and using additional methods to obtain consent may help to prevent early dropout from studies (O'Neil & Penrod, 2001; O'Neil, Penrod, & Bornstein, 2003). The biases discussed above can also be reduced by using probabilistic surveys that draw from well-defined populations such as professional or business groups with published e-mail addresses, in-house surveys of identified agency personnel, listserv members, members of professional associations, university professors, or alumni groups (Gunn, 2002; Shannon et al., 2002) .

Self-administered mail surveys are generally carried out with individuals who have been identified from lists of relevant candidates for the study, such as members of professional health care organizations, hospital employees, or health plan enrollees. Lists may be the best or, in some instances, the only way to identify these individuals. Coverage problems with such lists may result because they are not kept current, so that new people who would be eligible for the study are not included. In addition, other people's names may be left out or lost because of poor record keeping, some names may be duplicated on the list, and some that seem like duplicates may in fact not be. Researchers should be aware of these issues in evaluating a list of individuals to whom questionnaires will be mailed for a study. In fact, before actually launching the study, researchers may want to include a subset of the list in a pilot or pretest of study procedures to see what problems they will encounter. With respect to computerized self-administered questionnaires—because not everyone has access to computers and many people have a strong case of computer anxiety—the timely and broad application of this method may be limited to surveys of establishments or selected groups of individuals (professionals, patients, or students, for example).

As we will see later (Chapter Seven), there are methods for statistically adjusting for this noncoverage of certain groups to make the telephone and Internet survey sample more representative. Nevertheless, such adjustments cannot eliminate all possible biases that may result because of the underrepresentation of these groups in the sample.

Response Rates. Response rates refer to the proportion of people or organizations selected and deemed eligible for the study that actually completes the questionnaires (see discussion of response rates in Chapter Seven). The respective modes of data collection differ in their methods of calculating and interpreting these rates.

There may be problems in calculating the response rates for personal interview surveys if it is difficult to determine whether a household or individual is eligible for the study because of refusal or unavailability to complete a screening questionnaire to determine eligibility. These problems are, however, not unique to in-person interview methods.

The computation of response rates for random digit dialing telephone interviews is particularly troublesome; there may be a large number of telephone calls that are never completed because users may use screening techniques to cut off calls from automated devices, callers may use caller ID or other call screening devices, or they may choose to use only a cell phone instead of a landline phone (Frankel, 2004). Thus, wider use of answering machines, beepers, and cell phones complicates the determination of eligibility for telephone surveys. If budget constraints limit the number of callbacks, it will not be possible to determine whether these numbers are eligible ones—working residential telephone numbers, for example, rather than businesses or nonworking numbers. These issues complicate the computation of response rates for telephone interviews compared with personal interviews.

Analogous problems exist in computing the response rates for self-administered mail and Internet questionnaires. Pen-and-pencil questionnaires may not be filled out and returned because the intended respondent refused to answer the questionnaire or because he or she was deceased or had moved and left no forwarding address. A respondent could be legitimately excluded as being ineligible for the study if his or her status were known. In the case of Internet surveys, an e-mail can be returned because of an incorrect e-mail address. Or the e-mail may have been delivered to the correct address and the respondent refused to reply to the message. Or the person may have decided not to bother or overlooked it after opening it up. For some e-mail users, if they don't reply to a message immediately and it moves further down in their e-mail listing, it may cease to exist—unlike a piece of mail, which will at least sit on the desk or countertop to serve as a more direct physical reminder to reply.

The response rates for personal interviews tend to be the highest, followed by telephone, self-administered (particularly mail), and then Internet questionnaires. This means that of those determined or estimated to be eligible for a survey, more tend to respond to the in-person approach. This higher response is attributed to a number of factors, particularly the greater persuasiveness of personal contacts in eliciting cooperation, the smaller probability of breaking off the interview in person compared with interviews conducted over the telephone or the Internet, and the interviewer's ability to follow up with the respondent in person (Couper, Blair, & Triplett, 1999; Groves & Couper, 1998; Scriven & Smith-Ferrier, 2003; Solomon, 2001).

The response rates in federally sponsored national health surveys conducted using the personal interview approach have ranged from 63 to 71 percent (an average of 66 percent) for the Medical Expenditure Panel Survey to over 95 percent for the National Health Interview Survey (Ezzati-Rice & Cohen, 2004). Response rates for the state-level Behavioral Risk Factor Surveillance System surveys differ across states and have ranged from 48 to 59 percent for telephone interviews and from 52 to 72 percent for mail questionnaires in selected states (Link & Mokdad, 2004). Organization-sponsored Internet surveys response rates vary widely, depending on the sampling and follow-up procedures employed (Scriven & Smith-Ferrier, 2003).

In general, response rates tend to be lower in "cold contact" surveys, in which respondents have no prior knowledge that they will be contacted for a study, than in "warm contact" surveys, where respondents are sent a letter, called, or contacted in person before being approached for the actual interview. This tends to be true not only for in-person, telephone, or mail surveys but also for Internet surveys. Solomon (2001) found that the use of personalized e-mail cover letters, follow-up reminders, prenotification of the intent to survey, and simpler survey formats tended to increase Internet survey response rates.

There is evidence that young people, the elderly, the poor and poorly educated, the uninsured, and individuals who have certain disabilities (such as hearing loss) or tire easily may be less likely to participate in telephone surveys. This may have substantial implications for the representativeness and accuracy of estimates derived from telephone-based health surveys of these groups (Corey & Freeman, 1990; Donovan, Holman, Corti, & Jalleh, 1997; Kristal et al., 1993; Mishra, Dooley, Catalano, & Serxner, 1993; National Center for Health Statistics, 1987).

Those most likely to respond to mail questionnaires are often educated professionals with a substantial interest in the subject matter of the study. Surveys of Internet use have suggested that users also tend to be more educated than others, which is quite likely to result in the underrepresentation of socially disadvantaged groups in such studies (Kehoe & Pitkow, 1996).

For example, Morris, Colditz, and Evans (1998) found differences by race in the response rate to a 152-item mail questionnaire that asked elderly community respondents sixty-five years and older about their nutritional habits. The respondents were sent a copy of the survey, along with a letter and a stamped, addressed letter. This was followed by two subsequent mailings to nonrespondents over a four-week period. This effort yielded an 81 percent response rate for whites and a 53 percent response rate for blacks. In addition to finding a lower response rate for blacks, they also found that blacks were more likely than whites to have at least fifteen incomplete items on the questionnaire.

While personal interviews have been seen as more likely to result in a higher response rate than other methods, there is some indication that a high response rate to telephone, mail, or Internet surveys may be getting harder to achieve. Personal interview response rates have declined in recent years because people have become fearful of admitting strangers into their homes, fewer women are at home during the day to participate in such studies, and more high-security buildings and gated communities preclude ready admittance. Telephone interview response rates have declined as well because people have been reluctant to answer their telephones in order to avoid telemarketer soliciting (Frankel, 2004). The increase in junk mail and Internet spam mail has also made respondents more reluctant to complete Internet surveys. The response rates for major national health surveys such as the National Health Interview Survey have remained high, but the costs per interview have continued to rise because of the numbers of return visits necessary to find people at home or to gain access to high-security buildings or communities.

Nonetheless, answering machines and caller-identification features available to telephone customers are also formidable barriers to reaching respondents on the telephone. Individual computer users are using blocking software and firewall software to screen out unwanted Web pages. This may also have the unintended effect of hindering researchers from using pop-up ad solicitations as a way of encouraging respondents to complete online surveys. Furthermore, to the extent that households increasingly use screening devices such as call blocking and placing their names on a "do not call" list for advertisers, lower response rates are likely to result for telephone surveys and Internet surveys. This consequence may be mitigated to some extent by sending advance letters and e-mails to potential respondents when addresses are available or can be obtained or by making use of the local news media to publicize and lend legitimacy to the study (Crabb, 1999; Dillman, 2000; Frankel, 2004; Oldendick, 1993; Oldendick & Link, 1994; Solomon, 2001; Tuckel & Feinberg, 1991).

In the late twentieth century, telephone and mail questionnaires were thought to offer advantages over personal interviews in contacting hard-to-reach respondents. For example, in the mid-1980s, Goyder (1985) argued that the "mailed questionnaire . . . and electronic variants such as the telephone survey and direct video interaction are perhaps the optimal methods for surveying postindustrial society; these methods are tailor made for reaching a socially disintegrated citizenry, ensconced in high-rise urban fortresses in which face-to-face contact has been delegitimated, yet still susceptible to the behavioral psychology of a carefully orchestrated series of impersonal contacts and follow-ups by survey researchers" (p. 248). More recently, Dillman (2000, 2002, 2004) has argued that due to growing concerns with the limitations of reaching respondents through telephone surveys, the use of systematically designed and implemented self-administered mail and Internet surveys may be an optimal way to obtain survey data in the future.

The implications of the differential response rates and coverage of different groups for the accuracy and representativeness of estimates are discussed in the following section.

Noncoverage and Nonresponse Bias. Noncoverage or nonresponse of certain groups means that estimates for the survey as a whole or for those groups in particular may not be accurate because of these groups' underrepresentation in the study. As noted earlier, comparisons of estimates on selected health status variables between the population with telephones and those without indicate that those who do not have telephones are as a group in poorer health and may, in some instances, be less likely to be insured or use health care services at as high a rate as those with telephones. If there is a substantial underrepresentation of people without telephones or with health and health care characteristics that differ significantly from others in the population, then the characteristics for the population as a whole and for these subgroups in particular may be biased. Many households without a telephone are temporarily (or episodically) so because they have not paid the telephone bill, for example. The number of households continuously without telephone service is generally much smaller in most communities (Blumberg et al., 2004; Keeter, 1995).

For national health surveys of the general population with relatively high coverage and response rates, the estimates for those who have telephones do not differ significantly from estimates for the U.S. population as a whole, including those with and without telephones. Furthermore, the direction of differences between subgroups does not appear to vary for those with telephones and the population as a whole, because most people have telephones and most people agreed to participate in these studies. However, if there is an interest in studying certain subgroups, such as the elderly or low-income Spanish-speaking residents along the Texas and Mexico border, the lower telephone coverage or response rates for these groups might combine to introduce substantial biases (inaccuracies) into the data for those who could be reached by telephone (Adams-Esquivel & Lang, 1987; Blumberg et al., 2004; Corey & Freeman, 1990; Donovan et al., 1997; Keeter, Miller, Kohut, Groves, & Presser, 2000). To the extent that coverage and nonresponse might also be issues for mail questionnaires in general or for selected subgroups, comparable biases could occur. Knowing whom you want to include in a study and whom you cannot afford to leave out, as well as their probable rates of coverage and response to different data collection methods, will provide guidance for choosing the survey method that will provide the most accurate and complete data for those groups (Dillman, 2000).

Accuracy in Selecting Respondent. As will be discussed in Chapter Six, which describes different approaches to drawing samples for a health survey, an interviewer can use several approaches to select one or more respondents from a family for the actual interview. With computer-assisted personal and telephone interviews, the accuracy of the interviewer's selection is enhanced. Computerized algorithms can be designed to reduce the mechanical or clerical errors made by interviewers during this process.

Both the personal and telephone interview approaches offer advantages over mail and Internet questionnaires in getting the right person. The researcher has no control over who actually fills out a questionnaire once it is mailed or e-mailed. An individual respondent might ask his or her spouse to fill it out and return it; a doctor or health professional may forward it to a secretary or administrative assistant to complete.

Design Effects. The design effects for a survey, discussed in more detail in Chapter Seven, mean principally that the more the survey departs from a simple random sample design (analogous to drawing numbers from a hat), the larger the sampling (standard) errors are likely to be. The sample designs used for identifying sample households geographically to conduct personal interviews (area probability samples) are often complex and involve a number of stages of selection and several clusters of sampling units—at the county, U.S. census tract, and block and household levels. The design effects for these studies are thus often quite high.

The random digit dialing approach used in many telephone surveys, in which a list of all possible numbers for a given area code and prefix (or exchange) is generated and called, has a very low design effect. Approaches to increasing the proportion of eligible (working, residential) numbers by screening groups of numbers generated in this fashion do increase the design effect of the telephone survey. However, the design effects for most telephone surveys are much lower than those for area probability personal interview–based surveys (Groves, 1989; Marcus & Crane, 1986). Sampling from lists of potential respondents for self-administered surveys is also relatively straightforward and, for the most part, has low design effects. In general, lower design effects are better, and the sample designs for telephone and self-administered surveys usually offer advantages over personal interview survey designs in this aspect of designing and conducting health surveys.

Formulating the Questions

Questions that involve complex concepts or complicated phrasing or response formats have generally been thought easier to handle in a face-to-face interview with the respondent. The assumptions are that interviewers can make more use of visual cues to determine if the respondent has understood the question and that the respondent feels freer to ask questions to clarify responses than over the telephone. With the advent of computer-assisted interviewing, however, complex questions can be more easily designed and handled over the telephone—and in CAPI interviews as well—because relevant probes, help menus, and complex skip patterns that depend on the respondents' answers to certain questions can be programmed into the questionnaire that the interviewer reads from the computer display screen.

Like CAPI surveys, Internet surveys also have the advantage of allowing screen-based probes based on the response to questions entered on the computer by the respondent. Internet surveys present additional issues that have not been a challenge in administering CAPI surveys, including the fact that the same questionnaire looks different on different computers, and responses that are provided by the respondent that seem to be confidential may in fact be retrievable from hidden files on either a local computer or a network hard drive (Gunn, 2002; Scriven & Smith-Ferrier, 2003).

Some of the concerns regarding the visual appearance of the questionnaires and related response options on the computer can be resolved by centering response scales on the users' computers or providing clearly visible "don't know/not applicable" options for the respondents (Morrel-Samuels, 2003). Other solutions include designing an instrument that can be displayed on a variety of computer systems as well as working with the computer technology team on a project to ensure that the data entered from a survey go to only one controlled location in the computer network. Given the complexities involved in the development and testing of such questions, a considerable investment of computer and programming time and resources may be needed to prepare an Internet survey.

Problems arise when questionnaires filled out by respondents without an interviewer to assist them contain complex questions. Respondents may not understand certain concepts or instructions unaided or may consider the task too difficult and decide not to fill out the questionnaire.

One type of question that has been used quite often in surveys is the open-ended question. Here, respondents are asked to provide answers in their own words rather than choose a response from a number of categories provided in the interview or questionnaire. Personal interviews are thought to provide the best opportunity to use these types of questions, because both respondents and interviewers feel freer to spend the time to provide and record these answers than they would over the telephone. It should also be noted that while open-ended questions can be completed on a computer, there is the possibility that one may run into data entry problems in using an online form (like not allowing enough space to accommodate a response or the Web browser freezing during data entry) that can hinder the completion of an open-ended online survey question. While there is little evidence regarding the merits of using an open-ended online format, there is evidence that telephone interviews are shorter on average and that the amount of information recorded for open-ended questions is less than in the case of in-person interviews. It is not clear, however, that the accuracy or validity of the answers to open-ended questions is necessarily lessened over the telephone simply because people tend to give shorter answers (Bradburn, Sudman, & Wansink, 2004; Groves, 1989; Groves & Kahn, 1979).

As with complex questions, it is not advantageous to use open-ended questions and response formats on self-administered questionnaires because of respondents' possible unwillingness to take the time to answer them or because of their limited writing skills.

A limitation of telephone interviews compared with personal interviews or Internet surveys is that with the former, the interviewer can make use of visual aids (such as cards with response categories listed, containers to show the amount of some food product or beverage the respondent is asked to report the frequency of consuming, and so on). Conceivably such devices could be used in a self-administered questionnaire if their application in the study were made clear to the respondent. The use of audio (CD) or video (DVD) enhancements to a CASI approach may be of particular utility for people who are illiterate, have low reading levels, or do not speak English. They may also serve as a useful introduction to the survey process for respondents who are not familiar with the approaches used in survey research to collect data.

Somewhat different devices may be needed to facilitate complete and accurate responses to threatening or sensitive questions, such as those relating to sexual practices, drinking behavior, or drug use, compared with less threatening items, such as how often the respondent eats breakfast or went to the doctor in the previous year. One of the principal concerns with the advent of the telephone interview was whether equally accurate answers to the range of (threatening and nonthreatening) questions could be obtained with this approach compared with personal interviews.

Self-administered questionnaires are thought to offer the greatest anonymity to respondents, followed by telephone interviews and then personal interviews. It is assumed that the respondent enjoys greater anonymity over the telephone and is therefore more likely to report socially undesirable behaviors and less likely to feel pressure to provide socially desirable responses than he or she would in a personal interview. Cognitive psychology research literature in general and on health surveys in particular confirms that threatening or sensitive behaviors or characteristics, for example, are reported with equal or greater frequency over the telephone compared to personal interviews. Compared to respondents who complete an interview by telephone, however, those who completed a self-administered mail or Web survey more often tend to report that they are in poorer health or had more chronic conditions (Aquilino, 1994; Baker, Zahs, & Popa, 2004; Bradburn et al., 2004; Fowler, Roman, & Di, 1998; Hennigan, Maxson, Sloane, & Ranney, 2002; McEwan, Harrington, Bhopal, Madhok, & McCallum, 1992; Schwarz, Strack, Hippler, & Bishop, 1991; Tourangeau & Smith, 1996).

It may be the case that respondents in telephone or personal interviews provide what they think are socially desired responses to the interviewer's questions. To minimize this type of threat to validity, one needs to develop questions to address the issue of social desirability bias (Holbrook, Green, & Krosnick, 2003). (Principles for designing sensitive or threatening questions to minimize this type of response bias are highlighted in Chapter Eleven.)

A possible advantage of computerized self-administered questionnaires is that respondents may feel that the process is even more depersonalized and less threatening than a paper-and-pencil questionnaire, and therefore they may be more willing to answer candidly (Kiesler & Sproull, 1986; O'Reilly et al., 1994; Wright, Aquilino, & Supple, 1998).

More experimental research needs to be conducted comparing the respective methods for asking threatening and nonthreatening questions. However, the evidence to date suggests that personal, telephone, and self-administered approaches may produce comparable answers to nonthreatening questions but that the last method in particular offers advantages over the first two in asking about sensitive or threatening health or health care practices.

Formatting the Questionnaire

Advantages to carrying out a long interview in person are that the interviewer is better able to prevent a respondent from breaking off the interview and to deal with interruptions, respondent fatigue, or lagging motivation as the interview proceeds. In contrast, self-administered questionnaires should, as a rule, be kept short and simple to maximize respondents' willingness to fill out and return them.

Initially it was believed that telephone interviews needed to be brief because of the difficulty of keeping people on the telephone for extended periods of time. However, telephone surveys about health may have an advantage in this regard compared to surveys on other topics. Respondents are thought to be more interested in general in talking about their health than in talking about the brands of tires they use on their cars or whether they favor the Federal Reserve's current monetary policy, for example.

Evidence of whether computer-assisted interviews tend to shorten or lengthen the interview process is mixed. Results probably vary as a function of the particular computerized system adopted (Couper et al., 1998; Jones, 1999). Obviously both the personal and the telephone interview permit more control over the sequence in which a respondent answers the questions in a survey than does the self-administered questionnaire. When respondents fill out a questionnaire by themselves, they can conceivably answer the questions in any order they choose. Computerized modes of data collection enhance the consistency of the sequence in which questions are asked and answered. If this sequence is programmed into the interview, then the line of questioning can go in only the direction that the program permits.

Carrying Out the Survey

A distinct advantage of centralized telephone interviews is that they allow closer supervision of interviewers' performance in conducting the interview than is possible when individual interviewers are dispersed throughout an area. With computer-assisted telephone interviews in particular, the supervisor can listen in on the interview and actually view the screen through a remote supervisory monitor as the interviewer enters the respondents' answers. This greatly facilitates the supervisor's providing additional interviewer training or instructions as needed, assisting the interviewers if they encounter problems with certain respondents, and reducing the variability across interviews that can be a function of different interviewers' approaches to asking questions (Groves & Couper, 1998; Groves et al., 2002).

While one is not able to see or hear the persons involved in completing an on-line survey, it has some of the similar advantages created by a telephone survey in that the online transactions can be monitored by reviewing a log of the incoming and outgoing Internet traffic as well as monitoring the information recorded in the database. These monitoring activities can streamline the management of the survey while it is in the field as well as the data cleaning and editing activities that may occur after the data have been recorded in the online database.

Interviewer supervisors for large-scale personal interview field studies carried out by the major survey research firms are provided with computers for routinely reporting the status of their interviewers' progress in the field to their firm's headquarters. With the advent of CAPI systems, possibilities exist for recording or monitoring the personal interviews as well, thereby providing advantages similar to those found in centralized CATI systems (Thissen & Rodriguez, 2004).

The length of the data collection period must also be considered. Personal interview–based area probability studies require much longer periods for gathering data than do telephone interviews. Field interviewers may need to make several trips to a residence before they find someone at home. There is also a lag time in getting the completed interview logged and returned to the supervisor and ultimately to field or data-processing headquarters. With centralized telephone interviewing, it is possible to follow up with nonresponders at many different times during the day or at night, and there should be minimal lag time in getting the interview processed once it is completed. Because self-administered questionnaires are generally mailed, the field period for such studies is longer, and it is dictated by the initial response to the survey as well as by the number and intervals of planned follow-up efforts.

Computer-assisted modes of data collection promise to shorten the length of the field period for telephone and personal interviews because the data gathered during the interview can be immediately stored in the computer. However, more front-end work is required to develop and test the questionnaire before it goes into the field. Whether time is saved with computerized self-administered questionnaires would depend on the particular data-gathering system that is developed and the traditional mode of self-administration (mail or group) with which it is being compared (Fuchs, Couper, & Hansen, 2000).

Preparing the Data for Analysis

Once the data are collected, the next step is to make sure that they are complete and that any obvious mistakes made during the data-gathering phase are identified and corrected. The procedures for this next stage of processing are referred to as data "editing" or "cleaning" and are discussed in more detail in Chapter

Fourteen. Errors that may be identified include following the wrong sequence of questions so that the wrong questions are answered or that questions are left out or have values that are much too high (a thousand physician visits in the year) or low (a six-foot, six-inch adult male reported to weigh seventy-five pounds) either logically or relative to other information in the questionnaire.

Most errors of this kind occur in self-administered questionnaires on which the information may have been recorded in a haphazard or illegible fashion and there is no interviewer available to correct the respondent's mistakes. The quality of personal and telephone interviews is less likely to be affected by errors of this kind.

Computer-assisted modes of data collection and Internet data collection can expedite the data editing and cleaning process. Logical or other checks can be programmed in when the questionnaire is designed so that the interviewer or respondent is forced to correct inappropriate answers before proceeding.

Need for Imputation of Missing Values. Another problem arises when respondents refuse to answer certain questions or say they do not know the answer, or when a question is inadvertently left out by the interviewer or the respondent. Once again, this is most likely to be a problem with self-administered questionnaires. Methods for imputing (or estimating) values for the questions for which information is missing can be designed to provide a more complete data set for analysis (see Chapter Fourteen). These procedures, however, rely on certain assumptions about the appropriate basis for assigning values to cases for which the information is missing.

Research comparing the rates of missing values and other errors in computer-assisted and Internet methods of data gathering with traditional paper-and-pencil questionnaires generally document rates that are similar or lower for the computerized and Internet methods (Couper et al., 1998; Dielman & Couper, 1995; Groves & Nicholls, 1986; Martin, O'Muircheartaigh, & Curtice, 1993; Pettit, 2002; Schleyer & Forrest, 2000).

Speed of Turnaround. Principally because of the length of the respective field periods and the lack of centralized administration, personal and mail self-administered surveys are also likely to move through the data-processing phase of the study more slowly than telephone surveys or Internet surveys. Computerized data collection systems usually make the data coding, processing, and analysis steps simultaneous with the data collection phase of the study. Errors are identified and corrected while the data are being entered, and summary tallies are run on the data as batches of interviews are completed. This, of course, greatly reduces the data processing time required for the survey. However, much more time and effort are required at the beginning of the study to program and double-check all the features to be built into a computerized questionnaire and associated data-gathering and data-processing steps (Ball, 1996; Couper et al., 1998; House, 1985; Nicholls & Groves, 1986).

Costs

The price tag for a particular survey method may be the principal determinant of whether it can be feasibly employed. Personal interview approaches, for example, are more expensive than comparable telephone interview surveys or Internet surveys. Depending on the design of the respective types of studies, the overall costs for telephone interviews may be substantially less than those of in-person interviews.

The principal components accounting for the differences between the two approaches are the higher sampling and data collection costs for personal interview surveys. There are, after all, staff salaries and travel expenses to be paid when listing and contacting households selected for the study. No such costs are incurred when samples are drawn for telephone, Internet, or mail surveys, although funds are of course needed to generate or acquire the list of potentially eligible telephone numbers, e-mail addresses, or respondents and then to select those to be included in the final study. Direct data collection costs are less for telephone surveys than for personal interview studies, but the developmental costs may be higher for some computer-assisted surveys. Mail surveys are the least costly method of gathering survey data.

Summary

In summary, as shown in Table 5.1, the telephone and personal interview methods have more advantages than the mail questionnaire or Internet survey approach. The main differences between personal versus telephone interview or Internet survey methods are that noncoverage and nonresponse problems are greater in the latter. At the same time, however, costs are much lower, and there may be fewer disadvantages in carrying out the survey and coding and processing the data with telephone (especially CATI) interviews or Internet survey data collection. Sample coverage and response rates, question and questionnaire design, and data coding and processing issues may be more problematic with mail questionnaires and Internet surveys. But they offer a distinct advantage in terms of lower survey costs and have value as a relatively anonymous method for asking sensitive or threatening questions about health and health care behaviors.

Many health surveys incorporate more than one of these methods—personal interviews, telephone interviews, self-administered questionnaires, computer-assisted, and Internet surveys—into their study designs to lower survey costs or optimize the survey design advantages provided by a particular approach. Offering professionals and respondents for surveys of organizations or institutions such as hospitals or businesses a choice of response method is likely to increase the overall response rate to the study (Gallagher & Fowler, 2004; Parsons, Warnecke, Czaja, Barnsley, & Kaluzny, 1994; Spaeth & O'Rourke, 1994).

Researchers should consider not only the pros and cons of each method in deciding which approach to use but also how the methods might be meaningfully combined to minimize the costs or maximize the quality of their study.

Special Considerations for Special Populations

The who, what, where, and when questions posed at the start of this book take on renewed significance when researchers are choosing methods for gathering survey data. If the major topics to be addressed are sensitive and threatening ones (sexual or drug use practices), then more anonymous methods may be warranted in order to minimize the underreporting of these events. A survey of hard-to-reach or special populations (minority groups, prostitutes, intravenous drug users) would dictate consideration of the noncoverage or nonresponse biases that are likely to attend with different sampling and data collection designs. If timeliness and enhanced data quality are of particular concern, then computer-assisted interviewing approaches that permit the most rapid collection of high-quality data may be required (Marín, Vanoss, & Perez-Stable, 1990; Substance Abuse & Mental Health Services Administration, Office of Applied Studies, 2002).

Selected Examples

The California Health Interview Survey was a random digit dialing telephone survey of California households (UCLA Center for Health Policy Research, 2002a). The study was designed to produce reliable estimates for the state of California, most counties and some subcounty areas, and diverse racial/ethnic groups. Estimates of the number and characteristics of adults, children, and adolescents without access to care or health insurance can be generated from this study. Estimates of the prevalence of cancer screening, diabetes, asthma, and other health conditions and health behaviors can also be derived from this survey. All interviews were conducted using CATI.

The UNICEF Multiple Indicator Cluster Survey is a paper-and-pencil personal interview survey that was designed for administration in many countries (UNICEF, 2000, n.d.). Data from the study can be used to generate and compare estimates of household composition, availability of water, sanitation issues, salt iodization, issues of reproductive health and family planning for women, nutritional and immunization issues for children, and measurements of material and infant mortality across participating nations.

The National Dental Malpractice Survey was conducted to estimate dental malpractice experience and to test hypotheses regarding the practice characteristics that predict dental malpractice experience (Milgrom et al., 1994). The survey was based on a widely regarded and used approach to mail survey design developed by Don Dillman and his colleagues (discussed in more detail in Chapters Twelve and Thirteen). In an era where there is a need to balance survey costs with achieving a significant response rate, the notion of using a well-articulated survey design and implementation approach such as Dillman's tailored design method offers a very promising option (Dillman, 2000).

Guidelines for Minimizing Survey Errors and Maximizing Survey Quality

The strengths and weaknesses of the alternative approaches to gathering survey data summarized in this chapter highlight the importance and utility of a total survey design framework and associated consideration of the errors that are likely to result from the complex of decisions required in designing a survey. The responses to comparable questions, and related estimates, may vary across different methods (or modes) of data collection. If these effects differ in a particular direction for a given mode, they would be viewed as systematic mode effects (see Table 5.2).

No decision is perfect. Errors are inevitable. Trade-offs accompany the array of decisions required to design and conduct any survey—there may be high response rates but low coverage of drug users in the community from convenience samples of those participating in drug rehabilitation programs or large sampling errors for relatively rare groups in the study population, such as Vietnamese resi-

TABLE 5.2. SURVEY ERRORS: SOURCES AND SOLUTIONS— CHOOSING THE METHODS OF DATA COLLECTION.

	Systematic Errors: Mode Effects	Variable Errors: Mode Effects
Solutions to Errors	Evaluate the validity of responses for different modes of data collection.	Evaluate the trade-offs in terms of likely errors and costs for different modes of data collection.

dents living in a clinic's service area. To make conscious and informed decisions that enhance data quality, however, survey designers must take a clear-eyed look at what the trade-offs are likely to be, enlightened by a clear understanding of what the survey is primarily intended to accomplish and sound knowledge of the particular strengths and limitations of the data-gathering alternatives available to them.

Supplementary Sources

For a discussion of the pros and cons of personal interviews compared with mail questionnaires, see Dillman (1978, 1991, 2000) and Salant and Dillman (1994). For comparisons with telephone interviewing methods, see Groves (1990) and Groves et al. (1988). Couper et al. (1998) provide a useful overview of computer-assisted interviewing approaches, and Jones (1999) reviews adaptations required for Web-based surveys.

CHAPTER SIX

DECIDING WHO WILL BE IN THE SAMPLE

Chapter Highlights

1. The four basic types of probability sample designs—simple random sample, systematic random sample, stratified sample, and cluster sample—have different features that can be used to minimize costs and reduce sampling errors in surveys.
2. Major types of nonprobability sample designs are purposive, quota, chunk, and snowball sampling.
3. Four criteria for evaluating sample designs are the likely precision (variable sampling error) and accuracy (bias) of the resulting estimates (means or proportions, for example), as well as the complexity and efficiency (cost of minimizing errors) in implementing the design.
4. Four primary types of designs—area probability, random digit dialing, list, and Internet-based samples—have been used extensively in conducting personal household interviews, telephone interviews, mail surveys, and self-administered e-mail or Web surveys, respectively.
5. Probability sampling procedures for locating and sampling rare populations of people include screening, disproportionate sampling, network sampling, and dual-frame sampling.

6. **The main procedures used in sampling respondents within households include the Kish, Troldahl-Carter-Bryant, Hagan and Collier, last or next birthday methods, or a combination of these approaches.**

Sampling is used to decide who will be included in a survey because gathering information on everyone in a population (as is done in the U.S. census) is beyond the scope and resources of most researchers. There will always be random variation in estimates of the characteristics of a population derived from a sample of it because of fluctuations in who gets included in any particular sample. Estimates derived from conducting a census of the entire population of interest would not have these random sampling errors but would be prohibitively expensive to carry out on a frequent basis. Sampling makes gathering data on a population of interest more manageable and more affordable. It enables the characteristics of a large body of people or institutions to be inferred, with minimal errors, from information collected on relatively few of them.

As with all other aspects of designing and conducting a survey, attention must be given to ways of minimizing the sources of variable and systematic errors during sampling. The discussion that follows is intended to (1) underline the importance of relating the sample design to the research question being addressed in the study, (2) describe different types of sample designs, and (3) delineate criteria for evaluating alternative designs in the context of economically minimizing survey errors.

Relating the Sample Design to the Research Question

The constant point of reference for any major decisions about the practical steps in carrying out a survey should be the research questions that the study is principally intended to address. The framework introduced in Chapter Two for formulating the research question for the study (see Table 2.2) can also serve as a guide for the sample design process: the questions it asks are *what* and *who* is the focus of the study, *where* and *when* it is being done, and *why*. In the example provided in Chapter Two, the focus was on the cigarette-smoking behaviors (*what*) of high school seniors (*who*) in a large metropolitan high school (*where*). The timing and frequency of data collection (*when*) varied, depending on the study design and whether the emphasis was on describing or explaining this behavior or the impact of interventions to alter it (*why*). A clear indication of with whom, where, and when the survey will be done are essential for specifying the sample design for the study.

Target Population or Universe

The target population for the survey is the group or groups about which information is desired. This is sometimes referred to as the study *universe*. It is the group to which one wishes to generalize (or make inferences) from the survey sample. Sample inclusion criteria (such as the civilian noninstitutionalized population of the United States or adults ages eighteen and over) or exclusion criteria (persons living in group quarters or those who speak neither English nor Spanish) are directly reflective of the target population for the study.

Different research designs have fundamental and compelling implications for identifying and sampling from the target population. Cross-sectional designs dictate a look at whether the designated time period for identifying the population (such as clinic users) represents the population over time (patients who had visited the facility over the past year sampled from medical records) or at a specified point in time (patients seen at the clinic on designated days sampled from visit logs). Group-comparison designs argue for careful attention to ensuring that the groups that are being compared (racial and ethnic minorities) are systematically and adequately included in the sampling plan. Longitudinal designs must anticipate issues of whether the same or different people will be followed and what additional steps will need to be taken to ensure the comparability of the data gathered over time.

Sampling Frame

The *sampling frame* is the list of the target population from which the sample will be drawn. It is, in effect, the operational definition of the study universe (target population), the designation in concrete terms of who will be included, where they can be located, and when the data will be collected. In the school example, it would be the list of seniors (*who*) enrolled in city high schools (*where*) at the beginning or end of the school year (*when*).

There are often problems with the sampling frames available to researchers. A list provided at one point in time may fail to take into account students who drop out of school or new students who have enrolled by the time the study begins. There may be clerical errors in the list; for example, the same student's name may be inadvertently repeated on the list and the names of other students omitted. These and other sampling frame problems are common when trying to match the definition of the desired target population for the study to an actual list of eligible candidates—regardless of the data collection method used (in person, by telephone, or through the mail). We will see in later discussions that different types of problems with the sampling frame may be more severe with certain types of sample designs than with others, such as the difficulty of determining whether a sampled telephone number is an eligible working residential number rather than a cell phone or business when the line is always busy or no one ever answers the call.

Distinctions are sometimes drawn between the intended (target) population and the actual (study) population because of these sampling frame limitations. Basically, however, the researcher should try to match the basis and process for selecting the sample as closely as possible to the definition of the desired target population or universe for the study. Otherwise the sample is likely to be plagued with substantial noncoverage biases, that is, individuals who should be included but are not.

Sampling Element

The *sampling element* refers to the ultimate unit or individual from whom information will be collected in the survey and who therefore will be the focus of the analysis. The sampling elements for the study should be clearly specified in defining the target population or universe (individuals, households, families, or institutions, for example). In the preceding example, the sampling elements are high school seniors.

In complex sample designs, the researcher may need to go through several stages to get at the ultimate sampling element of interest. These successive stages may involve selecting several sampling units, such as cities, blocks within the cities, and households, to obtain the ultimate sampling unit: noninstitutionalized residents of a particular state or of the entire United States, for example. The designation of who to include in the study is also determined by the other aspects of the research question (what, where, when, and why the study is being done). Defining the precise individuals you want to collect information about or from is a central decision that will affect all subsequent approaches to that individual (person or institution), as well as the ways in which the data that are gathered on that sampling unit will ultimately be processed and analyzed.

Sample Design

The decision most critical to shaping the steps in the sample selection process is determining the type of *sample design* to be used. There are two principal types of sample designs: *probability* and *nonprobability* designs. The basic distinction between the two is that the former relies on the laws of chance for selecting the sampling elements, while the latter relies on human judgment.

The probability of entering the sample is directly determined by the sampling fraction used in selecting cases for probability-based designs, where the sampling fraction is equal to the sample size (n) divided by the size of the study universe (N), or n/N. In the example of the high school seniors, a probability sampling method could involve entering the identification numbers for all seniors registered at the school on a computer ($N = 300$) and then creating a program to draw a desired sample of sixty students ($n = 60$) by selecting every fifth name after some randomly assigned starting point. The sampling fraction (or chance) of a student coming into the sample would then be one in five (60/300). A nonprobability sampling approach would be to ask the principal or a group of teachers at the school which students it would be best to include, based on their knowledge of who smokes and their assessment of which students would be willing to cooperate with the project. The probability of coming into the sample on this relatively ad hoc basis cannot be determined.

Nonprobability sampling methods may be of several kinds. *Purposive samples* select people who serve a certain purpose, such as a focus group of employed mothers for a study of employed mothers' needs for child care services. *Quota samples* focus on obtaining a certain number of designated types of respondents—for example, women between fifteen and forty-four years of age who are shopping in a drugstore. A *chunk sample* is simply a group of people who happen to be available at the time of the study—the people in the waiting room of a big-city emergency room on the night that a researcher decides to collect data on why patients are there and how long they have to wait. Samples can also be drawn from people who volunteer, such as students who respond to an advertisement to participate in a study of the effects of a low-fat diet on weight loss. *Snowball sampling* is a type of purposive chain sampling that is quite useful when members of a population, such as drug users, are extremely hard to identify. The sampling starts with the identification of one or a small number of potential participants who are representative of the population of interest, who then identify other potential respondents who meet the same inclusion criteria. The chance (probability) of any given individual being chosen, using any of these nonprobability sampling approaches, cannot be empirically estimated. However, methods for enhancing the prospects of obtaining unbiased estimates of population characteristics based on nonprobabilistic sampling approaches are discussed later in this chapter.

The main reason for sampling from a population is to collect information on a subset of individuals or institutions that represents (or is similar to) the entire population of interest. With probability sampling techniques, there are well-developed statistical methods for estimating the range of error and the level of confidence that the results for any particular sample are likely to have in reflecting the real population value. Thus, probability sampling methods allow the researcher to have greater confidence when generalizing to the study's target population.

Nonetheless, nonprobability sample surveys serve a number of useful purposes. Such studies permit in-depth investigations of groups that are difficult or expensive to find, such as drug users, prostitutes, or homeless runaways. When probability methods for sampling these groups are largely unaffordable or unfeasible, nonprobability sampling approaches permit cases that are illustrative, even if not fully scientifically representative, of the study population to be included in the study. In the early stages of designing standardized surveys, they are helpful in developing and testing questions and procedures with respondents similar to those who will be included in the final study. They also serve to generate hypotheses that could be more fully explored in larger-scale, probability-based sample surveys.

Alternative probability-based sampling methods are described in the following section.

Types of Probability Sample Designs

The principal probability sample designs—*simple random sample, systematic random sample, stratified sample,* and *cluster sample*—present different approaches that are often used in combination in carrying out a survey. The simple and systematic random sample approaches represent relatively simple designs. The stratified and cluster sample approaches are used in complex multistage surveys. In practice, most complex survey designs involve combinations of all four sampling methods. Each of the methods will, however, be discussed in turn, so that their respective advantages and disadvantages can be delineated. (See Figures 6.1 and 6.2.) In the next section, examples of different types of probability samples—for personal, telephone, mail, and Internet surveys—are presented to explain how these approaches can be used in combination.

Simple Random Sample

A simple random sample is selected by using a procedure that gives every element in the population a known, nonzero, and equal chance of being included in the sample. The methods used most often for drawing simple random samples are lottery or random numbers selection procedures. In either case, before the sample is drawn, every element in the sampling frame should be assigned a unique identifying number. With the lottery procedure, these numbers can be placed in a container and mixed together; then someone draws out numbers from the container until the required sample size is reached.

A random numbers sample selection device produces a series of numbers through a random numbers generation process. Each number is unique and independent of the others. Random numbers generation and selection software or published random numbers selection tables can be used in drawing simple random samples. (See an example of a random numbers table in Figure 6.1.)

To select the identification numbers of the cases to be included in the sample, the researcher must first choose a random place to start on these tables (for example, by closing her eyes and putting her finger on the page, with the number on which her finger lands becoming the starting point). There should also be decision rules, specified in advance, for moving in a certain direction and choosing numbers (for example, she chooses the first two digits of the five-digit random numbers identified by moving from right to left across every row and column of the table after the random starting point, skipping any numbers that fall outside

FIGURE 6.1. TYPES OF PROBABILITY SAMPLE DESIGNS—RANDOM SAMPLES.

Type of Design	*Selected Examples of Drawing Sample*
Simple Random Sample (Select sample through randomly drawing numbers, such that every element in the population has a *known, nonzero, and equal* chance of being included.)	*Random Numbers Table* 91567 42595 27958 30134 04024 17955 56349 90999 49127 20044 46503 18584 18845 49618 02304 92157 89634 94824 78171 84610 14577 62765 35605 81263 39667 98427 07523 33362 64270 01638 34914 63976 88720 82765 34476 70060 28277 39475 46473 23219 53976 54914 06990 67245 68350 76072 29515 40960 07391 58745 90725 52210 83974 29992 65831 64364 67412 33339 31926 14883 08062 00358 31662 25388 61642 95012 68379 93526 70765 10592 15664 10493 20492 38391 91132

	Page 1	Page 2	Page 3
Systematic Random Sample (Select a starting point on a list randomly and then every *n*th unit thereafter, such that every element in the population has a *known* chance of being included.)	1 2 3* 4 5 6*	7 8 9* 10 11 12*	13 14 15* 16 17 18*

the range of IDs assigned to elements in the sampling frame). The researcher then matches the numbers generated by means of this process with the ID numbers for each element in the sampling frame. The elements with ID numbers that match those chosen from the random numbers table will be included in the sample. This process would continue until the desired sample size is reached. This type of systematic approach to the sample selection process is needed to ensure a fully randomized selection of cases.

Systematic Random Sample

Systematic random sample procedures represent an approximation to the simple random sample design. The process is similar to that found in the probability sampling approach that was used for drawing a sample of high school seniors: the researcher selects a random starting point and then systematically selects cases from the sampling frame at a specified (sampling) interval.

The determination of the starting point and sampling interval (k) is based on the required sample size. If, for example, a sample of one hundred students is desired out of a list of one thousand, then the sampling interval would be determined by dividing the total number on the list (sampling frame) by the desired sample size ($k = 1,000/100 = 10$). This means that the researcher should count down ten cases after starting from the case chosen as the random starting point within the first to tenth interval (between the first and tenth cases on the list) and continue to identify every tenth case until the one hundred cases are selected. In the example in Figure 6.1, the sampling interval is three: one of every three of the eighteen cases on the list will be selected, resulting in a sample of six cases.

Stratified Sample

The stratified sample approach is used when there is a particular interest in making sure that certain groups will be included in the study or that some groups will be sampled at a higher (or lower) rate than others. With the stratified sampling approach, the entire sampling frame is divided into subgroups of interest, such as city blocks that have high concentrations of Hispanics versus those that have few; health professionals who are members of their national professional association versus those who are not; or lists of telephone numbers that have been called previously and are known to be working numbers versus those that have not been called previously. This information could be obtained in advance from census data by matching professional association membership lists against lists of licensed professionals in the geographical area covered by the study, or through databases available from commercial survey sampling firms of telephone numbers that have been previously screened for residential or working number status, respectively. The researcher uses a simple random or systematic random sampling process to select cases from the respective strata. Some individuals would be selected from every stratum into which the sample is divided. (See Figure 6.2.)

The principal reason for dividing the sample into strata is to identify the groups that it is crucial to include based on the purposes of the study. If there are few members of the groups of interest in the target population, a simple random or systematic random sample may result in none or a very small number of these cases being included simply because there is a very small probability that such individuals will be sampled.

Dividing the population into strata and then sampling from each of these strata ensures that cases from all the groups of interest will be included. The proportion of cases selected (sampling fraction) in each stratum should be high enough to capture a sufficient number of cases to carry out meaningful analyses for each group. Another approach to obtaining enough cases for groups that may represent a relatively small proportion of the population as a whole is to draw a

FIGURE 6.2. TYPES OF PROBABILITY SAMPLE DESIGNS—COMPLEX SAMPLES.

Type of Design	Selected Examples of Drawing Sample		

Stratified Sample (Divide population into *homogeneous strata* and draw random-type sample separately for *all strata*.)

Proportionate: same sampling fraction in each stratum

Disproportionate: different sampling fraction in each stratum

Stratum A	Stratum B	Stratum C
A1*	B1*	C1
A2	B2	C2*
A3*	B3*	C3
A4	B4	C4*
A5*	B5*	
A6		

Cluster Sample (Divide population into *heterogeneous clusters* and draw random-type sample separately from *sample of clusters*.)

Cluster 1	Cluster 2	Cluster 3
A1*	A2*	A3*
B2	C4	A6
B3*	C3*	B5*
C1	B4	B1
A5*	C2*	A4*

higher proportion of cases from that stratum relative to the other strata. Proportionate sampling selects the same proportion of cases from each stratum, while disproportionate sampling varies the proportion (sampling fraction) across strata.

For example, the researcher might decide to sample college professors who are members of a national professional association at a higher rate than professors who are not members by taking one out of five (20 percent) individuals in the member stratum and one out of ten (10 percent) in the nonmember stratum. In this case, members would be sampled at twice the rate of nonmembers. The precise sampling fractions to be used in each stratum should reflect some optimum allocation between strata, based on the amount of variability across cases (standard error) and the cost per case in each stratum (Kish, 1965).

Cluster Sample

The cluster sample method also involves dividing the sample into groups (or clusters). However, the primary purpose of cluster sampling is to maximize the dispersion of the sample throughout the community in order to represent fully the diversity that exists there while also minimizing costs. This method has traditionally been used in national, state, or community surveys of people who live in certain geographical areas. Clusters of housing units (for example, city blocks containing fifty houses) are identified during the sample design process. Then these clusters are sampled, and either all or a subsample (seven to ten) of the households in the sampled clusters are sampled from each cluster (or city block). Information regarding the size and number of relevant clusters is obtained from census data, or, in the instance of countries or geographical areas where these data are not available or are out of date, the information may need to be obtained in advance of drawing the sample by having field workers go out to list or estimate the location and number of relevant clusters (blocks or households, for example).

This approach substantially reduces the travel costs between interviews. A simple random sample of households throughout the country or even within a moderate-size community would be prohibitive because of the distances between sampling units, the time and effort expended in following up with people who were not at home at the time of the first visit, and so on. We will see later that there are also advantages in sampling clusters of telephone numbers and using these clusters as the basis for identifying sets of telephone numbers that are most likely to yield working residential numbers.

However, it is quite likely that a cluster of houses or telephone numbers taken from one neighborhood may include people who are more like one another (racially, socioeconomically, and so on) than they are like a cluster of people identified in another neighborhood. As a result, there tends to be more diversity or heterogeneity between than within clusters. We will see that this may result in higher sampling errors in cluster sample designs than in random and stratified ones.

Criteria to Evaluate Different Sample Designs

Four primary criteria may be applied in evaluating alternative sample designs: precision, accuracy, complexity, and efficiency.

Precision refers to how close the estimates derived from a sample are to the true population value as a function of variable sampling error. The standard errors of the estimates (derived from the sample variance) provide an estimate of variable sampling error. Smaller standard errors reflect greater precision. Variable error always exists when a sample is drawn because the estimates (means or proportions, for example) for different randomly selected subsets of cases of the same size are likely to differ simply due to chance. Standard errors can be reduced by drawing larger samples and trying to minimize other sources of variable error in the study, such as the unreliability of survey questions. Standard errors are higher for smaller samples and more complex (especially cluster) designs. Such designs may, however, be necessary in order to ensure the efficiency and affordability of the study.

Accuracy refers to how close the estimates derived from a sample are to the true population value as a function of systematic error or bias. The accuracy of survey estimates can be measured by the use of criterion validity analysis methods described in Chapter Three. Bias results when certain groups or individuals who are eligible to be included are systematically left out because of problems with designing the sampling frame (excluding new residential construction) or implementing the intended sampling procedures (talking to the person who happens to answer the telephone rather than randomly selecting a survey respondent).

Complexity refers to consideration of the amount of information that must be gathered in advance of doing the study, as well as the number of stages and steps that will be required to implement the design. Cluster sampling approaches represent the most complex types of designs. Examples of more complex (combined) designs are described later in this chapter. *Efficiency* refers to obtaining the most accurate and precise estimates at the lowest possible cost.

Theoretically, sampling (variable) error cannot be computed for nonprobability sampling designs since the assumptions required for computing it are not met (random selection from a known population with a hypothesized mean and variance). Systematic error (noncoverage bias) is likely to be particularly problematic for nonprobability designs because simple convenience or availability as the primary bases for selection may lead to a highly unrepresentative set of cases. The complexity and costs (although not the efficiency) are likely to be less for many nonprobability designs.

Table 6.1 compares the advantages and disadvantages of different probability designs. The simple random sample is the least complex design, but because of the simple randomization process (luck of the draw), some groups (especially those that represent a very small proportion of the population) may not be included at all or in large enough numbers. This design is relatively straightforward to execute but would not be efficient for certain purposes, such as drawing a sample of households throughout a metropolitan area.

The systematic random sample has many of the same advantages and disadvantages as a simple random sample. It would, however, be a particularly useful approach when complete and accurate lists of the eligible study population are available. Biases may nonetheless enter into the systematic sampling process if a periodic ordering of elements in the sample frame exists that corresponds to the sampling intervals for designating selected cases, such as every other case being a male veteran followed by his spouse's name, or every seventh house on the blocks in a new residential community being on a corner lot.

Stratified sampling offers a number of advantages. The researcher can ensure that certain groups are systematically included by using disproportionate sampling

TABLE 6.1. ADVANTAGES AND DISADVANTAGES OF DIFFERENT PROBABILITY SAMPLE DESIGNS.

Design	Advantages	Disadvantages
Simple random	• Requires little knowledge of population in advance.	• May not capture certain groups of interest. • May not be very efficient.
Systematic	• Easy to analyze data and compute sampling (standard) errors. • High precision.	• Periodic ordering of elements in sample frame may create biases in the data. • May not capture certain groups of interest. • May not be very efficient.
Stratified	• Enables certain groups of interest to be captured. • Enables disproportionate sampling and optimal allocation within strata. • Highest precision.	• Requires knowledge of population in advance. • May introduce more complexity in analyzing data and computing sampling (standard) errors.
Cluster	• Lowers field costs. • Enables sampling of *groups* of individuals for which detail on individuals themselves may not be available.	• Introduces more complexity in analyzing data and computing sampling (standard) errors. • Lowest precision.

if needed. There is likely to be a lower variable sampling error principally because the standard error is computed based on a weighted average of the within-stratum variance, which has less variability (is more homogeneous) by definition than the sample as a whole does. However, this design does introduce somewhat more complexity into implementing the sampling plan and analyzing the data than do either simple or systematic random samples.

Cluster sampling greatly increases the efficiency of sampling widely dispersed populations or areas, and it permits sampling of groups of individuals (households, schools, and so on) when information on the number and characteristics of the individuals (ultimate sampling elements) themselves is not directly available. But it is the most complex design and has the lowest precision, principally because the standard errors are based on the variation between what are likely to be relatively homogeneous clusters. (This issue will be addressed in more detail in Chapter Seven in discussing sample design effects.)

Putting It Together: Combined Designs

Most probability-based sample designs use combinations of the array of discrete approaches and procedures just reviewed. Four primary types of designs highlighted here—*area probability, random digit dialing, list,* and *Internet-based samples*—have been used extensively in conducting personal household interviews, telephone interviews, mail surveys, and self-administered e-mail or Web surveys, respectively. The sample design for the three studies highlighted in Resources A to C will be discussed later in this chapter as examples of alternative sampling approaches.

Area Probability Sample

In area probability samples, the emphasis is on selecting certain geographical areas containing the defined target population (the civilian noninstitutionalized population of a given country in the UNICEF Multiple Indicator Cluster Survey, for example) with a known probability of selection. With area probability sample designs, data are usually gathered from the households and individuals included in the resulting sample through personal interviews with everyone living in the household or with selected household members.

Sampling with probability proportionate to size (PPS) is an underlying component of many area probability designs. This approach combines elements of simple random, systematic, cluster, and stratified sampling. A notable public health application of PPS sampling procedures is in the World Health Organization Expanded Programme on Immunization. That program uses a PPS design for sampling villages and children to estimate the vaccination status of young children in developing countries. It is sometimes referred to as the 30×7 design because it traditionally entails sampling thirty clusters (such as villages) and selecting seven children of the required age within each cluster. This approach can, however, be adapted to whatever number and size of clusters is appropriate to maximize the efficiency of sampling dispersed target populations (Bennett, Woods, Liyanage, & Smith, 1991; Milligan, Njie, & Bennett, 2004). The principal advantage of the PPS approach is that the sample is self-weighting, that is, the resulting distribution of cases on characteristics of interest (such as households in high-, medium-, or low-income areas) directly mirrors the distribution in the study universe.

An example of the steps required to execute a PPS design is provided in Table 6.2. The first step is to estimate the desired sample size (n) needed to meet study design requirements (procedures for estimating sample sizes are discussed in Chapter Seven). In step 2, a desired cluster size is decided on (n_c). The criteria that come into play are the trade-offs between saving on data collection costs by sampling groups of households that are close together versus the fact that standard (sampling) errors will increase as the size of these clusters increases. Traditionally, cluster sizes range from seven to ten sampling elements in area probability samples. In step 3 the number of clusters ($c = 11$) needed to achieve the sample size is computed by dividing the desired sample size ($n = 77$) by the cluster size ($n_c = 7$). In this example, eleven clusters with seven households in each cluster are needed to yield the desired sample size of seventy-seven households.

Step 4 entails estimating the total number of sampling units in the study universe. This number is derived from census data in those countries for which they are available, updated as appropriate for estimated change since the last census. In areas for which this information is not available, estimates can be provided by knowledgeable people in the community or other relevant sources (tax or school rosters). In step 5, cumulative totals of housing units in the study universe ($N = 2,200$) are computed, and in step 6, the sampling interval (k) for identifying clusters is determined by dividing the number in the study universe (N) by the target number of clusters (c): $k = 2,200/11 = 200$. The blocks in which every two-hundredth household appears, based on the cumulative listing, will be designated as ones from which a cluster of seven households will be selected. The sampling interval (one out of two hundred) dictates that in step 7, a random starting point will be identified from the cumulative list of housing units within this interval (the fiftieth household was identified from a random numbers table as the starting point in this example). In step 8, the sampling interval (200) is added to this initial starting point (50) to identify a housing unit (250) from the cumulative listing. The block in which it appears is selected, and this process is repeated to identify the blocks

TABLE 6.2. SAMPLING WITH PROBABILITY PROPORTIONATE TO SIZE.

Steps	Example
1. Estimate the desired sample size (n).	77
2. Fix the desired cluster size (n_c).	7
3. Calculate the number of clusters (c) needed to achieve the desired sample size: n/n_c.	77/7 = 11
4. Estimate the total number of units in the universe (col. B, Table) from which the sample will be drawn (N).	2,200 Col. B, Table.
5. Calculate the cumulative total of the number of units across *all* clusters in the universe.	Col. C, Table.
6. Calculate the sampling interval (k) for selecting clusters from the universe: N/c.	2,200/11 = 200
7. Pick a random starting point (r) to select clusters within the designated sampling interval (step 6), using a random numbers table.	50
8. Calculate the selection numbers (HU #) for the blocks to be sampled by entering the random starting point, adding the sampling interval, and then repeating the process to identify sampled blocks: $r = HU_1$ $HU_1 + k = HU_2$ $HU_2 + k = HU_3,$ etc.	Col. D, Table.
9. Assign cluster numbers to each designated block.	Col. E, Table.
10. Confirm % in strata for sample agree with % in universe.	Col. B, E (%), Table.

A City blocks (or towns)	B Estimated number of housing units	C Cumulative number of housing units	D Selection number	E Cluster number
High				
A	100	100	50	#1.
B	50	150	—	—
C	75	225	—	—
D	150	375	250	#2.
E	200 (575/2,200 = 26%)	575	450	#3. (27%)
Medium				
F	250	825	650	#4.
G	125	950	850	#5.
H	50	1,000	—	—
I	100	1,100	1,050	#6.
J	50 (575/2,200 = 26%)	1,150	—	— (27%)
Low				
K	200	1,350	1,250	#7.
L	300	1,650	1,450, 1,650	#8., #9.
M	125	1,775	—	—
N	150	1,925	1,850	#10.
O	275 (1,050/2,200 = 48%)	2,200	2,050	#11. (46%)

from which the subsequent clusters (up to eleven) will be selected. In step 9, numbers can then be assigned to each cluster identified in step 8.

As mentioned earlier, the beauty of the PPS design is that it is self-weighting, that is, the distribution of characteristics (such as income) in the resulting sample is essentially the same as the distribution in the study universe. This is confirmed in the example provided, where the distribution of three strata in the study universe is mirrored in the distribution of cases (approximately one-quarter, one-quarter, and one-half, respectively) in the study sample.

Geographic information systems, which permit computerized mapping of household and population distributions as well as overlaying associated demographic or other characteristics, offer a promising technology for facilitating the design and implementation of area probability samples (Quantitative Decisions, 2000).

Random Digit Dialing

Three primary approaches are used to develop sampling frames of phone numbers for telephone surveys: *list-assisted frames, random digit dialing,* and *multiple frame* sampling methods (Casady & Lepkowski, 1998; Lepkowski, 1988; Mohadjer, 1988). Originally, list-assisted frames drew on numbers that were published in telephone books. Newer methods employ computerized databases of directory numbers supplemented by other sources that include both listed and unlisted telephone numbers, such as motor vehicle registration department lists. The primary supplier of these telephone number databases is Donnelley Marketing Information Services (Stamford, Connecticut), which publishes most U.S. telephone directories.

The random digit dialing approach is based on a randomly generated set of telephone numbers, starting with the area code and exchanges (central office codes) for the area in which one wishes to place the calls. Current and proposed area code and exchange combinations are available on BELLCORE data files produced by Bell Communications Research (Morristown, New Jersey). Once relevant area code and exchange digits are identified, a random numbers generation procedure is used to create the rest of the digits for the numbers to be used in the sample. With this approach, every possible telephone number in the area has a chance of being included in the study.

The efficiency of this sampling process can be increased by reducing the nonworking, business, or nonresidential numbers that are likely to be generated. The Waksberg-Mitofsky procedure was developed to facilitate identification of working residential numbers (Waksberg, 1978). In the first stage of sample selection with the Waksberg-Mitofsky procedure, primary sampling units are, in effect, clusters or blocks of a hundred numbers identified by the first eight digits of the phone number: (xxx) xxx-xx00 through (xxx) xxx-xx99. Additional prefixes are needed for international calling. If the first randomly generated number in this block of one hundred numbers is an eligible (working, residential) number when called, then the entire block of numbers will be included in the sample. Otherwise that block will be eliminated from the sample. In the second stage of selection (within the selected blocks of one hundred numbers), the remaining series of numbers in the blocks (PSUs) selected are called until the desired sample size is reached.

Criticisms of the Waksberg-Mitofsky procedure have focused on problems and delays at two stages. At the first stage, there are problems and delays in identifying eligible households because of difficulties in getting through to the parties to whom the number is assigned. At the second stage, many numbers within an eligible cluster identified at stage 1 must be called for what turns out to be a relatively low yield of working residential numbers. Multiple frame sampling methods are used to address these problems through, for example, using information from list-assisted frames to stratify BELLCORE area code-exchange clusters by their likely yield of working numbers or calling more than one number within a cluster as a basis for disproportionately sampling clusters that are likely to yield a higher proportion of working numbers (Casady & Lepkowski, 1998; Potthoff, 1987; Tucker, Lepkowski, & Piekarski, 2002). Telephone samples can be purchased from commercial firms such as GENESYS (Fort Washington, Pennsylvania) and Survey Sampling (Fairfield, Connecticut). Address labels can be obtained for the telephone numbers to be called through commercial suppliers such as Tele-Match (Springfield, Virginia) for the purpose of sending advance letters to potential respondents.

New sampling issues have emerged in the successful design and execution of telephone surveys with the increasing availability of cell phones as well as a variety of means for screening out callers (such as voice mail and caller ID). These issues relate to how best to construct a sampling frame when cell phones are generally person rather than household or geography based, the differential availability of cell phones by different demographic subgroups (young adults and minorities, for example), and the issue of multiple probabilities of selection due to having multiple (landline and cell) telephones (Blumberg, Luke, & Cynamon, 2004; Frankel, 2004; Kuusela & Simpanen, 2005).

List Sample

The first step in list sample surveys is to identify a list of potentially eligible respondents, make some judgments about the completeness of the list, consider any problems that may be encountered when sampling from the list (duplicate names, blank or incomplete information on certain individuals, names of people who are deceased or who moved out of the area, and so on), and decide whether the respondents meet the eligibility criteria defined for the study. Once eligibility has been determined, it is necessary to derive the sampling fraction and systematically sample prospective participants on the list.

Internet Samples

A central issue in the design and conduct of Internet surveys is the likely coverage of a target population of interest through the Internet. Although computer and related Internet availability is growing worldwide, certain groups (such as professionals) are more likely than others (such as low-income individuals or households) to have access. In some cases, lists of the eligible target population may not be available. In those instances, nonprobability, snowball sampling approaches could be used to obtain Web-based responses, but the resulting sample cannot be deemed representative of a well-defined target universe. When lists of the target population are directly available, systematic mail or e-mail contacts could be used to provide secure ID access to a Web site for the administration of the survey.

With the growing complexity of conducting telephone surveys combined with declining rates of cooperation with both telephone and personal interview surveys, self-administered surveys, particularly those based on e-mail or Web survey design, are promising and cost-effective alternatives (Baker, Zahs, & Popa, 2004; Dillman, 1998, 2000; Link & Mokdad, 2004; Sudman & Blair, 1999).

Regardless of the frame or technologies used in drawing survey samples, the criteria of *precision, accuracy, complexity,* and *efficiency* are still central in evaluating existing and emerging methods.

Procedures for Selecting the Respondent

The preceding discussion has reviewed the major steps in designing probability samples of individuals. In this section, alternative procedures for the selection of individuals at what is usually the ultimate stage of sampling is described—that is, how to choose the individuals to interview once contact with a household has been made and not everyone who lives there is to be interviewed.

There are four principal probability-based approaches to respondent selection. Two use random selection tables after detailing the composition of the household (Figure 6.3) and two screen for respondents by means of characteristics that are fairly randomly distributed in the population (such as the person who had a birthday most recently) (Table 6.3).

FIGURE 6.3. PROCEDURES FOR SELECTING THE RESPONDENT—SELECTION TABLES.

Procedure

Methodology

Kish Tables
(Ask about all potentially eligible individuals in the household, list them, and then use Kish tables.)

Question: Please state the sex, age, and relationship to you of all persons xx or older living there who are related to you by blood, marriage, or adoption.

List all persons age 18 and over in dwelling unit

Relationship to Head (1)	Sex (2)	Age (3)	Adult (4)	Check (5)
HUSBAND	M	52	2	
WIFE	F	50	4	✓
SON	M	23	3	
DAUGHTER	F	19	5	
HUSB. FATHER	M	78	1	

Number persons 18 or over in the following order:

Oldest male, next oldest male, etc.; followed by oldest female, next oldest female, etc. Then use selection table below to choose respondent.

Selection Table D

If the number of adults in the dwelling is:	Interview the adult numbered:
1	1
2	2
3	2
4	3
5	4
6 or more	4

Troldahl-Carter-Bryant (TCB) Tables

(Ask how many persons live in the household, how many of them are women, and then use TCB selection charts.)

Questions: (1) How many persons *xx* years or older live in your household, including yourself?
(2) How many of these are women?

Row B	Col. A			
	Number of Adults in Household			
Number of Women in Household	1	2	3	4 or more
0	man	youngest man	youngest man	oldest man
1	woman	woman	oldest man	woman
2		oldest woman	man	oldest man
3			youngest woman	man or oldest man
4 or more				oldest woman

The intersection of column A and row B determines the sex and relative age of the respondent to be interviewed.

Kish Tables

The first approach was designed by sampling statistician Leslie Kish for use in area probability-based personal interview surveys (Kish, 1965). With this approach, the interviewer requests the names, ages, and (as appropriate) other information for all the members of the household, who are then listed on a household listing table in the order specified. Generally the household head (or whoever is answering the question) is listed first, followed by the other family members from oldest to youngest (see Figure 6.3). Once everyone living in the household has been identified and listed in a specified order, the number of the person to interview can be determined. These listing and respondent selection procedures have been greatly enhanced by computerized data collection methods.

Kish (1965) generated a series of eight selection tables that reflect different designations of the person to choose, given different numbers of people in the household. Each table was to be used with a certain proportion of the cases in a sample. Selection Table D in Figure 6.3 is an example of one such table. These tables can be directly programmed into computer-assisted systems or generated by computer using procedures Kish developed. Each ultimate sampling unit then has a preassigned Kish table to use as the basis for deciding whom to interview.

The Kish respondent selection process is a systematic way to ensure that all relevant members of the household are identified and have a chance of being included in the sample. There has been concern with the application of the Kish procedure in telephone surveys, however, where there is a greater probability than in personal interviews that certain respondents (such as women or the elderly) will break off the interview immediately if they feel they are being asked an intrusive or tedious series of questions. The other approaches to respondent selection have been designed to address some of these perceived disadvantages of the Kish approach for telephone surveys.

Troldahl-Carter-Bryant Tables

With the Troldahl-Carter-Bryant (TCB) procedure, only two questions are asked: (1) How many persons of a certain age (as appropriate to study objectives) live in the household? and (2) How many of these individuals are of a certain gender (Czaja, Blair, & Sebestik, 1982)? As with the Kish approach, there are alternative selection tables that can be computerized or assigned to a predetermined proportion of the interviews for deciding which age-sex respondent to choose.

Originally the second question in the TCB procedure asked for the number of males in the household. Research conducted by Czaja, Blair, and Sebestik (1982), however, suggested that the rate of nonresponse was higher when this approach was used and, furthermore, that the proportion of women living alone was also underrepresented. When the respondent was asked about the number of women in the household with the TCB approach, the results for the Kish and TCB methods were very similar. With the TCB approach, however, there may be a tendency to underrepresent individuals between the oldest and youngest in households in which there are more than two individuals of the same sex. Furthermore, there is a general tendency to underrepresent males in telephone surveys because they are less likely to be at home at the time of the call.

Hagan and Collier Method

The Hagan and Collier method of respondent selection is an effort to simplify even further the process for identifying which individuals to interview (Hagan & Collier, 1983). With this approach, the interviewer asks to speak, for example, with the youngest (or oldest) adult male. If there is no male in the household, the interviewer asks for the corresponding female. The researcher must provide precise instructions to the interviewer regarding how to proceed if no one in the household fits that description. There are then some ambiguities in directly implementing the Hagan and Collier approach, and no extensive methodological research is available that compares this to other methods of respondent selection.

Last or Next Birthday Method

An approach that has been widely used in telephone surveys in particular is the last or next birthday method of respondent selection. With this approach, the person answering the telephone is asked who in the household had a birthday most recently (last birthday method) or is expected to have one next (next birthday method). This person is then chosen for the interview. (An example of the application of the last birthday method of respondent selection is provided in Table 6.3.)

Everyone in the household presumably has the same probability of being asked to participate, though as with all other respondent selection procedures, reporting error on the part of the respondent who supplies the information on which the selection is based could lead to the exclusion of some persons who should be included.

Neither the Hagan and Collier nor the next or last birthday approach explicitly asks for the number of people in the household. This information is needed to determine the probability that any particular individual will be selected and to apply weights to the sampled cases so that they accurately reflect the composition of all the households included in the sample.

**TABLE 6.3. PROCEDURES FOR SELECTING THE RESPONDENT—
RESPONDENT CHARACTERISTICS.**

Procedure	Methodology
Hagan and Collier method: (Ask to speak with one of four types of age-sex individuals and if no one of that gender, ask for counterpart of opposite gender.)	Question: I need to speak with (youngest adult male/youngest adult female/oldest adult male/oldest adult female) over the age of *xx,* if there is one.
Last/next birthday method: (Ask to speak with the person who had a birthday last *or* will have one next.)	Question: In order to determine whom to interview, could you please tell me, of adults *xx* years of age or older currently living in your household, who had the most recent birthday? I don't mean who is the youngest, just who had a birthday last.

Methodological research on the various methods of respondent selection has documented higher rates of break-offs during the screening process using the Kish method. There is evidence, however, that errors in identifying the correct sample person may be more likely among minority (especially African American and Hispanic) respondents using the last birthday approach. A promising alternative is to ask the screener respondent how many adults are in the household; if two adults are present, use a random selection procedure, or if more than two, employ the birthday screening method (or Kish procedure if the birthdates are not known) to select a study respondent (Binson, Canchola, & Catania, 2000; Lavrakas, Stasny, & Harpuder, 2000; Rizzo, Brick, & Park, 2004).

Special Considerations for Special Populations

A significant problem in many surveys, and in health surveys in particular, is that the researcher wants to study subgroups that appear with low frequency in the general population, such as selected minority groups, individuals with certain types of health problems or disabilities, patients of a particular clinic or health facility, homeless people, or drug users. This is a particular challenge in national, state, and local surveys that are concerned with generating estimates for key subgroups, such as racial/ethnic minorities. There has been a great deal of interest and effort on the part of sampling statisticians to develop cost-effective approaches to increasing the yield of these and other target groups in health surveys (Andresen, Diehr, & Luke, 2004; Kalton & Anderson, 1986; Sudman & Kalton, 1986; Sudman, Sirken, & Cowan, 1988). One of these methods has been touched on already in this chapter: disproportionate sampling within selected strata. Figure 6.4 describes and provides examples of this and other approaches for sampling rare populations.

Screening

Screening for the subgroups that will be the focus of a study involves asking selected respondents whether they or their households (as appropriate) have the characteristic or attribute (X) of interest. If they answer yes, they are included in the study. If not, they (or some proportion who say no) are dropped from the study.

This approach can be used quite effectively with either area probability or telephone surveys. Adaptations of the Waksberg-Mitofsky approach to screening clusters of telephone numbers can be employed, for example, in screening for selected population subgroups (Blair & Czaja, 1982; Waksberg, 1978, 1983). In these approaches, a screening question is asked of the first working residential number in a block of telephone numbers (PSU) to see if the sampling unit meets the screening criteria (an African American or Hispanic respondent, for example). If it does not, that PSU will be excluded from further calling; if it does, calling will proceed in that PSU. This assumes that there is a higher probability that more eligible households will be clustered in the PSU that met the screening criterion than in those blocks of numbers that did not meet the criterion. This assumption is more likely to be met for certain sets of characteristics than for others.

In area probability designs, interviewers can similarly contact households and ask respondents the screening question as a basis for deciding whether to proceed with interviews in those families. Although area probability screening of this kind is very expensive, the telephone application of this approach has a definite cost advantage over the in-person one. A mail questionnaire would be another cost-effective method for identifying potentially eligible units. Higher nonresponse rates with this method would, however, increase the possibility of bias in identifying who is ultimately eligible for the study.

A particular problem with the screening approach is the possibility of false negatives, which occur when people who say no to the screening question may in fact have the attribute and might even admit to this later if included in the study and asked the same question again in the course of the interview. The rates of false negatives should be taken into account in thinking through the design of the screening question and in decisions about whether to exclude from the final study all or only a portion of those who say no initially. In general, some proportion of those who say no to the screening question should be included in the sample anyway to permit the rate of false negatives to be estimated.

FIGURE 6.4. PROBABILITY SAMPLE DESIGNS
FOR SAMPLING RARE POPULATIONS.

Type of Design	Methodology	Examples
Screening (Ask respondents whether they/ household have the attribute X and drop those from sample that do not.)	Do you have the attribute X? Yes → Include in Sample No → Drop from Sample	Do you have a chronic illness? Yes → Include No → Drop

Disproportionate Sampling (Assign a higher sampling fraction to stratum that has attribute X.)

Stratum A	Stratum B	Stratum C
A1X	B1	C1X
A2X	B2	C2
A3X	B3	C3
A4	B4X	C4
A5	B5	C5
A6	B6	C6

Sampling Fraction =   3/6   1/6   1/6

Percent black in PSU:
Stratum A: High
Stratum B: Low
Stratum C: Low

Network Sampling (Ask respondents if they know others in *family network,* defined in certain way, who have attribute X.)

Do you have family who have attribute X?

Yes → (1) How many?

(2) Who and where are they?

No → Terminate Interview

Do you have a parent with cancer?

Yes → (1) Mother, father, or both?

(2) Name(s) and address(es)?

No → Terminate Interview

Dual-Frame Sampling (Use a second sampling frame containing elements with attribute X to supplement original frame.)

Frame #1			Frame #2		
1X	7	13	1X	7X	13X
2	8	14X	2X	8X	14X
3	9	15	3X	9X	15X
4X	10	16	4X	10X	16X
5	11	17	5X	11X	17X
6	12X	18	6X	12X	18X

Frame #1:
Area probability sample of clinic's service area

Frame#2:
List sample of clinic patients

Disproportionate Sampling

A second approach to oversampling certain groups of interest, displayed in Figure 6.4, is the disproportionate sampling within strata discussed earlier. In the example in Figure 6.4, as in the design of the California Health Interview Survey, there is an interest in sampling the stratum with a higher concentration of minorities (X). The sampling fraction (number of sample cases divided by number of cases in stratum) in the stratum (A) that has a high proportion of minorities (3/6) is set at three times that of the other two strata (1/6). The optimum allocation of cases between the strata should take into account the expected variability and cost per case within the respective strata. The fact that the sampling fraction is varied across strata will also need to be taken into account in combining cases from the respective strata for analysis. These weights will need to be employed in the analysis and perhaps special analysis software or procedures used to account for the complex nature of the sample design. This will be discussed in Chapter Seven in describing the procedures for weighting survey data gathered by means of disproportionate sampling techniques and adjusting for design effects resulting from cluster sample designs.

Commercially available telephone databases contain linked zip code, census tract, and associated demographic data from the U.S. Census and other sources that can be used in stratifying telephone exchanges for the purpose of disproportionately sampling selected population groups based on place of residence or selected demographic characteristics (race or income, for example) in random digit dialing surveys (Survey Sampling International, 2005).

Network Sampling

Another method that has been developed and applied in health surveys is network or multiplicity sampling. Health survey sampling statisticians have in fact contributed significantly to developing this approach (Czaja & Blair, 1990; Czaja, Snowden, & Casady, 1986; Czaja, Trunzo, & Royston, 1992; Czaja et al., 1984; Sudman & Freeman, 1988).

Network sampling asks individuals who fall into a sample (drawn by means of conventional probability sampling methods) to use certain counting rules in identifying relatives or friends who have the attribute of interest, most often some medical condition or disability. Respondents are then asked to indicate how many people they know with the condition and where they live. The researcher can follow up with the individuals named or use the information provided to generate prevalence estimates for these conditions in the population.

With network sampling, the probability of any given individual being named is proportional to the number of different households in which the originally sampled persons and the members of their networks, defined by the specified counting rules, reside. This information provides the basis for computing so-called multiplicity estimators for network samples. These estimators reflect the probability that respondents will be named across the multiplicity of networks to which they belong. As with the screening approach, there may be response errors on the part of informants about the occurrence of the condition in their network and in the accuracy of the size of the network they report. The costs of following up with individuals named by the original respondents will also add to the overall expense of the study. Establishment of counting rules for determining the size of the network and construction of the associated multiplicity estimators is a relatively complex procedure. This approach requires consultation with a sampling expert.

Dual-Frame Sampling

Dual-frame sampling uses more than one sampling frame in the design of the sample for the study. In general, one of the frames is expected to have a higher or known concentration of the subgroup of interest, which can then be combined with the other frame to enhance the yield of those individuals in the study as a whole. In the example provided in Figure 6.4, the researcher could conduct an area probability sample of residents in a clinic's service area to gather information on the need for and satisfaction with medical care among community residents. If the study design also calls for comparisons of the access and satisfaction levels of community residents who have used the clinic versus those who have not, it may be necessary to supplement the area probability sample with a list sample of patients who have actually used the clinic.

As with the multiplicity sampling procedure, it is important in dual-frame designs to consider carefully the probabilities that individuals from the respective frames will come into the sample and to construct appropriately the weights and procedures for computing estimates based on combining the respective samples.

Sampling Mobile Populations

The preceding approaches are the principal methods used for sampling rare and elusive groups. Additional problems arise in identifying universes of highly mobile populations, such as migrant workers, the homeless, or visitors to a health care facility or provider. Nonprobability sampling methods offer one alternative, although significant noncoverage biases may exist in studies employing these approaches.

Increasing attention is being given to the adaptation of conventionally non-probabilistic sampling methods, such as snowball sampling, to boost the prospects of obtaining unbiased estimates of population characteristics as well as to increase the efficiency of locating hard-to-reach or hidden populations. In a *random walk* procedure, for example, after obtaining the names of other members of a hidden population, one is selected at random, added to the sample, contacted by the researcher, and asked to give referrals, from which one is randomly selected and so on, for a desired number of waves. In a more efficient variation on this approach, *respondent-driven sampling,* members of the hidden population are asked to do the recruiting of potential study respondents by giving numbered coupons to candidate respondents. Any member of the hidden population coming in with such a coupon is given a monetary reward, as is the person from whom the coupon was obtained (Heckathorn, 1997, 2002; Thompson & Collins, 2002).

Probability-based procedures have been developed to attempt to sample mobile and elusive populations. These include methods for sampling in time and space and capture-recapture methods, among others. With the first approach, specific blocks of time at given locations are identified, and these are then used to form primary sampling units for a first stage of sampling. At the second stage, systematic random samples of elements (visitors, for example) are drawn within selected time-space blocks (clusters). In the capture-recapture method, which was originally developed for counting wildlife populations, two independent observations are taken at approximately the same time to count the population of interest. The number of individuals observed each time, as well as the number observed at both periods, is used to estimate the size of the total population as a basis for deriving a relevant sampling fraction (or fixing a probability of selection) for the sample. Although both theoretical and practical problems exist with these methods, they offer promising alternatives to largely nonprobabilistic designs (Kalsbeek, 2003; Kanouse et al., 1999; Muhib et al., 2001; Stueve, O'Donnell, Duran, Doval, & Blome, 2001).

Selected Examples

The three studies used as examples in this book (Resources A, B, and C) represent three different approaches to sampling—area probability, random digit dialing, and list samples—for personal, telephone, and mail surveys, respectively. The sample design of the UNICEF Multiple Indicator Cluster Survey is variable across countries, but the emphasis is on multistage probability proportionate to size (PPS) household sampling, with information collected on household, mothers, children under age five, and children ages five to fifteen (UNICEF, n.d.). The California

Health Interview Survey is based on a list-assisted random digit dialing sample, with the random selection of one adult respondent and if present in the household, one child (under age twelve) and one adolescent (ages twelve to seventeen). The survey makes extensive use of list sampling frames and disproportionate sampling to obtain sufficient cases to generate precise estimates for an array of racial/ethnic subgroups (UCLA Center for Health Policy Research, 2005). The National Dental Malpractice Survey is based on a list sample of general practicing dentists in the United States in 1991, drawn from a list of dentists in private practice provided by the American Dental Association (Washington State University, Social and Economic Sciences Research Center, 1993). The list contained both dentists who were and were not members of the American Dental Association. The sample designs for these three studies involve different aspects or combinations of the methods just described.

Guidelines for Minimizing Survey Errors and Maximizing Survey Quality

Table 6.4 summarizes the major sources of systematic and variable errors and related solutions during the sample design process. Noncoverage bias may be a particular issue in Internet or telephone surveys in which selected subgroups of the target population are not adequately represented in the sample frame available for identifying potential study participants. In these cases, multiple sample frames and related mixed modes of data collection (such as e-mail and telephone strategies) may be required to more adequately represent the target population in the study.

Allowing interviewers to arbitrarily select respondents or to interview whoever is available at the time of contact could lead to the significant over- or underrepresentation of selected groups in the survey, such as males or working-age adults. A variety of systematic respondent selection procedures (or some combination of them) could be used to facilitate the random selection of study subjects (see Figure 6.3 and Table 6.3).

Complex sample designs, especially multiple-stage cluster designs, can lead to higher sampling variability. Such procedures may be required to reduce the overall cost of the study. Researchers need to be aware of likely error and cost tradeoffs in designing their samples, as well as the implications for estimating the sample size and analyzing the data, taking the complex nature of the sample design into account. The procedures for estimating the sample size and related adjustments for the analyses of data based on complex survey samples are discussed in Chapter Seven.

TABLE 6.4. SURVEY ERRORS: SOURCES AND SOLUTIONS— DECIDING WHO WILL BE IN THE SAMPLE.

	Systematic Errors		*Variable Errors*
	Noncoverage Bias (Frame Bias)	**Noncoverage Bias (Respondent Selection Bias)**	**Design Effects**
Solutions to Errors	Match the sample frame to the target population. Use multiple sample frames, if needed, to more fully capture the target population of interest.	Employ methods for randomly selecting the study respondents.	Try to balance the complexity (especially the cluster nature) of the sample design needed to address the study objectives in relationship to survey costs.

In summary, P-A-C-E off the steps carefully in designing the survey sample, that is, *P*ay *a*ttention to both *c*ost and *e*rrors. *P*recision (random error), *a*ccuracy (systematic error), *c*omplexity, and *e*fficiency, as well as the match of the sample design to the survey objectives, are the key criteria to keep in mind in evaluating the pros and cons of different designs or combinations of design alternatives.

This chapter has provided an overview of the alternatives for deciding *who* should be selected for the sample. Chapter Seven presents techniques for estimating, adjusting, and evaluating *how many* should be included.

Supplementary Sources

For an overview of sample designs in general, see Kish (1965) and Levy and Lemeshow (1999). For health surveys in particular, see Cox and Cohen (1985).

CHAPTER SEVEN

DECIDING HOW MANY
WILL BE IN THE SAMPLE

Chapter Highlights

1. The research questions, objectives, and associated research design are the fundamental bases for computing the sample size needed to reliably carry out a study.
2. Design effects reflect the extent to which the sampling error for a complex sample design differs from that of a simple random sample of the same size.
3. Survey response rates are based on the number of completed interviews as a proportion of those cases drawn in the original sample that were verified (or estimated) to be eligible for the study.
4. Sample weighting procedures involve assigning more (or less) weight to certain cases in the sample to adjust for disproportionate sampling or the differential noncoverage or nonresponse to the survey by different groups.
5. Researchers may want to obtain software for computing sample sizes and associated weighting and variance adjustments for complex sample designs, given the ready availability of such software commercially and in the public domain.

Simultaneous with deciding who to include in a sample is the decision about how many respondents to include. This chapter discusses how to determine the study sample size, the response rates, the appropriate weighting of sample cases, and the errors associated with sampling them in a particular way.

Relating the Sample Size to the Study Objectives and Design

As indicated in Chapter Two, the study objectives and associated research design are the primary anchors and guides for the conduct of a survey, including the computation of the desired sample size for the study. The essential focus of descriptive designs is to estimate or profile the characteristics (parameters) of a population of interest. Analytical designs are directed toward testing hypotheses about why certain characteristics or relationships between variables are observed. Experimental studies examine whether a given program or intervention had an intended (or hypothesized) impact. Analytical and experimental designs entail comparisons between groups, often over time, as a basis for exploring the explanations for why an outcome or effect was observed in one situation (for individuals exposed to certain health risks or those randomly assigned to an experimental group) but not in others (among unexposed individuals or members of the control group).

The discussion provides a general overview of the sample size estimation process as well as formulas and examples for common designs and types of estimates. Formulas for other types of designs, tables of sample sizes based on these computations, and computer software for determining sample sizes under certain study designs and assumptions are readily available (for example, see Borenstein, Cohen, & Rothstein, 2000; Cohen, 1988; Kraemer & Thiemann, 1987; Lemeshow, Hosmer, Klar, & Lwanga, 1990; Levy & Lemeshow, 1999; Lipsey, 1990; Lwanga & Lemeshow, 1991). Statistical software packages, such as STATA, SAS, SPSS, and EpiInfo, also have procedures for computing sample size estimates. Lemeshow et al. (1990) and Lipsey (1990) were the principal sources for the formulas for computing sample sizes used in Tables 7.1A, 7.1B, and 7.3. The logic and rationale for estimating required sample sizes must be clearly understood, regardless of the specific technologies used in deriving them. Exhibit 7.1 compares the major steps and criteria to use in estimating the sample size for descriptive and analytical or experimental designs.

Computing the Sample Size for Descriptive Studies

A sample is used as a basis for estimating the unknown characteristics of the population from which it is drawn. The standard error is a measure of the variation in the estimate of interest (for example, the proportion of low-income minority women who had seen a doctor during the first trimester of their pregnancy or the mean number of visits for prenatal care overall) across all possible random samples of a certain size that could theoretically be drawn from the target population or universe (women living in a particular community). The estimates for all the samples that could (hypothetically) be drawn can be plotted and expressed as a *sampling distribution* of those estimates. As the size of the samples on which the estimates are based increases, sampling theory suggests that this distribution will take on a particular form, called a *normal sampling distribution* (see Figure 7.1).

FIGURE 7.1. NORMAL SAMPLING DISTRIBUTION.

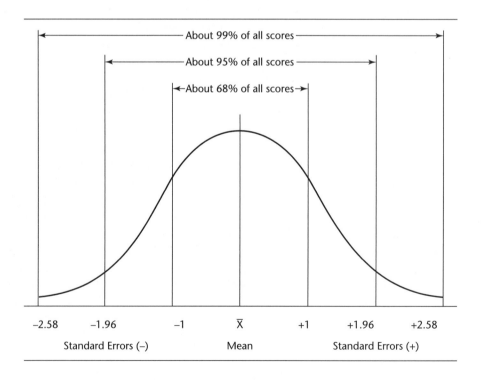

If the means of all possible simple random samples of a certain size that could be theoretically drawn from a population were averaged, the result would equal the actual mean (μ) for the population as a whole. The standard error (SE) is the standard deviation (or amount of variation on average) of all the possible sample means from this population mean. The greater the variation in the population mean from sample to sample, that is, the larger the standard error associated with this distribution of sample values, the less reliable the estimate can be said to be.

Standard errors may be high because (1) there is a great deal of variation in the elements of the population being studied (wide variations in whether different subgroups go for prenatal care, for example) or (2) the size of the sample used is too small to obtain consistent results when different samples of this size are drawn. Knowing that the distribution of values for all possible samples drawn from a population is theoretically going to take on the shape of a normal sampling distribution is useful in making inferences about a population from sample data. As Figure 7.1 indicates, for a normal sampling distribution, 68 percent of the sample means obtained from all possible random samples of the same size will fall within the range of values designated by plus or minus 1.00 standard error of the population mean, 95 percent will fall within plus or minus 1.96 standard errors, and 99 percent within plus or minus 2.58 standard errors.

In practice, it is not possible to draw all possible samples from a population. Researchers instead draw only one sample, and for large samples, they assume a normal sampling distribution of the estimates of interest (percentages and means) and compute the standard error for the estimate from this one sample. Based on the assumption of a normal sampling distribution, they can then estimate the probability of obtaining a particular value for a sample mean by chance, given certain characteristics (mean, variance) of the population.

Some values (those at the ends or tails of the normal distribution) would rarely occur—only 5 percent of the time, for example, for values further than two standard errors from a hypothesized population mean. If the estimate obtained in the study falls at these extreme ends of the distribution, researchers could conclude that the hypothesized population mean was probably not the true value given the small chance of its being found for a sample drawn from that population if the hypothesis were true. Ninety-five percent of the time this assumption would be correct.

The general steps for estimating the sample size for descriptive designs where estimating population parameters is the goal are summarized in Exhibit 7.1. The first step in estimating the sample size for a descriptive study is to identify the major study variables of interest. These are reflected quite directly in the research questions regarding *what* is the focus of the study (visits for prenatal care). Then thought must be given to the types of estimates that are most relevant for summarizing

EXHIBIT 7.1. CRITERIA FOR ESTIMATING THE SAMPLE SIZE BASED ON THE STUDY DESIGN.

Design:	Descriptive	Design:	Analytical or Experimental
Objective:	To estimate a parameter.	Objective:	To test a hypothesis.
Framework:	Sampling distribution	Framework:	Power analysis

Steps: (Descriptive)

1. Identify the major study variables.
2. Determine the types of estimates of study variables, such as means or proportions.
3. Select the population or subgroups of interest (based on study objectives and design).
4a. Indicate what you expect the population value to be.
4b. Estimate the standard deviation of the estimate.
5. Decide on a desired level of confidence in the estimate (confidence interval).
6. Decide on a tolerable range of error in the estimate (precision).
7. Compute sample size, based on study assumptions.

Steps: (Analytical or Experimental)

1. Identify the major study hypotheses.
2. Determine the statistical tests for the study hypotheses, such as a t-test, F-test, or chi-square test.
3. Select the population or subgroups of interest (based on study hypotheses and design).
4a. Indicate what you expect the hypothesized difference (Δ) to be.
4b. Estimate the standard deviation (σ) of the difference.
4c. Compute the effect size (Δ/σ).
5. Decide on a tolerable level of error in rejecting the null hypothesis when it is *true* (alpha).
6. Decide on a desired level of power for rejecting the null hypothesis when it is *false* (power).
7. Compute sample size, based on study assumptions.

information regarding these variables (such as the proportion of women in the population who had been for care during the first trimester of their pregnancy or the mean number of visits in total for prenatal care). Third, the study design directly dictates the number of groups and time period over which the data are to be gathered. Group-comparison designs that focus on estimating the differences between groups (African American and Hispanic women, for example) would require a look at the number of cases needed in each group for meaningful comparisons between them. Longitudinal designs, which focus on estimated changes over time, would require at least as many cases as cross-sectional designs, which estimate the characteristics of the population as a whole, but fewer than group-comparison designs.

The basis for estimating the sample size for a given design also assumes that the value (step 4a) or the associated standard deviation (step 4b) for the estimate of interest can be specified or obtained. The next steps entail deciding on the level of confidence (step 5) the investigator would want to associate with the range of values that may contain the true population value (parameter) as well as what would be the desired level of precision (or deviation) around the estimates that are derived from a sample of a specified size (step 6).

Table 7.1A provides the specific formulas and examples of sample size estimation for a number of common descriptive designs and types of estimates.

Design: Cross-Sectional (One Group); Estimate: Proportion

The investigator might estimate that around half ($P = .50 = 50$ percent) of the women in the study population are likely to go for prenatal care during the first trimester. It might be deemed reasonable to report an estimate that is precise within plus or minus 5 percent of this value (desired precision, $d = .05$), that is, 50 percent of the women in the study population plus or minus 5 percent (45 percent to 55 percent) visited a doctor during the first trimester. These estimates should, however, be based on previous research or knowledge of the study population. An example with .50 as the estimate is used here because a .50/.50 split in the proportion that did/did not have a characteristic tends to yield the largest sample size requirements.

As seen in Figure 7.1, the researcher could be confident that 95 percent of the time the sample estimates will fall within 1.96 standard errors ($Z_{1-\alpha/2}$) of the specified population value, if it were the true value. The standard error for a proportion is

$$SE_p = \sqrt{P(1-P)/n} \quad \textit{where,} \; P = \text{estimate of proportion} $$
$$\text{in the population}$$

The precision ($d = .05$), or tolerable deviation of values around the estimate, can be expressed in terms of units of standard errors [$d = Z_{1-\alpha/2}(SE_p)$]. The formula for expressing the desired precision in units of standard errors essentially serves as the basis for deriving (or solving for) the sample size (n) needed to produce this acceptable range of error at a given level of confidence:

TABLE 7.1A. SAMPLE SIZE ESTIMATION— DESCRIPTIVE STUDIES: SELECTED EXAMPLES.

Design and Estimates	Formula	Example
Cross-Sectional (One Group)		
Proportion	$n = \dfrac{z^2_{1-\alpha/2}P(1-P)}{d^2}$ *where,* P = estimated proportion d = desired precision	$n = \dfrac{1.96^2 \times (.50)\,(.50)}{(.05)^2} = 384$
Mean	$n = \dfrac{z^2_{1-\alpha/2}\sigma^2}{d^2}$ *where,* σ = estimated standard deviation d = desired precision	$n = \dfrac{1.96^2 \times (2.5^2)}{1^2} = 24$
Group-Comparison (Two Groups)		
Proportion	$n = \dfrac{z^2_{1-\alpha/2}[P_1(1-P_1)+P_2(1-P_2)]}{d^2}$ *where,* P_1 = estimated proportion (larger) P_2 = estimated proportion (smaller) d = desired precision	$n = \dfrac{1.96^2[(.70)(.30)+(.50)(.50)]}{.05^2} = 707$
Mean	$n = \dfrac{z^2_{1-\alpha/2}[2\sigma^2]}{d^2}$ *where,* σ = estimated standard deviation (assumed to be equal for each group) d = desired precision	$n = \dfrac{1.96^2[2 \times (2.5^2)]}{1^2} = 48$

Note:

$Z_{1-\alpha/2}$ = *standard errors* associated with *confidence intervals*:

1.00	68%
1.645	90%
1.96	95%
2.58	99%

Source: Lemeshow, Klar, & Lawanga (1990).

$$d = z_{1-\alpha/2}(SE_P) \qquad \textit{where, } d = .05 = 1.96 \times SE_P, \text{ when } \alpha = .05$$
$$d = z_{1-\alpha/2}[\sqrt{P(1-P)/n}]$$
$$d^2 = z^2_{1-\alpha/2}P(1-P)/n$$
$$n = z^2_{1-\alpha/2}P(1-P)/d^2$$

In the example in Table 7.1A, 384 cases are needed to estimate that the population value is .50 plus or minus .05 with a 95 percent level of confidence if the sample estimate is between .45 and .55.

In Table 7.1B, selected other examples of the sample sizes required to estimate a proportion with a desired level of precision based on the formula for a cross-sectional (one-group) design and assuming a 95 percent level of confidence are provided. The number of cases required increases as the proportion begins to approach .50 (meaning that the sample divides fairly evenly on the estimate or characteristic of interest) and the desired level of precision (the tightness of the allowable range around the estimate) is made more stringent (smaller) (Marks, 1982).

TABLE 7.1B. SAMPLE SIZE ESTIMATION— DESCRIPTIVE STUDIES: SELECTED EXAMPLES.

Estimated Proportion (P)	Desired Precision (d)									
	.01	.02	.03	.04	.05	.06	.07	.08	.09	.10
.01	381	96	43	24	16	11	8	6	5	4
.02	753	189	84	48	31	21	16	12	10	8
.03	1,118	280	125	70	45	32	23	18	14	12
.04	1,476	369	164	93	60	41	31	24	19	15
.05	1,825	457	203	115	73	51	38	29	23	19
.06	2,167	542	241	135	87	61	45	34	27	22
.07	2,501	626	278	157	101	70	52	40	31	26
.08	2,828	707	315	177	114	79	58	45	35	29
.09	3,147	787	350	197	126	88	65	50	39	32
.10	3,458	865	385	217	139	97	71	55	43	35
.15	4,899	1,225	545	307	196	137	100	77	61	49
.20	6,147	1,537	683	385	246	171	126	97	76	62
.25	7,203	1,801	801	451	289	201	148	113	89	73
.30	8,068	2,017	897	505	323	225	165	127	100	81
.35	8,740	2,185	972	547	350	243	179	137	108	88
.40	9,220	2,305	1,025	577	369	257	189	145	114	93
.45	9,508	2,377	1,057	595	381	265	195	149	118	96
.50	9,605	2,402	1,068	601	384	267	197	151	119	97

Note: Design—Cross-sectional (one group); estimate: proportion; confidence interval—95 percent. See formula for this design in Table 7.1A, on which the computations of the sample sizes in this table are based.

Design: Cross-Sectional (One Group); Estimate: Mean

The investigators might also be interested in estimating the average number of visits women had during their pregnancy to within plus or minus one visit ($d = 1$). The projected numbers of visits for prenatal care may range from zero to ten, with some women not expected to go at all and others having as many as ten visits. The standard error for the sample mean is

$$SE_m = \sigma / \sqrt{n} \quad \textit{where, } \sigma = \text{standard deviation of variable in the population}$$

The basis for deriving the desired n to yield this precision with a given level of confidence parallels that used in estimating the sample size for proportions:

$$
\begin{aligned}
d &= z_{1-\alpha/2}(SE_m) \\
d &= z_{1-\alpha/2}\sigma/\sqrt{n} \\
d^2 &= z^2_{1-\alpha/2}\sigma^2/n \\
n &= z^2_{1-\alpha/2}\sigma^2/d^2
\end{aligned}
\qquad \textit{where, } d = 1 = 1.96 \times SE_m, \text{ when } \alpha = .05
$$

The standard deviation (σ) for the variable of interest will not necessarily be known in advance of doing the study. However, it may be estimated from previously published research and pilot tests or pretests with the target population or related groups. It may also be estimated using the range of likely answers, that is, by dividing the expected range (ten) by four (to reflect the four quartiles of a distribution) to yield an estimated standard deviation of 2.5 for this particular estimate (Marks, 1982).

Applying the formula for estimating the sample size for means in the example in Table 7.1A, twenty-four cases are needed to estimate the number of visits (plus or minus one visit), with a 95 percent level of confidence assuming a standard deviation of 2.5.

Design: Group Comparison (Two Groups); Estimate: Proportion

The researchers may also be interested in having an adequate number of observations to estimate the differences in the proportions (who went for care) for different groups (Hispanic and African American women, for example). Based on knowledge of the subgroups of interest or previous research, they may assume that only 50 percent of Hispanic women will go for prenatal care in the first trimester compared with 70 percent of African American women—a 20 percent difference. The researchers would like to be able to detect this magnitude of difference within a reasonable range of variability ($d = .05$, or. $20 +/-.05$ = a range of .15 to .25) with 95 percent confidence.

In estimating the sample size required for estimating differences in the proportions, the standard errors of the proportions for both groups (P_1 and P_2) must be taken into account (see the example in Table 7.1A). The sample size is then obtained using the following formula:

$$n = z^2_{1-\alpha/2}[P_1(1 - P_1) + P_2(1 - P_2)]/d^2$$

In the example in Table 7.1A, 707 cases are needed in each group to detect a difference of 20 percent between the groups with a 95 percent level of confidence.

Design: Group Comparison (Two Groups); Estimate: Mean

The researcher may also assume that the average numbers of prenatal care visits are likely to differ for Hispanic and African American women in the target community. They would like to be able to estimate this difference with a reasonable level of precision ($d = 1$ visit) and confidence (95 percent). The formula for estimating the sample size for group-comparison designs is comparable to that for the one-group case, but it uses the combined (or pooled) standard deviation ($2\sigma^2$) for the two groups:

$$n = z^2_{1-\alpha/2} [2\sigma^2]/d^2$$

In this example, the standard deviation (σ) for the means for the respective groups is assumed to be the same (2.5). Based on this formula, in the example in Table 7.1A, at least forty-eight cases would be needed in each group to estimate a difference between the groups to within plus or minus one visit at a 95 percent level of confidence assuming a standard deviation of 2.5 for the sample mean for each group.

Tables for estimating the sample sizes for the types of estimates and designs summarized in Table 7.1A are available in Lemeshow et al. (1990) and Lwanga and Lemeshow (1991).

Computing the Sample Size for Analytical and Experimental Studies

Whereas descriptive studies focus on *what* the characteristics (or parameters) of a population are, analytical and experimental studies attempt to understand *why*. Descriptive studies attempt to provide precise estimates, while analytical and experimental studies test specific hypotheses. The hypotheses may be derived from theory or practice regarding the relationship between or the impact of certain variables (such as attitudes and knowledge regarding prenatal care or interventions to enhance pregnant women's access to services) on others (the appropriate use of prenatal care).

The theory or assumptions underlying these types of studies generally predict that there will be a statistical association between the variables or significant differences between groups being compared on a characteristic of interest. To set up a statistical basis for testing these assumptions, two types of hypotheses are stated: a *null hypothesis* (Ho) and an *alternative* (or research) *hypothesis* (Ha). The null hypothesis essentially states that there is no association between the variables or differences between groups. The alternative hypothesis states the associations or differences that are expected if the first hypothesis (of no difference) is rejected. The latter more directly mirrors the theoretical or substantive assumptions on which the study is based.

The likelihood of rejecting the null hypothesis is greater the stronger the relationship is between variables (knowledge of risks during pregnancy and prenatal care use) or the greater the differences between groups (Hispanic and African American women) that actually exist. However, these relationships can be very difficult to demonstrate empirically if a large amount of sampling or measurement error characterizes the data gathered to test the hypotheses. From a sampling point of view, the key concern is having a large enough number of cases to minimize the variable sampling (standard) error in the estimates. As discussed earlier in this chapter and displayed directly in the standard error formula $[\text{SE} = \sigma/\sqrt{n}\,]$, sampling error can be reduced by increasing the sample size (denominator) or minimizing the random errors in the data collection process (reducing the numerator, by either enhancing the reliability of study measures or adapting or standardizing the interviewing and data collection process). A larger sample size would be required if the differences to be detected are small (but nonetheless substantively significant) and the random errors around the estimates large.

Table 7.2 displays the likely outcomes of the hypothesis-testing process, which parallels sensitivity and specificity analysis in evaluating the validity of alternative screening procedures (see Chapter Three). In reality, either the null hypothesis

TABLE 7.2. TYPE I AND TYPE II ERRORS.

Sample	Population	
	Group 1 and 2 differ (Ho is *not* true)	**Group 1 and 2 do not differ (Ho is true)**
Significant difference (reject Ho)	Correct conclusion Probability = $1 - \beta$ (power) (*true* +)	Type I error Probability = α (alpha) (*false* +)
No significant difference (do *not* reject Ho)	Type II error Probability = β (beta) (*false* −)	Correct conclusion Probability = $1 - \alpha$ (confidence) (*true* −)

(Ho) or the alternative hypothesis (Ha) is true, but not both. Inaccuracies and imprecision in the data-gathering process could nonetheless result in a failure to empirically confirm the underlying empirical reality.

A Type I error results from falsely *rejecting* the null hypothesis when the hypothesis is actually *true*. Type I error is reflected in the significance level (α) used for delineating values that are very unlikely if the population estimate is a given value (μ) but are nonetheless still possible. The probability of *not rejecting* the null hypothesis when it is *true*, that is, the sample estimate appears within a reasonable range of frequently appearing values given that the hypothesized population parameters are true, is reflected in the confidence interval ($1 - \alpha$) set around this estimate. If the number of cases is quite large, as in administrative data sets such as claims records, a difference may be statistically but not substantively significant (such as a difference of twenty-five dollars in the total cost of hospitalizations for Medicare versus Medicaid patients with a given diagnosis).

Type II error (β) refers to the reverse error: *failing to reject* the null hypothesis when it is actually *false*. This type of error becomes particularly critical to consider when differences are assumed to exist but are very small or the errors around the estimates are large. Each alternative hypothesis has a different probability of being accepted or rejected as a function of the differences and errors that are assumed for each. This presents special challenges in thinking through the substantively meaningful relationships that can be affordably detected. The lower the likelihood is of a Type II error (β), that is, the less likely one is mistakenly to fail to reject the null hypothesis, the greater the power ($1 - \beta$) of the test is said to be. The probability of both Type I and Type II errors decreases as the sample size increases, primarily because the estimates obtained from larger samples are more reliable (have less random sampling variation).

Approaches to estimating sample sizes required to test hypotheses meaningfully require a specification of the null and alternative hypotheses, the expected values for the key estimates as well as the likely sampling variability around them, and suitable levels of significance and power. A widely used convention is to set the significance level at 5 percent ($\alpha = .05$) and power at 80 percent ($1 - \beta = .80$), although these may certainly be varied, depending on the desired trade-offs in terms of the respective types of errors (Type I and Type II error), as well as costs.

The alternative hypotheses (Ha) may be stated as either a one-tailed or two-tailed option. One-tailed hypotheses state that associations or differences between groups are likely to be in a certain direction (one group will have more or fewer visits for prenatal care than another, that is, Ha: $\mu_1 < \mu_2$). Two-tailed tests simply state that the groups are not the same or equal (Ha: $\mu_1 \neq \mu_2$), but they do not dictate the direction of the difference. The sample size requirements for one-tailed hypotheses (based on tests for differences in one direction) are lower than for two-tailed tests (that test for differences in both directions). A one-tailed test is recommended when one has a large measure of confidence in the likely direction of a difference because of a logical or biological impossibility of it being otherwise or because of knowledge of previous research in the area.

In experimental designs, there is a particular interest in detecting the effect (or difference) between experimental and control groups. The effect size (Δ / σ), which essentially reflects the hypothesized difference (Δ) between groups, standardized (adjusted) for the average (or pooled) variation (σ) between groups, provides a basis for calculating the sample size for these types of designs (Cohen, 1988; Lipsey, 1990). This method may also be used in estimating the sample size requirements for analytical designs.

The general steps for estimating the sample size for analytical and experimental designs are summarized in Exhibit 7.1. The first step entails stating the primary null (Ho) and alternative (Ha) hypotheses to be tested. The second and third steps dictate consideration of the statistical procedure to be used in testing the study hypotheses, based on the types of estimates (means, proportions, odds ratios) being considered (step 2) and the underlying design (such as an analytical group-comparison, case-control, or experimental design) on which the study is based (step 3). These steps directly dictate the types of analysis it is most appropriate to conduct given the hypotheses and associated design: a t-test or analysis of variance (ANOVA) tests of the differences between means or a chi-square test of differences between proportions between two groups in analytic group-comparison or experimental designs, or the computation of an odds ratio for case-control studies, for example (see Chapter Fifteen).

The fourth step entails providing specific hypothetical values for the estimates of interest (means, proportions, or odds ratios), the likely sampling variation in each, and the computation of the effect size when this approach is to be used in estimating the required sample size. For some estimates (proportions and odds ratios), the sampling variability is implicitly computed in the formulas or approaches used in deriving the sample size estimates, and for others (means), this would have to be estimated from previous studies or from the range of the distribution of values on the variable (described earlier).

Steps 5 and 6 entail setting reasonable levels of Type I error and power for economically detecting hypothesized differences.

Analytical and experimental studies require that statistical procedures such as a t-test, F-test, or chi-square test be employed to test the study hypotheses regarding whether there are differences between groups. Descriptive studies estimate the actual magnitude of these differences. As a result, the sample size requirements for descriptive studies are generally higher. In applied public health and health services research, researchers are generally interested in establishing whether a relationship exists between variables, but less concerned with estimating the precise magnitude of the difference. The power analysis procedures underlying analytical and experimental studies are then most often used in establishing the sample size requirements for surveys that entail comparisons between groups.

Table 7.3 provides the specific formulas and examples of sample size estimation for a number of common analytical or experimental designs and types of estimates. Tables for estimating the sample sizes derived from the formulas provided here for analytical designs are available in Lemeshow et al. (1990) and Lwanga and Lemeshow (1991). The approach to effect size estimation for experimental designs is principally derived from Cohen (1988), Kraemer and Thiemann (1987), and Lipsey (1990). Selected charts from Lipsey, on which the power analysis for the examples of experimental designs is based, are reproduced in Figure 7.2.

Design: Group Comparison (Two Groups), Ho: $P_1 - P_2 = 0$

The investigators may have specific hypotheses in mind with respect to likely differences between groups (Hispanics and African Americans) in the proportion (of women) who went for (prenatal) care. The first example in Table 7.3 demonstrates two approaches to estimating the sample size required to test alternative hypotheses regarding the magnitude of these differences, assuming a certain power (80 percent) and Type I error or level of significance (.05): (1) a computational formula and (2) effect size estimation.

The example assumes an alternative hypothesis (Ha: $P_1 - P_2 \neq 0$) in which $P_1 = .70$ and $P_2 = .50$. To solve the equation, these estimates (.70, .50), their average

TABLE 7.3. SAMPLE SIZE ESTIMATION—ANALYTICAL AND EXPERIMENTAL STUDIES: SELECTED EXAMPLES.

Design and Hypothesis	Formula	Example
Group Comparison (Two Groups) $Ho: P_1 - P_2 = 0$ $Ha: P_1 - P_2 \neq 0$	*Formula* $$n = \frac{\{z_{1-\alpha/2}\sqrt{2\bar{P}(1-\bar{P})} + z_{1-\beta}\sqrt{P_1(1-P_1)+P_2(1-P_2)}\}^2}{(P_1-P_2)^2}$$ *where,* $\bar{P} = (P_1+P_2)/2$ P_1 = estimated proportion (larger) P_2 = estimated proportion (smaller)	$$n = \frac{\{1.96\sqrt{2(.60)(.40)} + .842\sqrt{[(.70)(.30)+(.50)(.50)]}\}^2}{(.70-.50)^2}$$ $n = 93$
	Effect size $ESp = \phi_1 - \phi_2$ *where,* ESp = effect size for proportions ϕ_1, ϕ_2 = arcsine transformation for proportions (groups 1,2)	$ESp = 1.982 - 1.571 = .411$ $n = 93$ (see Figure 7.2)
Group Comparison (Two Groups) $Ho: \mu_1 = \mu_2$ $Ha: \mu_1 \neq \mu_2$	*Formula* $$n = \frac{2\sigma^2[z_{1-\alpha/2}+z_{1-\beta}]^2}{(\mu_1-\mu_2)^2}$$ *where,* σ = estimated standard deviation (assumed to be equal for each group) μ_1 = estimated mean (larger) μ_2 = estimated mean (smaller)	*Formula* $$n = \frac{2(2.5)^2[1.96+.842]^2}{(6-4)^2}$$ $n = 25$
	Effect size $ES\mu = \dfrac{\mu_1-\mu_2}{\sigma}$ *where,* $ES\mu$ = effect size for means μ_1, μ_2 = estimated means (groups 1,2) σ = pooled standard deviation $$\sigma = \sqrt{\frac{\sigma_1^2+\sigma_2^2}{2}}$$	*Effect size* $ES\mu = \dfrac{6-4}{2.5} = .80$ $n = 25$ (see Figure 7.2)

Case Control
Ho: OR = 1
Ha: OR ≠ 1

Formula

$$n = \frac{\{z_{1-\alpha/2}\sqrt{2P^*_2(1-P^*_2)} + z_{1-\beta}\sqrt{P^*_1(1-P^*_1)+P^*_2(1-P^*_2)}\}^2}{(P^*_1-P^*_2)^2}$$

where,

(NOTE: "*" here and above refers to proportion (P*) exposed in case-control design.)

P^*_1 = proportion exposed in cases, i.e.,

$$= \frac{(OR)P^*_2}{(OR)P^*_2+(1-P^*_2)}$$

P^*_2 = proportion exposed in controls

OR = odds ratio

$$n = \frac{\{1.960\sqrt{2\times0.3\times0.7}+0.842\sqrt{0.4615\times0.5385+0.3\times0.7}\}^2}{(0.4615-0.3)^2}$$

n = 130

where,

(NOTE: "x" here and above refers to multiplication of terms or "multiplied by.")

$P^*_1 = 2\times0.3/[2\times0.3+0.7]=0.4615$

$P^*_2 = .30$

OR = 2

Note:

$Z_{1-\alpha/2}$ = *standard errors associated with confidence intervals:*

1.00	68%
1.645	90%
1.96	95%
2.58	99%

$Z_{1-\beta}$ = *standard errors associated with power:*

.524	70%
.842	80%
1.282	90%
1.645	95%
2.326	99%

Sources: Lemeshow, Hosmer, Klar, and Lwanga, 1990; Lipsey, 1990.

$[(P_1 + P_2)/2 = (.70 + .50)/2 = .60]$, and the standard errors (z) associated with a designated confidence interval and power must be specified. For a 95 percent confidence interval, $Z_{1-\alpha/2} = 1.96$, and for power of .80, $Z_{1-\beta} = .842$. Based on the first example in Table 7.3, around ninety-three cases are needed in each group.

The effect size for proportions is estimated by the differences in the arcsine transformations of the respective proportions. Figure 7.2A provides the arcsine transformations for proportions (arcsine of .70 = 1.982; arcsine of .50 = 1.571). The resulting difference in the estimates used in this example (.411) reflects the estimated effect size (ES_p). Figure 7.2B can then be used to estimate the sample size required in each group to obtain a given level of power (say, 80 percent) with a significance level of .05. In this example, the curve for an effect size of .41 crosses the row for a power of .80 (or 80 percent) at a sample of size around ninety-three, thereby confirming the previous results based on the formula.

Design: Group Comparison (Two Groups), Ho: $\mu_1 = \mu_2$

The second example in Table 7.3 assumes an alternative hypothesis (Ha: $\mu_1 \neq \mu_2$) in which μ_1 equals six visits and μ_2 equals four visits. To solve the equation, these estimates, their estimated standard deviations (2.5 for both groups), and the standard errors associated with a designated confidence interval (95 percent, $Z_{1-\alpha/2} = 1.96$) and power (80 percent, $Z_{1-\beta} = .842$) must be specified. Based on the formula using this example, approximately twenty-five cases are needed in each group.

The effect size for means (ES_μ) is based on the difference between the means estimated for each group $(6 - 4)$ divided by their pooled standard deviation $[\sigma = \sqrt{(\sigma_1^2 + \sigma_2^2)/2} = 2.5]$. The resulting effect size is .80. Using Figure 7.2B once again, the curve for an effect size of .80 crosses the row for a power of .80 (or 80 percent) at a sample size of twenty-five, assuming a .05 level of significance, thereby confirming the previous results based on the formula.

The power chart in Figure 7.2A assumes independent samples. When estimating the sample size requirements for related samples (those in which the same individuals are interviewed over time or groups are purposefully matched on selected characteristics), the researcher may want to assume a somewhat larger effect size in using this power chart. This is because the resulting effect size (Δ/σ) is larger for the same hypothesized difference (Δ), due to the sampling error (σ) being smaller in these types of designs.

Some rules of thumb for estimating likely effect sizes in analytical and experimental designs when they are not known or cannot be computed directly are as follows:

FIGURE 7.2. SELECTED RESOURCES FOR POWER ANALYSIS.

A. Arcsine Transformations (φ) for Proportions (P)

P	φ	P	φ	P	φ	P	φ
.01	.200	.26	1.070	.51	1.591	.76	2.118
.02	.284	.27	1.093	.52	1.611	.77	2.141
.03	.348	.28	1.115	.53	1.631	.78	2.165
.04	.403	.29	1.137	.54	1.651	.79	2.190
.05	.451	.30	1.159	.55	1.671	.80	2.214
.06	.495	.31	1.181	.56	1.691	.81	2.240
.07	.536	.32	1.203	.57	1.711	.82	2.265
.08	.574	.33	1.224	.58	1.731	.83	2.292
.09	.609	.34	1.245	.59	1.752	.84	2.319
.10	.644	.35	1.266	.60	1.772	.85	2.346
.11	.676	.36	1.287	.61	1.793	.86	2.375
.12	.707	.37	1.308	.62	1.813	.87	2.404
.13	.738	.38	1.328	.63	1.834	.88	2.434
.14	.767	.39	1.349	.64	1.855	.89	2.465
.15	.795	.40	1.369	.65	1.875	.90	2.498
.16	.823	.41	1.390	.66	1.897	.91	2.532
.17	.850	.42	1.410	.67	1.918	.92	2.568
.18	.876	.43	1.430	.68	1.939	.93	2.606
.19	.902	.44	1.451	.69	1.961	.94	2.647
.20	.927	.45	1.471	.70	1.982	.95	2.691
.21	.952	.46	1.491	.71	2.004	.96	2.739
.22	.976	.47	1.511	.72	2.026	.97	2.793
.23	1.000	.48	1.531	.73	2.049	.98	2.858
.24	1.024	.49	1.551	.74	2.071	.99	2.941
.25	1.047	.50	1.571	.75	2.094		

FIGURE 7.2. SELECTED RESOURCES FOR POWER ANALYSIS, *continued.*

B. Power Chart for σ = .05, Two tailed or σ = .025, One-Tailed

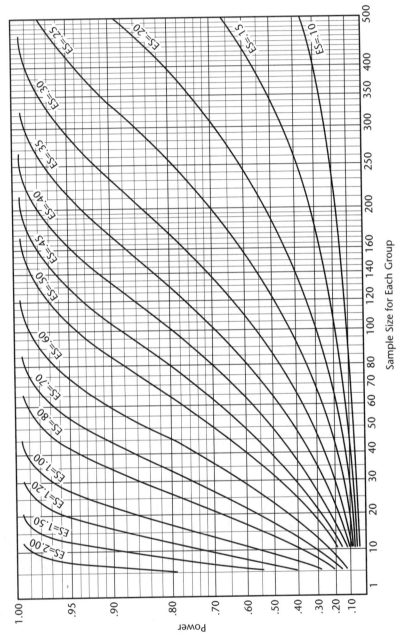

Source: Both charts in Figure 7.2 are reprinted from Lipsey, M. W., *Design Sensitivity: Statistical Power for Experimental Research,* pp. 88, 91, copyright © 1990 by Sage Publications, Inc. Reprinted by permission of Sage Publications, Inc.

If Effect Size Is Estimated to Be,	*Then, Effect Size =*
Small	$< .50$
Medium	$\geq .50–.79$
Large	$\geq .80$

Design: Case-Control (Two Groups), Ho: OR = 1

The final example in Table 7.2 is based on a case-control design in which the alternative hypothesis is that the odds ratio (OR) is not equal to one, meaning that the risk of disease occurrence (hypertension) is greater for the group that has a given risk factor (smokers) compared with those who do not. In this example, smokers are hypothesized to have twice the risk of nonsmokers (OR = 2.0). The hypothesized OR should be based on previously published or clinical research documenting the role of the risk factors of interest as a predictor of who has the disease and who does not. The proportion of smokers in the control group (P^*_2) is estimated to be .30. The proportion of smokers among cases must be derived based on the estimated OR and proportion exposed (smokers) among the controls. The formula requires that these estimated and derived values, as well as the standard errors used to designate the power and significance level, be entered (Lemeshow et al., 1990).

In this example, 130 cases and an equivalent number of controls are needed to detect an OR of 2.0, assuming 30 percent of the controls and 46 percent of the cases are smokers, a power of 80 percent, and a significance level of .05. If one is not sure of the exposure rate of the controls, estimated rates of exposure in the controls (.30) and cases (.46) could be averaged (.38) and used for P^*_2 in the formula for computing the sample size. This would yield a somewhat higher sample size requirement (an estimated n of 141 rather than 130 in this example).

Design: Analytical Using Multivariate Analyses

Sometimes analytical, hypothesis-testing studies make use of multivariate statistical procedures, such as linear or logistic regression. (See Chapter Fifteen for a fuller discussion of these and other procedures.) In that case, a criterion that could be used to estimate the required sample size is as follows:

Criterion

For logistic or linear regression, the required sample size for each model is 10 to 15 cases per variable entered into the model.

Example

n = Number of variables * 15

$n = 20 * 15$

$n = 300$

For example, a maximum of 20 variables might be entered as predictors in the model. In that case, there should be a minimum of 10 to 15 cases in the sample per variable, resulting in a maximum of 300 cases needed.

Sample Size Requirements for Addressing All of the Study Objectives

Studies may entail a mix of descriptive and analytical objectives. Descriptive objectives focus on providing specific estimates on a concept of interest (such as the prevalence of a given disease or the percentage of women who had gone for prenatal care in the first trimester) with a given level of precision. Analytical or experimental objectives assume that statistical procedures will be employed to test and accept or reject selected research hypotheses with a given level of confidence and power. Given that descriptive objectives require precise estimates and the other types of objectives simply either a yes or no response to rejecting or accepting the study hypotheses, the sample size requirements for descriptive objectives are generally higher than for analytical or experimental objectives.

The essential anchor for estimating the sample size requirements for a study is the study objectives. Different types of objectives may dictate different sample sizes. The steps in arriving at a final sample size estimate are summarized below:

1. Select the sample size estimation procedure that best matches each study objective.
2. Compute the sample size required to address each objective.
3. Based on the sample sizes required to address each of the objectives, appropriate sample size adjustments, as well as time and resource constraints, recommend an overall sample size. (The types of additional adjustments that may be required are discussed more fully later in this chapter.)
4. Discuss possible limitations in terms of statistical precision or power in addressing any specific study objectives, given the recommended sample size.

It is important to assess the sample size requirements for stated study objectives prior to either designing a new survey or conducting secondary analyses of an existing data set.

Computing the Design Effect for the Sample

The size of the sampling errors is also affected by the design of the sample itself. The variances (the standard deviations squared) of estimates obtained from stratified or cluster sample–based designs generally differ from those based on a simple random sample. The ratio of the variance of the complex sample (VAR_{cs}) to that of a simple random sample (VAR_{srs}) is used to quantify the design effect (DEFF) of a specific sample design (Kalton, 1983): $DEFF = (VAR_{cs})/(VAR_{srs})$. Design effect adjustments are required only for studies that entail some form of cluster sampling. If the design effect for the study is not taken into account up front in estimating the required sample size, the number of cases resulting may not be sufficient for obtaining the desired level of precision and power. It will be important to keep good documentation identifying the clusters and strata (if relevant) from which cases are drawn, to facilitate the use of statistical software and procedures for adjusting for design effects.

Some rules of thumb governing the likely estimated magnitude of design effects are as follows:

If DEFF Is Estimated to Be,	Then, DEFF =
None	1.0
Low	> 1.0–1.3
Medium	1.4–1.9
High	≥ 2.0

The reason that variances (and thereby design effects) are higher in cluster sampling (such as the probability proportionate to size) designs is that the sampling variance includes the variation between clusters, in addition to the variability between respondents within a given cluster. A cluster tends to be groups of households or blocks in a given neighborhood, and therefore the characteristics of respondents within the cluster may be relatively homogeneous (for example, in terms of socioeconomic status), but may differ significantly from respondents in clusters taken from other neighborhoods. The more homogeneous the respondents are within clusters and the larger the number taken from each cluster, the higher the design effect is.

Related assumptions can be used in an alternative approach to estimating the likely design effect for a study: $DEFF = 1 + (b - 1)\ roh$, where $DEFF$ = design effect, b = cluster size, and roh = rate of homogeneity (intracluster correlation):

None = 0

Low = ≤ .10

Medium = .11–.19

High = ≥ .20

Some variables (such as age and gender) may have very low rates of homogeneity within a cluster (that is, there is great diversity within the cluster), while others (such as race) may have high rates of homogeneity. If the latter is the case and that characteristic or variables related to it are a focus of the study objectives, then a higher design effect should be assumed in estimating the target sample size for the study. The choice of the size of the clusters to be taken should be based on considerations of the likely homogeneity within clusters, as well as the number of cases that could be efficiently handled by an interviewer or data collector assigned to each cluster. In many field studies, clusters generally include seven to ten households (or other relevant sampling units). (See Bennett, Woods, Liyanage, & Smith, 1991, for a fuller description of cluster sample surveys and related implications for the design effect.)

A design effect of 1.3, for example, means that the variance for any estimate based on the sample is 30 percent higher than that derived from a simple random sample. This would reflect a design in which there is a relatively low design effect. To adjust for the design effect in computing standard errors for more complex sample designs, the standard errors of a given estimate (50 percent) can be computed by means of the formula for a simple random sample (5 percent for a sample of one hundred cases) and then multiplied by the square root of the design effect (1.3). This will result in a standard error of the estimate ($5 \sqrt{1.3} = 5.7$), which more appropriately reflects the complex sample design used in the study.

In a stratified design, cases are drawn from all the strata into which the population has been divided. The standard error for a stratified sample is based on the weighted average of the standard errors within each stratum. There will, in fact, be less diversity within each of these relatively homogeneous strata than across the sample as a whole. The net result of taking the weighted average of the standard errors of these relatively homogeneous strata is that the standard errors for a stratified design will be less than those that result from a simple random sample of the same population.

In contrast to a stratified sample, with a cluster design, only a sample of clusters is drawn from all the clusters into which the population has been divided. The computation of the standard errors for a cluster design is based on a weighted average of the standard errors between the clusters selected for the sample. The more internally homogeneous (or correlated) the cases are within the respective clusters, the more heterogeneous the means between clusters are likely to be. The net result of taking the weighted average of the standard errors between relatively homogeneous clusters, then, is that the standard errors for a cluster design will be higher than those based on a simple random sample of the same population. The design effects associated with cluster-type designs may result in their standard errors being two or three times greater than those of a simple random sample.

Most complex survey designs involve combinations of simple random samples and stratified and cluster-type sampling approaches. These designs may also include differential weighting of the sample elements. The design effect for these types of designs—the ratio of the variances on key estimates for the particular sample to that of a simple random sample—will lie somewhere between that of pure stratified and pure cluster-type sample designs.

Statistical procedures have been developed to estimate the standard errors or variances and, from them, the design effects for certain types of sample designs. These procedures include *balanced repeated replication, jackknife repeated replication,* and *Taylor series approximation.* Lee, Forthofer, and Lorimor (1986, 1989) provide an overview of these three alternatives to the analysis of complex sample survey data with particular reference to several large-scale health surveys. These procedures are available in standard software packages to facilitate the computation of relevant design effects.

The packages that have been most widely available to general users include SUDAAN (Research Triangle Institute, North Carolina); PC–CARP (Department of Statistics, Iowa State University, Ames, Iowa); the CSAMPLE procedure within EPiInfo, developed for the Centers for Disease Control and Prevention (available from USD, Stone Mountain, Georgia); and WesVarPC (Westat, Rockville, Maryland). Statistical analysis software packages such as STATA, SAS, and SPSS have also added features for taking the complex nature of sample designs and related design effects into account.

Several sources have compared the program capabilities, computational efficiencies, cost, and user friendliness of a number of the standard software packages for computing variances for complex surveys (American Statistical Association, Section on Survey Research Methods, n.d.-a; Cohen, 1997; Kneipp & Yarandi, 2002). No one package is superior to the other. The choice depends on the analysis procedures of interest, the size of the database, the complexity of the sample design, and the expertise and resources available for the use of a given package.

Different subgroups and estimates in a study may also have different design effects, principally as a function of the degree of correlation (similarity) within groups that results from sampling clusters of these individuals. Varying design effects for different groups should be taken into account in determining the sample size required for these groups and in adjusting the standard errors of estimates for them during analysis.

Additional Adjustments in Computing the Sample Size

Once the sample size is computed based on considerations of the study's research questions and design, additional adjustments to this estimated sample size are still needed to ensure that the desired target number of cases is obtained (see Table 7.4).

TABLE 7.4. ADDITIONAL ADJUSTMENTS IN COMPUTING THE SAMPLE SIZE.

Criteria	Example
1. Adjust for the size of the population.	$n/(1 + (n - 1)/N)$ $n = 384$; $N = 250,000$ *therefore* $n = 384/(1 + (384 - 1)/250,000)$ $= 384$
2. Adjust for the estimated sample effect.	**nadj * DEFF** DEFF = 1.3 *therefore* $n = 384 \times 1.3 = 499$
3. Adjust for the expected response rate.	**nadj/Response rate** Response rate = .80 *therefore* $n = 499 \div .80 = 624$
4. Adjust for the expected proportion eligible.	**nadj/Proportion eligible** % Eligible = .90 *therefore* $n = 624 \div .90 = 693$
5. Compute survey costs.	**Estimated cost/case = $50** *therefore* Total estimated cost = 693 $\times$ $50 = $34,650

Note: This example assumes a beginning sample size of 384, based on the study objectives.

Step 1: Adjust for the Size of the Population

Generally a sample represents a very small proportion of the overall target population. But if a sample constitutes a relatively high proportion of the target population, there is likely to be less sampling error because the study sample is more like the target population.

The proportion that a sample (n) represents of the target population (N) is reflected in the sampling fraction: n/N. The finite population correction (fpc) is another way of expressing the extent to which the sample (n) represents a small or large proportion of the population (N): $fpc = (1 - n/N)$, where n = sample size and N = population size.

Selected examples of different finite population correction factors, based on the sampling fraction, are as follows:

- Where $n = 100$, and $N = 10,000$
  $n/N = 100/10,000 = .01$
  $fpc = 1 - .01 = .99$
- Where $n = 100$, and $N = 300$
  $n/N = 100/300 = .333$
  $fpc = 1 - .333 = .667$

In the first example, the sample size of 100 represents a very small proportion (.01) of the population ($N = 10,000$), and the finite population correction is therefore large. In the other example, the opposite is the case, and the fpc is therefore smaller.

The implication of the fpc for the sampling variability and related standard error (SE) is reflected in the following adjustment to the standard error underlying a given sample:

Formula

$SE = sqrt\ [(1 - n/N) * s^2/n]$

Implications

The higher the proportion a sample represents of the population (n/N) (for example, $100/300 = .333$), then the lower the fpc (for example, $1 - .333 = .667$) and the SE of estimates based on the sample.

Therefore, fewer cases are needed in the sample because of its greater precision (lower SEs).

To address the fact that the de facto universe for a study might be quite small ($N = 100$, for example) and the sample size estimated using conventional sample size formulas for a given level of precision or power may be high ($n = 384$), an adjustment to the estimated size could be made based on the finite population correction factor:

Formula for Sample Size Adjustment Based on fpc

$nadj = n/(1 + (n - 1)/\text{N})$, where n = computed sample n and $\mathcal{N}$ = size of population

Example

$nadj = 384/(1 + (384 - 1)/100)$

    $384/(1 + (383)/100)$

    $384/4.83$

    80

If the universe size is large (100,000 or greater), the finite population correction is likely to be inconsequential and no adjustment based on the size of the population would be required. In the example in Table 7.4, no adjustment is assumed because of the large population from which the sample was drawn ($\mathcal{N} = 250,000$).

Step 2: Adjust for the Estimated Sample Design Effect

The sample sizes resulting from the computations described in Exhibit 7.1 assume that the sample design is a simple or systematic random sample. If this is not the case, it will be necessary to estimate what the anticipated design effect will be, that is, the impact a more complex design will have on the sampling errors in the survey. Since the actual design effect for a study cannot be computed until after the data are collected, it has to be approximated by examining the design effects for comparable estimates in other studies. The sample size estimate is then multiplied by this factor to increase the size of the sample, since the "effective" sample size will be smaller, given the complex nature of the design. Multiplying the 384 cases derived for the first example in Table 7.1A by an estimated design effect of 1.3 (for a design involving some cluster sampling, such as a random digit dialing survey that entails oversampling of selected groups) yields an estimate of 499 cases. This number of cases adjusts for the fact that the design will not be a simple random sample.

Step 3: Adjust for the Expected Response Rate

The next step involves dividing the sample size derived from the preceding steps by the estimated response rate for the study. By thus inflating the number of cases, the investigator adjusts for the fact that a certain proportion of the sample will not respond. An 80 percent response rate is assumed for the example in Table 7.4 (499/.80 = 624 cases).

Step 4: Adjust for the Expected Proportion of Eligibles

This step is similar to the preceding one in that the number of cases derived in step 2 is divided by the expected portion of cases that will be found to be eligible for the survey once they are contacted. The estimated figure here is around 90 percent of the cases (624/.90 = 693 cases). This may be realistic for a list sample survey, in which 10 percent of the individuals are deceased or have moved out of the area since the list was compiled. It would be much lower (25 percent, for example) for a random digit dialing survey, in which a large number of randomly generated telephone numbers (say, 2,500) may have to be called to find working residential numbers. The number that must be generated initially (original sample n) in this case would be 624/.25 = 2,496.

Step 5: Compute Survey Costs

This series of steps can be repeated for the major estimates being considered in the analyses, the resulting range of sample sizes reviewed, the costs per case estimated, and the final sample size determined. This last decision is made on the basis of the number of cases it would be ideal to have, whether this number fits with the study budget, and what compromises might have to be made to match the design to the dollars available for the survey.

The results of the computations in Table 7.4 suggest that approximately 700 (693) cases are required to have 95 percent confidence that the hypothesis that about half (50 percent) of the women in the target population went for prenatal care in the first trimester is true, should the value for the sample drawn from the community fall anywhere in the range of 45 to 55 percent. Using a hypothetical estimate of the cost per case of $50, approximately $35,000 would then be required to carry out the survey.

Calculation of Response Rate

An important approach to evaluating the implementation of a particular sample design is the level of success in contacting and collecting information from the individuals or elements to be included in the study. This involves calculating a *response rate* (RR)—the percentage or proportion of the cases eligible for the survey with whom interviews or questionnaires were actually completed: $RR = (C/n_{eligible})$. A variety of approaches have been used in computing survey response rates. In an effort to standardize the assumptions and computations used within the industry, the Council of American Survey Research Organizations (1982) developed specific alternatives for computing these rates, which have been accepted and endorsed by professional associations such as the American Association for Public Opinion Research (2004). The response rate being used here essentially corresponds to the RR3 formula, in which the proportion of cases with unknown eligibility is estimated. As will be discussed in the following section, some of the cases that were originally selected for the sample may turn out to be ineligible for a variety of reasons and can therefore legitimately be excluded from the denominator in computing the final response rate.

Table 7.5 portrays the basic elements to be used in computing an overall response rate for area probability, random digit dialing, and list samples. It draws on the case studies of these different types of sample designs that were described earlier, as well as on the hypothetical sample of 693 cases derived in Table 7.4.

Step 1: Specify the Original Sample Size

The first item of information to consider in computing an overall response rate for a survey is the size of the original sample: the total number of elements originally included in the study, which is 693 cases in this example.

Step 2: Subtract Known Ineligible Units

From the original sample are subtracted the elements found ineligible for the survey as the study proceeds ($n = 64$). In area probability samples, this would include housing units that are verified to be unoccupied; households such as businesses or institutional housing that do not fit the criterion of being private residences and are excluded from the definition of the universe; and households that do not fit some screening criterion relevant for the study, such as having family incomes below a certain level or elderly persons living there. For telephone surveys, telephone numbers generated through a random digit dialing process that are found to be nonworking numbers or business telephones when called would be deemed ineligible. In list samples of individuals, persons who had died by the time of the survey or, if appropriate, moved outside the area encompassed in the study's target population would be declared ineligible and deleted from the denominator in computing the response rate.

Step 3: Estimate Unknown Ineligible Units

As Table 7.5 indicates, a problem in each of these types of sampling procedures is that it is often difficult to determine with certainty whether a particular sampling element is ineligible for the study. For example, in area probability samples, if no

TABLE 7.5. CALCULATION OF RESPONSE RATE.

Elements in Response Rate	Type of Sample Design			Example
	Area Probability	**Random Digit Dialing**	**List**	
1. Original Sample Size	No. of housing units	No. of assigned phone numbers	No. of elements on list	693
less Ineligible Units				
2. *Known*	Unoccupied unit Institutional housing Doesn't fit screening criteria	Nonworking number Nonresidential number Doesn't fit screening criteria	Deceased Moved outside area Doesn't fit screening criteria Duplicate listings	64
3. *Unknown* (estimate based on proportion of known ineligibles)	Never home	Ring/no answer/ machine Line busy	Moved/no forwarding address	5 ――
equal 4. Eligible Units				624
less 5. Noninterviews	Refusal Break off Too ill (in hospital) Senility/physical problem Language barrier Away for entire field period Never home (estimate)	Refusal Break off Too ill (in hospital) Senility/physical problem Language barrier Ring/no answer/ machine (estimate) Line busy (estimate)	Not returned Moved/ no forwarding address (estimate)	125 ――
equal 6. Completed Interviews				499

$$\text{7. Response Rate} = \frac{\text{No. of Completed Interviews}}{\text{No. of Eligible Units}} = \frac{499}{624} = 80\%$$

Note: The numbered elements in computing the response rate refer to steps more fully discussed in the text.

one is ever home when the interviewer makes repeated visits at different times throughout the field period and he or she is unable to determine from neighbors or a landlord whether the housing unit is occupied, then the eligibility of that particular housing unit for the study may be indeterminate (or unknown). The problem of determining eligibility may be even more of an issue for telephone numbers generated through the random digit dialing process if there is never an answer when certain numbers are dialed or the line is always busy. If eligibility for a list sample is linked to the individual's place of residence, questionnaires returned with no indication of the person's forwarding address will be problematic in determining whether that potential respondent continues to be eligible for the study. In these cases, the researcher will have to develop some decision rule for estimating the number of elements for which eligibility cannot be determined directly.

A criterion that can be used in estimating whether those who could not be reached are ineligible is to assume that the proportion who are not eligible is comparable to the proportion of those who could be reached that were not eligible. This proportion can be used in approximating the number of cases with unknown status who should be excluded because they are probably ineligible for the study. There may be biases in using this estimate, however, if those who could not be contacted differed in systematic ways (were older, had lower incomes, and so on) from those who were contacted.

There were 55 cases for which eligibility was not known in the original sample of 693 cases. There were then 638 cases in the sample (693 − 55) for which eligibility was known. Of these 638 cases, 64 (10 percent) were found not to be eligible. Applying this same percentage to the 55 cases for whom eligibility was not known directly, we would estimate that 10 percent (or 5) of these cases would not be eligible for the survey. The remaining 50 cases were assumed to be eligible but were not interviewed.

Step 4: Compute Eligible Units

The number resulting from subtracting the number of actual and estimated ineligible units ($n = 69$) from the original sample ($n = 693$) is the number of eligible units for the study ($n = 624$), which constitutes the denominator for computing the study's response rate.

Step 5: Specify Noninterviews

Interviews may not be obtained for a number of reasons. The respondents may refuse to participate in the study or break off the interview once it begins. They may be too ill to participate, have mental or physical limitations, or not be fluent in the language in which the interview is being conducted, which would inhibit or limit their participation. Some people may be away during the entire field period. Those who were never home or those in telephone and list sample surveys for whom eligibility could not be determined for other reasons but were estimated to qualify or be "eligible" ($n = 50$, using the approach discussed above) would be included as noninterviews as well. The total number of eligibles with whom interviews were not completed in the example in Table 7.5 was 125.

Step 6: Specify Completed Interviews

The numerator for the response rate is the number of elements eligible for the study with whom interviews or questionnaires are actually completed ($n = 499$).

Step 7: Compute the Response Rate

The final response rate is the proportion that the number of completed interviews represents of the number of units known (and estimated) to be eligible for the study, which is $499/624 = 80$ percent in the example in Table 7.5.

Weighting the Sample Data to Reflect the Population

We saw in the discussion of approaches to sampling rare populations in Chapter Six that the investigator may want to sample some subgroups in the population at different rates to ensure that there will be enough of these individuals without having to increase the overall size of the sample, thus adding to the costs of the study. Also, there may be problems once fieldwork begins if some groups are less likely to respond than others.

Ideally, the researcher wants the sample to mirror as closely as possible the population as a whole. Adjustments for ensuring this correspondence between the distribution of the sample and the population on characteristics of interest involve procedures for *weighting the sample* so that it resembles the population from which it was drawn. Weighting is a process of statistically assigning more or less weight to some groups than others so that their distributions in the sample correspond more closely to their actual distributions in the population as a whole (Yansaneh, 2003).

Two primary types of weighting procedures are discussed here and outlined in Tables 7.6 and 7.7. The first set of procedures includes adjustments that can be used if decisions were made when the sample itself was drawn originally that caused it to look different from the population as a whole, such as sampling certain groups at higher (or lower) rates (Table 7.6). These include *expansion weights* to

**TABLE 7.6. WEIGHTING THE SAMPLE TO ADJUST
FOR DISPROPORTIONATE SAMPLING.**

Strata/Weight	African American	Hispanic	Total
Population (*N*)	90,000 (90%)	10,000 (10%)	100,000 (100%)
Sample (*n/N*)	1/100 = 900 (81.8%)	1/50 = 200 (18.2%)	1,100 (100%)
Expansion weight (*N/n*)	100/1 * 900 = 90,000 (90%)	50/1 * 200 = 10,000 (10%)	100,000 (100%)
Relative weight (total *N*/total *n* = 100,000/1,100 = 90.9)	100/90.9 * 900 = 990 (90%)	50/90.9 *200 = 110 (10%)	1,100 (100%)

reflect the actual number and distribution of cases in the population and *relative weights* to readjust the weights to the number of cases to the actual sample size, while maintaining the relative distribution of subgroups within the population.

The second set of procedures is undertaken to adjust for differential nonresponse or noncoverage for different groups in the population (Table 7.7). These include class- or group-specific adjustments based on the respective groups' *response rates*, and *poststratification* weighting, which assigns weights to certain subgroups within the sample to bring the distribution of these subgroups in the sample into closer conformity with their known distribution in the population.

Weighting to Adjust for Disproportionate Sampling

The cases may also be weighted to reflect either the actual size of the population from which they are drawn or the number of cases in the original sample.

Weighting to Population Size: Expansion Weights

The sampling fraction (*n/N*) is the proportion of cases drawn for the sample (*n*) as a proportion of the total number of elements in the population (*N*). With multistage designs, the overall sampling fraction for a case is a product of the sampling fractions at each stage of the design. If we want the number of people in the sample to mirror the number they represent in the population, we can compute expansion weights for each case based on the inverse of the sampling fraction. This approach is illustrated in Table 7.6, in weighting the data for a study in which Hispanics were sampled at twice the rate of African Americans.

The sampling fraction for the samples (n) of 900 African Americans and 200 Hispanics, out of 90,000 and 10,000 of these groups in the population (N), respectively, would be 900/90,000 = 1/100 and 200/10,000 = 1/50. Multiplying the number of cases in the sample for each group by the inverse of its sampling fraction would yield the number of each group in the *population:* 900 × (100/1) = 90,000 and 200 × (50/1) = 10,000. This is one way of getting back to the actual distribution of each group that exists in the population, even though one group may have been sampled at twice the rate of another. Otherwise the relative distribution of the cases in the sample (900/11,000 for African Americans; 200/11,000 for Hispanics) would not accurately mirror their distribution in the population.

An example of the use of this approach when only one person is selected to be interviewed in a household (with four people, for example) is to weight the case of the selected sample person by the inverse (4/1) of the proportion this one case represents of everyone in the household (1/4) so that the sample data accurately reflect the composition of all the households in the population from which the sample was drawn. The assignment of these weights can be carried out through specifying weight procedures in standard statistical packages such as STATA, SAS, and SPSS that permit values relevant for specific subgroups to be assigned to the individuals in those groups.

If the population from which a particular sample is drawn is quite large, however, the researcher may not want to use this approach. With standard statistical analysis packages, large sample sizes resulting from weighting the data in this fashion could render the tests of statistical significance virtually meaningless because the computations do not reflect the actual number of observations on which the estimates are based and, with large enough sample sizes, virtually all estimates or the relationships between them are statistically significant.

Weighting to Sample Size: Relative Weights

One way to deal with this problem is to adjust the expansion weights to produce a relative weight that downweights the number of cases to be equal to the actual sample size while maintaining the appropriate distribution of cases produced by the expansion weights. (See "relative weight" in Table 7.6.) The relative weight is constructed by computing the mean of the expansion weights and then dividing the expansion weights for each case by this mean.

The sum of the expansion weights for each group equals the total population $[\Sigma \, (w_i \times n) = N]$. Referring to the example in Table 7.6:

$$\Sigma \, (w_i \times n) = (100 \times 900) + (50 \times 200)$$
$$= 90{,}000 + 10{,}000$$
$$= 100{,}000$$

To compute the mean expansion weight, divide the sum of the expansion weights (N) by the number of cases in the sample (n): $100{,}000/1{,}100 = 90.9$. As illustrated in Table 7.6, the relative weight is then computed by dividing the expansion weight for each case by this mean expansion weight. Dividing the expansion weight for a given individual by this mean weight yields weighted numbers of cases that are equivalent to the total unweighted sample size but are appropriately readjusted for the relative distribution of each group within the target population:

Relative Weight	N	%
$90{,}000/90.9 =$	990	90%
$10{,}000/90.9 =$	110	10%
Total	1,100	100%

The total number of cases that appears in any particular analysis when this weight is applied reflects the actual number of cases in the study sample ($n = 1{,}100$), not the population as a whole ($N = 100{,}000$). The advantage of applying this additional weighting procedure is that it allows the tests of statistical significance to be based on the number of cases from which the sample estimates being examined were actually derived.

The researcher should be sure that all the relevant information required for constructing the final sample weights is fully documented in the course of the study and, when appropriate (such as whether a case represents a Hispanic respondent or not), coded on the record for each case.

Weighting to Adjust for Nonresponse or Noncoverage

Problems occurring during the sample design and execution process can cause the characteristics of a sample to differ from the population it was intended to represent. Differential coverage or response to a survey by different subgroups can, for example, account for such differences. Two types of weighting procedures to adjust for these possible sources of bias in the distribution of sample cases are *response rate* and *poststratification weighting*. Self-weighting samples based on proportionate sampling designs may still require these weighting adjustments to deal with noncoverage or nonresponse bias.

Response Rate Weighting Adjustments

To adjust for differential response rates (or nonresponse) for each group, the expansion weight computed to adjust for the disproportionate sampling fractions for each group is divided by the group's response rate (see Table 7.7). For example, if the response rates for African American and Hispanics in a study are determined to be 80 percent and 70 percent, respectively, then the expansion weight could be divided by .80 or .70 to adjust for the differential nonresponse before computing the relative weight.

Class- or group-specific response rate weighting adjustments assume that the original sample can be stratified into different groups for which response rates can be computed.

Poststratification Weighting

Once the sample design is executed and the sample appropriately weighted to adjust for disproportionate sampling or nonresponse of different groups, distributions on selected characteristics of the sample can be compared with characteristics of the population of interest obtained from other sources (census data, clinic records, insurance claims files). If substantial differences are found, then poststratification

TABLE 7.7. WEIGHTING THE SAMPLE TO ADJUST FOR NONRESPONSE OR NONCOVERAGE.

Strata/Weight	African American (*RR* = 720/900 = .80)		Hispanic (*RR* = 140/200 = .70)	
Response rate weight (applied to relative weight)	720 * (100/90.9)/.80 = 720 * 1.1/.80 = 720 * 1.375 = 990		140 * (50/90.9)/.70 = 140 * .55/.70 = 140 * .786 = 110	
Poststratification weight	**Poor**	**Nonpoor**	**Poor**	**Nonpoor**
Population (%)	5%	60%	15%	20%
Sample (%)	3%	72%	5%	20%
Weight	*1.66*	*0.83*	*3.00*	*1.00*

Note: The resulting poststratification weights are noted in italics.

weights can be applied to the sample to cause it to look more like the population from which it was drawn.

These weights are termed *poststratification weights* because they are assigned after ("post") designing the sample itself, based on grouping the sample into groups ("strata") for which distributions for the population as a whole are available (see the example in Table 7.7). Ratios are then constructed by comparing the percentages of the population known to be in each stratum with the percentages reflected in the sample itself. The resulting ratios are the poststratification weights assigned to each case in the sample based on the characteristics used for defining the various strata.

As with the other weighting procedures, each case that appears in the sample then is weighted to increase or decrease its contributions, as appropriate, so that the resulting distribution of cases of this kind in the sample is similar to distributions in the population as a whole. In the example in Table 7.7, poor Hispanics are given a poststratification weight of 3.00 because they appear to be underrepresented in the sample compared with their known distribution in the population. In contrast, nonpoor African Americans are given a poststratification weight of .83 because they appear to be overrepresented in the sample.

The poststratification weight factor would be multiplied by any other previous weights. Poststratification weighting adjustments assume that a source is available to use as the basis for describing the distribution of the population on the respective characteristics. Census data are often used in making poststratification adjustments for national surveys. A comparable source of information may not be available to investigators, particularly in local surveys. Such adjustments will also not fully correct for biases resulting from substantial nonresponse or noncoverage problems with the sample or for other differences not explicitly incorporated in the poststratification weights.

Special Considerations for Special Populations

Stratification and the disproportionate sampling of concentrated clusters of selected target groups may introduce substantial economies in identifying and sampling rare and special populations, but these practices may also yield significant *dis*economies in the overall efficiency of the sample design due to increased nonresponse bias or sampling (standard) errors relative to costs. The procedures introduced here and in the previous chapter provide useful diagnostics and devices for addressing the sources of variable and systematic errors that are likely to plague surveys of special populations in particular.

Selected Examples

The California Health Interview Survey (CHIS) was designed to include a sufficient number of minority (Hispanic, African American, American Indian/Alaskan Native, Asian American) individuals to yield reliable estimates for these populations and subpopulations within these groups. There were also selected counties and municipalities for which estimates were to be generated that required targeting an adequate number of cases to represent these areas. The overall response rate for the CHIS 2001 was based on the screening response rate (59.2 percent), that is, the proportion of households for which information could be obtained to determine eligibility for the study, multiplied by the selected adult respondent completion rate (63.7 percent). The response rate resulting (37.7 percent) was relatively low. The corresponding rates for the CHIS 2003 were slightly lower than those for the 2001 survey: screening response rate (55.9 percent), adult completion rate (60.0 percent), and overall (33.5 percent). Expansion weights and nonresponse and poststratification weights are all components of the CHIS weighting procedures to adjust for disproportionate sampling as well as low response rates and corollary insufficient representativeness of the sample (UCLA Center for Health Policy Research, 2002e, 2005). Analyses based on the CHIS must use software such as SUDAAN or other procedures available in statistical analysis software packages such as STATA to adjust the tests of statistical significance for the design effects resulting from the complex nature of the sample design.

The UNICEF Multiple Cluster Indicator Survey recommended the use of the probability proportionate to size (PPS) cluster sampling scheme in participating countries. Detailed instructions were provided regarding how to carry out the PPS procedures (UNICEF, 2000, n.d.). Given that the distribution of cases in the study based on a PPS design should reflect their proportionate representation in the population as a whole, no weighting for disproportionate sampling was required unless there was explicit oversampling or undersampling of selected subgroups. Nonresponse and poststratification weights may, however, still be needed if high rates of nonresponse or noncoverage result in carrying out the study. The design effect does need to be taken into account in estimating the initial sample size for the studies, as well as in adjusting the sample variances during the analyses of the data.

The National Dental Malpractice Survey entailed the least complex sample design. The response rate for the study was also among the highest (76.7 percent) reported for surveys of dentists in the United States (Washington State University, Social and Economic Sciences Research Center, 1993). It essentially represented a random sample of practicing dentists in the United States. No design effect or weighting adjustments were therefore needed in estimating the sample size or in analyzing the survey data, once collected.

Guidelines for Minimizing Survey Errors and Maximizing Survey Quality

Know your fractions: they do, in fact, sum to a large part of the whole in the sample size estimation process. The standard error ($SE = \sigma/\sqrt{n}$), for example, is a key formula that parsimoniously summarizes the average variable sampling error associated with estimates derived from samples of a designated size from a population with known (or at least hypothesized) characteristics. The larger the denominator (sample size) and the smaller the numerator (average variation within a specific sample), the lower the variable error associated with the sample estimates. This formula also provides the foundation for deriving the sample size for many types of designs, that is, solving for "n" solves the "n."

The numerator and denominator and the quantity captured by their arithmetic relationship in computing the design effects, response rate, and weights are similarly little measures that say a lot about both the magnitude and management of variable and systematic errors associated with the number and distribution of sample cases.

This chapter has reviewed procedures for computing sample sizes and analyzing the data to minimize the variable errors resulting from imprecision in estimating the standard errors for survey samples (see Table 7.8). Nonresponse and poststratification weighting adjustments help to reduce the systematic errors (or biases) resulting from high rates of nonresponse or noncoverage in sampling from the target population.

Controversies exist in the applied sampling field with respect to whether weighting and other complex design adjustments may in fact introduce more rather than fewer errors in the analyses of sample survey data (Korn & Graubard, 1991, 1995; Rao & Bellhouse, 1990). Furthermore, random coefficient linear regression models, also known as "hierarchical linear models," offer a new and promising alternative to traditional variance-adjustment approaches (based on sample design effects) for analyzing data based on multistage cluster sampling designs (Kreft, 1995). In any case, survey designers should be aware of the sampling issues discussed in this and the preceding chapter and be prepared to ask informed questions of a qualified sampling consultant, if necessary, to resolve how best to proceed.

TABLE 7.8. SURVEY ERRORS: SOURCES AND SOLUTIONS— DECIDING HOW MANY WILL BE IN THE SAMPLE.

	Systematic Errors			Variable Errors	
	Noncoverage Bias	Unit Nonresponse Bias	Weighting Errors	Standard Errors	Design Effects
Solutions to Errors	Construct and apply post-stratification weights.	Construct and apply non-response weights.	Construct and apply dispro-portionate sampling weights (*when applicable*).	Compute the sample size required to have a desired level of precision or power in addressing the study objectives. Apply adjustments to increase the sample size as needed.	When using complex, especially cluster sample, designs, incorporate design effects in estimating the required sample size and analyzing the data.

Supplementary Sources

Lemeshow, Hosmer, Klar, and Lwanga (1990) and Lwanga and Lemeshow (1991) provide formulas, tables, and examples for computing sample sizes for a variety of types of health studies. The use of effect sizes as a basis for sample size estimation is fully described in Cohen (1988), and software for executing this approach is documented in Borenstein, Cohen, and Rothstein (2000). Kraemer and Thiemann (1987) and Lipsey (1990) offer useful and practical adaptations of Cohen's method to an array of analytical and experimental study designs. Public domain software, such as DSTPLAN, is available for estimating sample sizes (American Statistical Association, Section on Survey Research Methods, n.d.-a; University of Texas M D Anderson Cancer Center, 2003; Statistics.com, n.d.). EXCEL spreadsheets could also be created, using the formulas provided in this chapter, to facilitate the computation of sample sizes for different types of study designs and estimates.

CHAPTER EIGHT

GENERAL PRINCIPLES
FOR FORMULATING QUESTIONS

Chapter Highlights

1. The development of survey questions should be guided by practical experience with the same or comparable questions in other studies, scientific experiments that test alternative ways of asking questions and the magnitude of the errors that result, and theoretical expectations about what ways of asking a question will produce what outcomes based on cognitive psychology and other conceptual approaches to total survey design.

2. The criteria for evaluating survey questionnaires include the clarity, balance, and length of the survey questions themselves; the comprehensiveness or constraints of the responses implied or imposed by these questions; the utility of the instructions provided for answering them; the order and context in which they are integrated into the survey questionnaire; and the response errors or effects that result from how the questionnaire is ultimately designed, as well as from the characteristics and behavior of the respondents who answer it, the interviewers who administer it to them, and the mode of data collection employed.

This is the first of four chapters that present guidelines for developing the survey questions and incorporating these questions (or items) into an integrated and interpretable survey questionnaire to be read or presented to respondents. It provides an overview of (1) the preliminary steps to take in identifying or designing the questions to include in a survey, (2) the theoretical approaches to use in anticipating sources of errors in these questions, and (3) general guidelines for question and questionnaire development to minimize errors that can result from the design of the questions or the questionnaire or from the way in which the questions are asked or the questionnaire is administered.

Preliminary Steps in Choosing Survey Questions

Survey researchers should use the principal research question and associated study objectives and hypotheses to guide the selection of questions for their survey. For example, what are the major concepts that the survey designers want to operationalize? Are they the main variables that will be used to describe the study sample and, by inference, the population from which it was drawn, or are they independent, dependent, or control variables to be used in testing an explicit study hypothesis? In other words, how will the concepts actually be used in the analyses, and what is the most appropriate level of measurement to employ in choosing the questions to capture (or operationalize) these concepts?

Second, survey researchers should not try to reinvent the wheel. After thinking through the concepts to be operationalized in their survey, they should begin to look for other studies that have dealt with similar topics and assemble copies of the questionnaires and articles that summarize the research methods and results of those studies.

Researchers should next determine whether formal tests of the validity and reliability of specific questions or scales of interest have been conducted. They should also look for any other evidence of methodological problems with these items, such as the rates of missing values or the degree of correspondence of responses to those questions with comparable ones asked in other studies. If possible, researchers should speak with the designers of these studies to gain additional information about how well questions worked in their surveys.

Using seasoned approaches not only provides researchers guidance as to the probable quality and applicability of the items for their own purposes but also enhances the possibility for substantive comparisons with these and other studies and adds to the cumulative body of methodological experience with survey items.

Third, the researcher should consider the type of question each item represents and the best way to ask that particular type of question. Are they questions about factual and objective characteristics or behaviors, nonfactual and subjective attitudes or perceptions, or some (subjective or objective) indicators of health status? How respondents think about these different types of questions will vary. For example, respondents may call on different frames of reference and feel different levels of threat in answering a question about the number of visits they made to a dentist in the year compared with one about their perceived risk of contracting HIV/AIDS. The rules for asking questions should take these different cognitive experiences into account in order to discover what the respondent really thinks about the issue.

Fourth, researchers should consider the extent to which the medium (personal interview, telephone interview, mail questionnaire, Internet, or computerized data collection mode) affects the message (what does or does not come across to the respondent) in the survey. Respondents in personal interviews are influenced by the implicit or explicit verbal and visual cues provided by the interviewer as well as by the questionnaire that the survey designer provides. With telephone interviews, the medium, and hence the message, is largely a verbal one. With mail, computerized self-administered, and Web-based questionnaires, the messages are entirely visual. The intent in designing any survey question is that the message the researcher intended to send comes across clearly to the respondent.

Fifth, and perhaps most important, survey designers should have some idea of the kinds of errors that can arise at each stage in developing survey questions and the approaches to use to minimize or eliminate such errors. There is an increasing interest in developing and applying theoretical frameworks for minimizing survey errors and maximizing survey quality. Principles for designing survey questions are still more often based on experience than on experiments. The following section presents the results of experiments and also discusses the vast body of experience available to designers of survey questions. The purpose of this section is to suggest how to minimize the errors that inevitably result when people are asked to describe what is in their heads.

Sources of Errors in Survey Questions

Smith (1987) pointed out that the emphasis in survey question design has shifted from relatively unstructured inquiries that closely approximated normal conversations in early surveys to the highly formalized, structured, and standardized protocols of most contemporary studies. According to Smith, these protocols reflect a "specialized survey dialect" far from the "natural language" of normal conversation (p. S105). Critics of standardized survey question design argue that meaning is lost and distortions and inaccuracies result when people are questioned in this way. Growing in prominence are conversational interviewing methods that allow interviewers to interact freely with the respondent and modify questions as needed to fit the respondent's situation in the interest of obtaining the most accurate responses.

One of the underlying issues in this debate is whether a standardized approach can meaningfully capture the experiences of respondents given that the formalized language of interviewing is not how they usually communicate (Beatty, 1995; Biemer & Lyberg, 2003; Molenaar & Smit, 1996; Suchman & Jordan, 1990). In fact, the art of asking questions, which requires creativity and ingenuity on the part of the survey designer to develop an item that speaks to the respondent in the way that the designer intended, has always been an important aspect of designing survey questions. In contrast, the science of formulating and testing hypotheses about whether what the question elicits from respondents is an accurate reflection of what they really *mean* or of the *truth* that the survey designer intended to learn has only begun to emerge. (Conversational interviewing techniques are more fully discussed in Chapter Thirteen.)

The first book to inventory the guidelines and principles to use in designing survey questions, aptly titled *The Art of Asking Questions,* appeared over fifty years ago (Payne, 1951). The principles presented in that book were based primarily on the experience of the author and others in designing and implementing questions in polls and public opinion surveys. However, they were also based on the results of so-called split-ballot experiments, in which different approaches to phrasing or formatting what were thought to be comparable questions were used with similar groups of respondents, and the results were then compared. The simplicity and wisdom of the suggestions in that book continue to make sense to many contemporary designers of surveys and polls and to be confirmed by more formal methodological research on survey question design (Biemer, Groves, Lyberg, Mathiowetz, & Sudman, 1991; Bradburn et al., 1979; Bradburn, Sudman, & Wansink, 2004; Converse & Presser, 1986; Dillman, 2000; Groves, 1989; Lessler & Kalsbeek, 1992; National Center for Health Statistics, 1999; Schuman & Presser, 1981; Schwarz, 1999; Schwarz & Sudman, 1992, 1994, 1996; Sudman, Bradburn, & Schwarz, 1996; Tourangeau, Rips, & Rasinski, 2000).

For example, a meta-analysis of 176 of the split-ballot studies conducted during the 1930s and 1940s suggested that the manner in which subjects responded to survey questions largely supports cognitive psychological research regarding response-order effects in surveys. It was found that respondents who participated in a study when the questions were read to them were more likely to choose the most recently heard item (a recency effect) when the question or the response choices were longer than when they were shorter. Other predicted patterns of primary and recency effects were not confirmed, which might have been due to the inherent limitations in analyzing secondary data that were not designed to systematically test these effects. The authors conclude, however, "The data from these early experiments nonetheless provide a partial, albeit limited, test of rival hypotheses and explanations of response-order effects in the literature" (Bishop & Smith, 2001, p. 479).

The primary impetus for formalized, empirical research on the accuracy of survey questions began with experimental work by investigators at the University of Michigan Survey Research Center. Their work involved comparisons of survey data and physician record data on health events and health care, as well as studies of the impact of interviewer characteristics and behaviors on responses to survey questions (Kahn & Cannell, 1957; University of Michigan Survey Research Center and National Center for Health Services Research, 1977).

With the publication of *Response Effects in Surveys,* Sudman and Bradburn (1974) made a major theoretical contribution to modeling the different aspects of the survey design processes and the various errors that can emerge. In that book, the authors introduced a framework that detailed the role of the interviewer, the respondent, and the task (principally the questionnaire and how it was administered) in the research interview. They also introduced the concept of *response effects* to reflect the differences between the answers obtained in the survey and the actual (or true) value of the variable that the question was intended to capture. These are differences that can result from the characteristics or the performance of the three principal components of the survey interview. An additional dimension for identifying likely response effects that has taken on greater prominence since Sudman and Bradburns's initial formulation are effects due to the mode of data collection: personal interview, telephone, mail self-administered, or Internet or other computerized adaptations. (See Chapter Five for a fuller discussion of likely mode effects or differences.)

Subsequent to Sudman and Bradburn's preliminary work, the concept of *total survey design* and an accompanying approach to estimating *total survey errors* from all sources in surveys came into prominence in the late 1970s. For example, Andersen, Kasper, Frankel, and Associates (1979) argued that errors in surveys were a function of both the inconsistency and the inaccuracy of data, which in turn resulted from problems with the design and implementation of the sampling, data collection, and data processing procedures involved in carrying out a survey.

Sudman and Bradburn's concept of response effects provided significant conceptual and methodological guidance for identifying and quantifying an important potential source of errors in surveys: people's responses to the survey questions themselves. These errors, it was thought, resulted from interviewers' or respondents' behaviors or the nature of the interview task itself. In 1979 these same researchers and their associates published *Improving Interview Method and Questionnaire*

Design, which summarized much of their own research on how to increase the accuracy of reports on sensitive topics, such as drug use, alcohol consumption, and sexual behavior, in surveys, using their response effects framework (Bradburn et al., 1979).

In 1980 the Panel on Survey Measurement of Subjective Phenomena was convened by the National Academy of Sciences to review the state of the art of survey research, with particular reference to how subjective (nonfactual) questions are asked in surveys (National Research Council, Panel on Survey Measurement of Subjective Phenomena, 1984). The panel concluded that the lines between subjective and objective questions in survey research cannot always be clearly drawn, since respondents' answers to even factual questions are filtered through their internal cognitive memory and recall processes. With questions on more subjective topics, such as respondents' knowledge about or attitudes on certain issues, understanding how they think about the topic may in fact be essential to designing meaningful questions to find out what they think about it.

There has been a growing interest on the part of survey methodologists in the design of empirical studies for identifying and quantifying the sources and magnitude of response effects (or errors) in surveys and in using this information to enhance survey quality (Biemer & Lyberg, 2003; Bishop & Smith 2001; Groves, Dillman, Eltinge, & Little, 2002; Schechter & Herrmann, 1997). In reviewing the state of health survey research methods, Couper (2004) suggested that examining response effects in surveys is still quite applicable today in spite of the infusion of technology such as cell phones and the World Wide Web into survey data collection activities.

Sudman and Bradburn (1974), in their initial formulation of the response effects concept, pointed out that determining the real (or "true") answer to survey questions is more problematical with nonfactual or attitudinal questions than with what are generally thought of as factual or objective questions. The latter assume there is some external, identifiable behavior or event that is being referenced in the question asked. Respondents' reports of these phenomena do not always necessarily agree with these "facts," however.

In estimating the accuracy of respondents' reports on factual questions of this kind, tests of criterion validity are applied (see Figure 3.2 in Chapter Three for a description of this procedure). With this approach, the facts that respondents report in the survey questionnaire (such as the number of times teenagers may report binging or purging during the year, or older adults report that they had heart disease, hypertension, or diabetes) are compared with a criterion source (a clinical assessment of eating disorders or a clinical diagnosis of heart disease, hypertension or diabetes) to estimate just how accurate their answers are. Estimates of respondents' false-positive or false-negative responses are then developed to quantify the magnitude of their overreporting or underreporting in the study (Field, Taylor, Celio, & Colditz, 2004; Ghaderi & Scott, 2002; Wu, Li, & Ke, 2000).

The accuracy of responses to nonfactual questions can, to some extent, be assessed by means of examining their construct validity—that is, the extent to which the results agree with the theory on which the concepts expressed in the question are based (see the discussion of construct validity in Chapter Three). However, it may not always be apparent whether it is the theory or the methods that are at fault if the results are not what was expected theoretically.

Efforts to assess the accuracy of nonfactual questions have therefore tended to rely more on split-ballot or other experiments in which different ways of asking subjective questions are used and the results compared. Inconsistencies in the results serve to warn the researcher that the questions may indeed convey different meanings to respondents. The more consistent the results are, the more confidence the researcher can have that the questions are substantively comparable (Biemer & Lyberg, 2003; Bradburn et al., 2004; Converse & Presser, 1986; Schuman & Presser, 1981).

Survey research methodologists have called for the development of a comprehensive theory or set of theories to provide more systematic predictions about which survey design decisions are going to lead to which outcomes and with what magnitude of error (Biemer & Lyberg, 2003; Bradburn, 1999; Dillman, 2000; Groves, 1989; Groves et al., 2002; Groves, Singer, & Corning, 2000). Understanding these conceptual frameworks can assist in developing a scientific knowledge base to draw on in designing and conducting surveys.

Contributions of Cognitive Psychology to Questionnaire Design

The theoretical perspectives and concepts of cognitive psychology are viewed as a promising starting point by survey methodologists concerned with developing a science of survey question and questionnaire design and a scientific way to estimate the errors associated with these procedures. In 1983, for example, the Committee on National Statistics, with funding from the National Science Foundation, convened an Advanced Research Seminar on the Cognitive Aspects of Survey Methodology (CASM) to foster a dialogue between cognitive psychologists and survey researchers on these issues. The proceedings of that conference, *Cognitive Aspects of Survey Methodology: Building a Bridge Between Disciplines,* pointed out how concepts and methodologies from cognitive psychology could be used to inform the design of surveys in general and health surveys in particular (National Research Council, Committee on National Statistics, 1984). This also led to a second CASM seminar in 1997, which focused on the future of CASM research as well as on innovative methods for improving research. The proceedings of that conference highlighted the increased adoption of cognitive methods in the design of survey questionnaires (National Center for Health Statistics, 1999).

Tourangeau (1984) pointed out that there are four main stages identified by the social information processing frameworks of cognitive psychology that can be used in describing the steps respondents go through in answering survey questions: (1) the *comprehension stage,* in which the respondent interprets the question; (2) the *retrieval stage,* in which the respondent searches his or her memory for the relevant information; (3) the *estimation/judgment stage,* in which the respondent evaluates the information retrieved from memory and its relevance to the question and, when appropriate, combines information to arrive at an answer; and (4) the *response stage,* in which the respondent weighs factors such as the sensitivity or threat level of the question and the social acceptability or probable accuracy of the answer, and only then decides what answer to give.

Another stage that was subsequently identified and precedes these stages of asking and responding to questions is that of encoding the knowledge that the question is intended to elicit—that is, the original obtaining, processing, and storing of this information in memory (Tourangeau et al., 2000). For example, experimental studies of the accuracy of parents' recall of their child's immunizations documented that parents were generally not able to report these immunizations accurately because they had not encoded or committed them to memory initially (Lee et al., 1999).

This framework identifying the various stages of retrieving information and responding to survey questions has gained considerable prominence as a basis for designing and evaluating survey questions in order to minimize the errors that are likely to occur at each stage (Biemer et al., 1991; Bradburn & Danis, 1984; Collins, 2003; Lee et al., 1999; McCarthy & Safer, 2000; Rasinski, Willis, Baldwin, Yeh, & Lee, 1999; Social Science Research Council, 1992).

Different types of survey questions may place different demands on the respondent at different stages of the response formulation process. The retrieval stage may be particularly important in asking respondents to recall relatively nonthreatening factual information because of the heavy demands such questions place on their memory of relevant events or behaviors. Survey questions may place special demands on individuals who are bilingual. Information that is encoded and stored in one language may be harder to recall and retrieve in another language, since they may be related to different stimuli. Furthermore, responses that a bilingual respondent may provide in one language may not match that of a second language (Hung & Heeler, 1998; Luna & Peracchio, 1999).

For certain attitudinal questions, the *judgments* that the respondents make about the issue (the third stage of the process) may be particularly critical as they think through how they will answer the question. For example, respondents may be more likely to have a strong response to an attitudinal question when the topic is important to them (Areni, Ferrell, & Wilcox, 1999).

When asked more threatening or sensitive questions, respondents may decide at the last (response) stage to sacrifice the accuracy of their responses to lower the psychic threat that results from giving answers that are not perceived to be socially acceptable ones (Tourangeau et al., 2000).

Research in cognitive psychology has focused on examining the processes by which information is recalled and retrieved, as well as examining the validity and reliability of the information that the respondent recalls. Concerns about the ability of respondents to accurately recall memories from the distant past (such as an adult's recollection of childhood sex abuse) have led to studies that examine the accuracy of information retrieved during an interview. For example, Wright, Gaskell, and O'Muircheartaigh (1998) examined the extent to which adults could recall circumstances surrounding a historical event that occurred more than a year earlier. They found that adults were more likely to be able to recall an important event if it was associated with something they perceived to be important or to which they had some emotional attachment. Principe, Ornstein, Baker-Ward, and Gordon (2000) examined the ability of three- and five-year-old children to recall what took place during a physical examination that occurred twelve weeks earlier. They found that the accuracy of the children's recall of the details of the exam was related to events midway between the date of the initial physical exam and the twelve-week interview. Those who, six weeks later, had an intervening interview about the visit or observed a videotape showing a child receiving a checkup were more likely to be able to recall the details of the initial exam.

Cognitive psychologists posit that there are schemata (frameworks or "scripts") that respondents have in their heads and subsequently call on in responding to stimuli, such as those generated by survey research questions (Markus & Zajonc, 1985). One of the devices used in experimental cognitive psychology laboratories to discover and define these scripts is to ask subjects to think aloud in answering questions that are posed by the researcher—that is, literally to say out loud everything that comes to mind in answering the question, which the researcher can then tape or otherwise record for subsequent analysis. These reflections thus become the data that the investigator uses to arrive at an understanding of the schemata inside people's heads that are called on in responding to different types of questions.

Furthermore, cognitive psychologists are concerned with more than how a question is asked and the process the respondent goes through in answering it. They are also concerned with the context in which the question is presented and how the associations with other events that respondents make as a result affect their interpretation (or processing) of the question and the information they call forth to answer it. The importance of the context in influencing the schemata called forth by respondents has also been applied in trying to interpret the impact that the context or order (as well as the phrasing) of questions within a survey questionnaire has on how people answer those questions.

The National Center for Health Statistics (NCHS), the U.S. Census Bureau, the U.S. Department of Agriculture, the Bureau of Labor Statistics, Statistics Canada, and ZUMA (Zentrum fur Umfragen, Methoden und Analysen), among others, have directly applied principles of cognitive psychology in the design of major national surveys. NCHS, for example, supports a Questionnaire Design Laboratory, which employs the concepts and methods of cognitive psychology to test items to be included in the NCHS continuing surveys (National Center for Health Statistics, 1999; Willis, 2004, 2005). (Also, see the Web sites of the National Center for Health Statistics and the other organizations for more information on the applications of cognitive psychology to the design of surveys.)

Methods for Developing Survey Questions

The science and art of developing survey questions has matured significantly as a result of advances in the application of the principles of cognitive psychology to question design, an increasing acknowledgment of the value of qualitative and ethnographic research methods, and marketing research techniques for developing questions that best speak the language and convey the meaning intended by respondents. Different question development strategies may point to different types of problems with the instrument and also vary substantially with respect to the costs associated with implementing them (Harris-Kojetin, Fowler, Brown, Schnaier, & Sweeny, 1999; Jobe, 2003; Lessler, 1995). An array of procedures is reviewed here. Investigators will not necessarily apply all of these in developing and testing survey items. However, they should be aware of them and consider which or which combination may be most fruitfully applied in ensuring that the questions they ask are both sensible and meaningful to respondents.

Group Interviews

Group interviews, and particularly *focus groups,* have been used extensively in marketing research to solicit the opinions of targeted subsets of potential customers for a new product or marketing strategy (Frey & Fontana, 1991; Krueger & Casey, 2000; Morgan, 1997). With the increasing recognition that the standardized and scientized language of surveys may not be readily understandable by many respondents, focus groups of (generally six to ten) individuals, like those who will be included in a survey (such as caregivers for the elderly, persons with HIV/AIDS, intravenous drug users, or women who are making treatment decisions regarding menopause), are invited to provide input at all stages of the instrument development process. For example, they may be asked to identify the issues that are of concern to the groups that are the primary focus of the study or what comes to mind when they think of the key study concepts (caregiver stress, safer sex, high-risk behavior, experiences or attitudes toward hysterectomy and hormone replacement therapy) in the early stages of instrument development; review and comment on actual drafts of the questionnaire; and suggest explanations or hypotheses in interpreting study findings once the data are gathered (O'Brien, 1993; Richter & Galavotti, 2000; Willis, 2004, 2005).

Ethnographic Interviewing

Ethnographic interviewing, borrowed from traditional qualitative research methods, may provide useful guidance at each stage of the instrument development process. In-depth individual interviews may be preferred to focus groups when there is a concern with the reluctance of certain types of respondents (teenagers or those who are less educated, for example) to speak up or to address particularly sensitive or personal topics in a group setting. These interviews may be relatively unstructured or structured in terms of the questions asked of participants. They are often supplemented with participant observation by the investigator, who spends time informally visiting with or observing individuals or groups like those who will be the focus of the study, such as teenage gang members or pregnant women who go to a public health clinic (Axinn, Fricke, & Thornton, 1991; Bauman & Adair, 1992; National Center for Health Statistics, 1999; Rubin & Rubin, 2005).

Participatory Action Research

One of the concerns raised about the development of studies in general and of survey questions in particular is that they involve a process that is somewhat divorced from community input (Israel, Schulz, Parker, & Becker, 1998). *Participatory action research (PAR)* focuses on using a community-driven partnership to design and execute a research project, as well as to disseminate findings back to a community (Brown, 2004; Call et al., 2004; Cornelius, Booker, Arthur, Reeves, & Morgan, 2004). In terms of the development of survey questions, one could use consumers and practitioners from the community to develop questions that they believe correspond with their experiences. Since this process is community driven, the role of the researcher would be that of providing technical expertise in the development of the survey questions to assist the group in balancing the need for questions that clearly reflect study concepts with the need for survey questions that are clearly interpretable to community members.

Other Cognitive Techniques

Other techniques that have been drawn from research in cognitive psychology in particular include *think-aloud strategies, laboratory and field experiments, behavior coding of interviews,* and *linguistic analysis of questionnaires.* With *think-aloud* strategies, respondents like those who will be included in the study are administered questions developed to measure study concepts and asked a series of specific probe questions at the time a question is asked (concurrent think-aloud) or at the end of the interview (retrospective think-aloud) regarding what they were thinking when they answered the questions and how they arrived at their answers.

Think-aloud strategies are particularly useful for surfacing the cognitive processes (the framework for approaching the question and basis for calling upon or weighing evidence) that respondents may employ at the various stages of responding to questions identified by cognitive psychologists. This approach has been used extensively in the NCHS Questionnaire Design Research Laboratory (QDRL) in evaluating questions for the NCHS–National Health Interview Survey (NHIS) supplements, as well as other government-sponsored surveys. A training manual was also developed by the NCHS QDRL to assist researchers in applying this approach (National Center for Health Statistics, 1994b, 2005d, 2005e; Willis, 2004, 2005).

A disadvantage of the think-aloud strategy is that it does not provide for the systematic manipulation and evaluation of alternative approaches to phrasing questions. Laboratory and field experiments attempt to address these weaknesses. In experimental studies, a particular theory or set of hypotheses is used to guide the development of distinct options for phrasing or ordering questions, and an experimental design is employed to carry out this study either in a laboratory setting or with respondents like those who will be included in the study through personal, telephone, or self-administered interviews (Fienberg & Tanur, 1989).

The National Center for Health Statistics has conducted or sponsored an array of experimental studies of this kind, which provide the foundation for much cognitive research on question and questionnaire design. Reports on these studies are published in the NCHS Vital and Health Statistics Series Number 6 (National Center for Health Statistics, 2005d) and NCHS Cognitive Methods Working Paper Series (National Center for Health Statistics, 2005e).

Investigators with limited resources or research design expertise may be reluctant to undertake such experiments in developing their own surveys. They should, however, be guided by the insights and guidance provided by the research that has been conducted in this area. The chapters that follow apply the findings from such studies in detailing the principles for formulating different types of survey questions.

Behavior coding entails a rigorous analysis of the behavior of interviewers and respondents, based on trained coders coding their behaviors by listening to live or taped interviews (Fowler, 1989; Fowler & Mangione, 1990; Oksenberg, Cannell, & Kalton, 1991; Willis, 2004, 2005). This is a relatively labor-intensive approach, and as a result it is generally based on only a small number of interviews. An alternative approach is to have interviewers focus on recording selected aspects of the respondents' behavior in the course of the interview, such as whether they ask to have the question repeated or clarified, interrupt the interviewer, or ask how much longer it will take. In either case, the resulting information can be quite useful in identifying and revising questions that seem to create problems for the interviewer or respondent.

Linguistic analysis of questionnaires focuses on using computer software to identify "questions that tax the cognitive abilities of the respondent, questions that entail a memory overload and questions where the answers cannot be retrieved because of semantic or syntactical ambiguity" (Martin & Moore, 1999, p. 64). Once these problem questions are identified, substitute words and phrases can be developed and retested for clarity using the same software (Graesser, Kennedy, Wiemer-Hastings, & Ottati, 1999).

All of these procedures are intended to develop questionnaires that are meaningful and relevant to diverse respondents and thereby minimize the likely response effects in administering and answering the questions.

Methods for Testing Survey Procedures

The development of a new product almost always involves a series of tests to see how well it works and what bugs need to be corrected before it goes on the market. The same standards should be applied in designing and carrying out surveys. *No* survey should *ever* go into the field without a trial run of the questionnaire and data collection procedures to be used in the final study. Failure to conduct this trial run is one of the biggest and potentially most costly mistakes that can be made in carrying out a survey. It is certain that something will go wrong if there is not adequate testing of the procedures in advance of doing the survey. Even when such testing is done, situations can arise that were not anticipated. The point with testing the procedures in advance is to anticipate and eliminate as many of these problems as possible and, above all, avert major disasters in the field once the study is launched. The survey design literature variously refers to this phase of survey development as a pilot study or pretest (Collins, 2003; Foddy, 1998; Presser & Blair, 1994). It may, in fact, encompass a range of activities, including evaluating (1) individual questions, (2) the questionnaire as a whole, (3) the feasibility of sampling and data collection procedures, and (4) the procedures for coding and computerizing the data, if time and resources permit. This last step is imperative for computer-assisted data collection methods, in which the procedures for gathering the data involve direct entry of the respondents' answers into a computerized data system.

Questions

Conventional survey pretests (or pilot studies) have often not incorporated formal procedures for developing and evaluating survey questions, but simply an open-ended debriefing with respondents or interviewers regarding problems they encountered with the draft questionnaire. Formal protocols for asking respondents about problems they had with particular questions are more effective in identifying such problems than are open-ended, general debriefings. Furthermore, it is easier for respondents to pinpoint problems with questions in which valid response alternatives are clearly left out than with questions that present more subtle conceptual difficulties, such as loaded, double-barreled, or ambiguous questions (Collins, 2003; Foddy, 1998; Hunt, Sparkman, & Wilcox, 1982; Presser & Blair, 1994).

The procedures derived from qualitative research methods and cognitive psychology already reviewed provide a much more disciplined look at the effectiveness of survey questions. At a minimum, the pretest should determine whether the words and phrases used in a question mean the same thing to respondents as to the survey designers. For example, is it clear to all respondents that "family planning regarding their children" refers to birth control practices and not to planning relative to their child's education or other aspects of their child's development (Converse & Presser, 1986)? Testing should also surface problem items such as loaded, double-barreled, or ambiguous questions or ones in which the entire range of response alternatives is not provided to respondents. A think-aloud strategy with respondents may be particularly useful to clarify what they were thinking of when answering the question.

One should also seriously consider excluding questions for which there is a very skewed distribution or minimal variation in the variable or for a particular subgroup of interest (for example, when 99 percent of the respondents give the same answer to a question). Although such a finding may be of substantive importance, it may also signal that the question is not adequately capturing the variation that does exist in the population on the factors it was intended to reflect.

If a large number of respondents refuse to answer a question or say they do not know how to answer it, this too suggests that the item probably should be revised and retested.

In developing questions, one may need to focus on the potential for respondent burden that may occur as a result of including too many individual items or lengthy scales into the instrument. This may require statistical analyses such as internal consistency reliability analysis, confirmatory factor analysis, the application of item response theory, or regression analysis as ways of identifying and eliminating redundant questions (Laroche, Kim, & Tomiuk, 1999; Moore, Halle, Vandivere, & Mariner, 2002). (Also see discussion of these and related procedures in Chapter Three.)

Questionnaire

Another important task during pretesting is to identify problems that exist with the questionnaire as a whole. How difficult and burdensome do the respondents perceive answering or filling out all the questions to be? Do the skip patterns between questions work properly? Are the transitions between topics logical? Is there evidence that respondents fall into invariant response sets in answering certain series or types of questions? Do large numbers of respondents break off the interview early or begin to express impatience or fatigue as the interview proceeds? The occurrence of any of these problems should be a signal to the survey designer that he or she needs to redesign all or part of the questionnaire.

Sampling Procedures

The third major aspect of a study that should be evaluated is the feasibility of the proposed sampling procedures. Complex procedures for oversampling certain groups (such as using screening questions or disproportionate, network, or dual-frame sampling methodologies) should be thoroughly tested to make sure that the field staff can accurately execute these procedures. Also, a large enough pretest will enable the researchers to estimate whether the probable yield of target cases using the proposed approach will be adequate. Within-household respondent selection procedures, particularly those that require interviewers to ask a number of questions or go through several different steps, should also be thoroughly tested before being incorporated into the final study.

Ideally the pretest should be carried out with a sample of people similar to those who will be included in the final study. Purposive rather than probability sampling procedures could be useful in netting enough members of subgroups for which special problems in administering the survey questionnaire are anticipated (poorly educated persons, members of non-English-speaking minorities, known drug users, and so on). There would then be an opportunity to see if problems do in fact arise in administering the survey to these groups and to come up with ways of dealing with them before implementing the final study.

Data Collection Procedures

Pretests can evaluate whether certain procedures can be satisfactorily carried out using the data collection method proposed. An important dimension to assess is the probable response rate to the study. During the final (or dress rehearsal) stage, all the initial contact and follow-up procedures that will be used in the actual study should be implemented and the results evaluated. Findings may indicate that the methods for prior notification of respondents have to be refined, the introduction to the interview redesigned, more intensive follow-up procedures developed, or cash incentives provided.

Data Preparation Procedures

A final technical aspect of the survey design that can be evaluated during the pretest phase is the feasibility of the procedures for coding and computerizing the data. The design and testing of the data entry, file structure, and storage systems for computerized data collection methods are integral parts of the questionnaire design process itself. Deciding early on in the project whether to use a computerized data entry system (for example, computer-assisted personal interviewing, computer-assisted telephone interviewing, computer-assisted self-interviewing, or a Web-based system) involves examining the merits of preprogramming data cleaning and editing procedures into such a data system (thus saving time later in the process) over the traditional approach of first collecting the data with a paper-and-pencil approach, entering the data into a statistical package, and then editing and cleaning the data afterward. While the former does not eliminate all the necessary steps in cleaning the data, it can enhance the quality of the data collection activity by capturing errors while one is in the field.

In addition, planning how the responses to answers obtained will be coded is useful in evaluating the cost and feasibility of a paper-and-pencil data collection strategy. It is also helpful during the pretest stage of either a computerized or a paper-and-pencil questionnaire to use an open-ended response format in asking questions for which the range of probable responses is not known. The results can then be used to design codes for the questions in the final study.

Survey Cost Estimates

If there is uncertainty about the possible cost of executing certain aspects of a study, the pretest results can be helpful in finalizing its overall budget.

The actual number of cases to include in the pretest should be guided by the resources available to the researcher as well as by the types of questions to be answered with these preliminary studies. A simple test of how well the questionnaire worked, for example, would require fewer resources than evaluations of the entire range of sampling, data collection, follow-up, and coding and data-processing procedures proposed for the final survey. It is generally much more expensive to make changes with computerized data collection procedures subsequent to pretesting, because of the time and expense in redesigning all the interdependent parts of the survey package. According to one rule of thumb, a dress rehearsal for the study should include between twenty-five and fifty cases. However, if statistical procedures are to be carried out with the pretest data (for example, test-retest reliability or internal consistency reliability analysis), then sample sizes required to carry out these procedures effectively need to be estimated (see Chapter Seven). It would be advisable for the researcher to divide this number of cases (or more cases, if resources are available) among several stages of testing so that there is ample opportunity to test all the changes that are made to the survey instrument or procedures before the fielding of the actual study. With federally sponsored surveys, fewer than ten questionnaires can be piloted or pretested without formal approval of the revised instrument by the Office of Management and Budget (National Partnership for Reinventing Government, 1998).

The section that follows presents the general principles for formulating survey questions that emerge from the practical, empirical, and theoretical mosaic of current health survey research design.

Basic Elements and Criteria in Designing Survey Questionnaires

The basic elements and criteria to consider in designing survey questions and integrating them into a survey questionnaire are summarized in Figure 8.1. The primary elements of a survey questionnaire are (1) the questions themselves, (2) the response formats or categories that accompany the questions, and (3) any special

FIGURE 8.1. BASIC ELEMENTS AND CRITERIA IN DESIGNING SURVEY QUESTIONNAIRES.

Elements	Illustrations	Criteria
Questions		
Words	HIV/AIDS	Clarity
Phrases	agree or disagree	Balance
Sentences	Do you agree or disagree that HIV/AIDS can be transmitted by shaking hands with a person with HIV/AIDS ?	Length
Responses		
Open-ended	_____	Comprehensiveness
Closed-end	xxxxxxxxxx . . . . 1 xxxxx . . . . 2 xxxxxxxxxxxxxx . . . . 3 xxx 4	Constraints
Instructions	(Instructions tell you what to do next or how to do it.)	Utility
Questionnaire	Survey Questionnaire 1. ☐☐☐☐☐ ? 　　　　xxxx (Skip to Q. 3) . 1 　　　　xxx . . . . 2 2. ☐☐☐ ?　(Record answer verbatim.) _____ 3. ☐☐☐☐☐☐☐☐☐☐☐ ? (Record number of times or circle 00 if none.) 　　　　None . . . . . . 00 　　　　No. of Times . . . . . . __	Order and Context
Questionnaire Administration	Mode: Administration Interviewer ↔ Task: Questionnaire ↔ Respondent	Response Effects

instructions that appear in the questionnaire or that are associated with a particular question to tell the respondent or interviewer how to address it.

Questions

Words, phrases, and *sentences* are the major elements used in formulating survey questions.

Words. Words are the basic building blocks of human communication. They have been likened to the atomic and subatomic particles that constitute the basis of all chemical elements. Question designers need to be aware that the words and phrases used in a survey questionnaire and the way in which they are combined into the questions ultimately asked can affect the meaning of the question itself (Bertrand & Mullainathan, 2001; National Research Council, Panel on Survey Measurement of Subjective Phenomena, 1984; Wänke, 1996).

The fundamental criterion to keep in mind when evaluating the words chosen to construct a survey question is their clarity. There are two major dimensions for assessing the clarity of the words used in phrasing a survey question: the clarity with which they express the concept of interest and the clarity with which they can be understood by respondents (Fowler, 1995; Schaeffer & Presser, 2003).

First, researchers should consider whether the word adequately captures or conveys the concept that the researcher is interested in measuring with the survey question. What is the substantive or topical focus of the question—on the disease of HIV/AIDS, for example—and what does the researcher want to learn about it—the respondents' knowledge about, attitudes toward, or behavior in response to the illness? This is the first-order responsibility of researchers in deciding what words to use—clarifying what they are trying to learn by asking the question.

The second dimension in deciding on the words to use in a survey question is whether the words chosen to express the concept are going to make sense to the *respondents.* Health survey designers often wrongly assume that survey respondents know more about certain concepts or topics than they actually do; the same designers may use words or phrases that have certain technical meanings that respondents do not fully understood.

Good advice in choosing the words to use in survey questions is, *Keep them simple.* Payne (1951), for example, suggested that one should assume an eighth-grade level of education of respondents in general population surveys. For other groups, such as well-educated professionals or low-income respondents, assumptions of higher or lower levels of education, respectively, would be appropriate. The readability of survey questions can be evaluated through specialized software available for this purpose as well as through grammar checking options available in major word processing packages,—for example, Microsoft Word (Microsoft Corporation, 2005) and WordPerfect (Corel, 2005).

Phrases. Just as the process of selecting words and putting them together to constitute phrases and sentences in designing survey questions is a cumulative one, criteria noted in Figure 8.1 can also be seen as relevant to apply at the subsequent stages in designing survey questions. For example, both the individual words that are chosen and how they are combined into phrases affect the clarity of their meaning conceptually and to the respondents themselves.

Another criterion that comes into play as the researcher begins to consider the combinations of words—or phrases—that could be used in developing survey questions is the relative balance among these words. The balance dimensions to consider in phrasing survey questions are threefold: (1) whether both sides of a question or issue are adequately represented, (2) whether the answer is weighted (loaded) in one direction or another, and (3) whether more than one question is implied in the phrasing of the question. Asking whether respondents agree with an item rather than implying but failing to provide the equivalent alternative when asking about attitudes toward a topic has been found to lead to different responses from those given when explicit alternatives are provided: "Do you agree or disagree that . . . . ?" versus "Do you agree that . . . . ?" (Bradburn et al., 2004; Payne, 1951; Schuman & Presser, 1981).

Another dimension of balance in the phrasing of survey questions is whether a question is explicitly loaded in one direction or another, such as "Don't you agree that . . . . ?" Such a question makes it quite hard for the respondent to register a response that is counter to the one implied. In another form of the loaded question, certain premises or assumptions are implied in how the question is asked: "How long have you been beating your kids?" Recent research on the phrasing of sensitive questions about such behaviors as alcohol or drug use suggests that a survey researcher's deliberately loading questions in this way may elicit more reporting of these kinds of behaviors. In the absence of validating data on such behaviors, overreporting of them is assumed to be more accurate than underreporting. In general, however, survey designers should be cautious in phrasing survey questions to make sure that they do not inadvertently encourage a respondent to answer in a certain way.

A third aspect in balancing the phrasing of survey questions is whether two questions are implied in what is meant to be one: "Do you agree or disagree that HIV/AIDS can be transmitted by shaking hands with a person with HIV/AIDS or through other comparable forms of physical contact?" Along with the vagueness of the phrase "through other comparable forms of physical contact," there seems to be an additional question that goes beyond asking simply about the results of "shaking hands with a person with HIV/AIDS." Questions that have more than one referent of this kind are called *double-barreled questions.* They shoot more than one question at the respondent simultaneously, making it hard for the respondent to know which part of the question to answer and for the survey designer to figure out which aspect of the question the person was actually responding to. The use of double-barreled questions and poorly written questions can increase the time it takes to respond to the question as well as the amount of clarification needed in order to answer a question (Bassili & Scott, 1996). It is also possible that as a result of these poorly written questions, the responses to the questions are not valid since it is difficult to determine exactly what the respondent is answering.

Sentences. Clarity and balance are criteria that can be used in evaluating survey questions as well as the words and phrases that compose them. In addition, the length of the resulting sentences becomes an important dimension in evaluating survey questions. Payne (1951) suggested that in general, the length of questions asked of respondents should be limited to no more than twenty words. Recent research has suggested, however, that shorter questions are not always better questions (Bradburn et al., 2004; Scherpenzeel & Saris, 1997). For example, in a meta-analysis of the variations of the quality of survey questions across different topics Scherpenzeel and Saris (1997) found that questions with a moderate introductory text (forty-one to seventy words) used in conjunction with long questions (more than ten words) generated a higher validity and reliability than other approaches.

People may be more likely to report both threatening and nonthreatening behaviors if the questions asked of them are somewhat long. The assumption here is that longer questions give respondents more time to assemble their thoughts and also more clues to use in formulating answers. But longer questions may work better in personal interviews than in telephone interviews or mail questionnaires. With telephone interviews, respondents may have trouble remembering all the points raised in a long question and be reluctant to ask the interviewer to repeat it. Respondents filling out a mail questionnaire may feel that the question looks too complicated or will take too long to answer. More guidance for deciding how long questions should be is provided in subsequent chapters.

Responses

In some ways, discussing the questions asked in surveys apart from the responses they elicit is an arbitrary distinction. The latter are directly affected by, and even in some instances embedded in, how the former are phrased. However, there are criteria for how to answer the question implied in the types of response categories provided or assumed in the question. These criteria are in addition to *what* the question is asking, which is implied by the choice of words and phrases for the sentence used in framing the question. Criteria that are particularly relevant to apply in evaluating how questions should be answered are the comprehensiveness and constraints associated with the response categories that are imposed or implied by the survey question.

The two major types of survey questions are *open-ended* and *closed-end* questions. They differ principally in whether the categories that respondents use in answering the questions are provided to them directly. An open-ended question is, "What do you think are the major ways HIV/AIDS is transmitted?" Respondents are free to list whatever they think is relevant.

Closed-end variations of this question provide respondents with a series of statements about how the disease might be transmitted and then ask whether they agree or disagree with each statement. Other forms of closed-end responses involve rating or ranking response formats. With a rating format, respondents can be asked to indicate, for each mode of transmission provided in the survey questionnaire, whether they think it is a very important, important, somewhat important, or not at all important means of transmitting the disease. With a ranking response, respondents can be shown the same list of, say, ten items and asked to rank them in order from one to ten, corresponding to their assessment of the most to least likely means of transmitting HIV/AIDS. The ranking format is generally harder for respondents.

The reliability and validity of rating scales tend to be higher for those for which the respondent is asked to mark (for example, circle) a score on a 4- or 5-point scale. Using finely graded longer scales (ranging from 1 to 10 or 1 to 100, for example) or asking respondents to write in their answer may lead to lower levels of stability and accuracy. Verbal scales (such as strongly agree, agree, uncertain, disagree, strongly disagree) can be adapted to numerical scales (ranging from 1 to 5, for example) for use in telephone surveys to facilitate the ease of both asking and responding to the question (Bradburn et al., 2004; Scherpenzeel & Saris, 1997).

The open-ended response format can lead survey respondents to provide a comprehensive and diverse array of answers. The closed-end response format applies more constraints on the types of answers respondents are allowed to provide to the question. Each approach has its advantages and disadvantages.

Open-Ended Questions. Using open-ended questions during the pilot or pretest stage of a study offers particular advantages. The researcher can take the array of responses provided in these test interviews and use them to develop closed-end categories for the final study. With this approach, the survey designer can have more confidence that the full range of possible responses is included in the closed-end question. However, it is much easier to code and process responses from closed-end questions. Using open-ended questions in this way can then optimize both the comprehensiveness of the answers obtained to questions during the development and testing phases of the study and the cost-effective benefits resulting from the constraints imposed by the closed-end response format of the final study.

Open-ended questions may still be necessary or useful in the final study if the researcher is interested in the salience or importance of certain issues or topics to respondents (Geer, 1991). Open-ended questions encourage respondents to talk about what is at the top of their heads or what comes to mind first when answering the question. To the extent that there is convergence in the answers respondents provide when this open format is used, the researcher can have confidence in the salience of these issues to study respondents.

Closed-End Questions.   Survey respondents tend to try to work within the framework imposed by the survey questionnaire or interview task. Providing respondents with only certain types of alternatives for answering a question may mean that some responses that are in respondents' heads are not fully reflected in their answers. The number and type of response categories, whether a middle (or neutral) response is provided for registering attitudes, whether an explicit "don't know" category is offered to respondents, and other choices will directly affect how they answer the questions (Biemer et al., 1991; Blair & Burton, 1987; Bradburn et al., 2004; Schuman & Presser, 1981; Sudman & Schwarz, 1989). As mentioned earlier, however, coding closed-end questions takes less time than coding open-ended ones and may be more reliable across respondents and interviewers as well. The impact and usefulness of these various closed-end response alternatives for different types of survey questions is discussed in more detail in subsequent chapters.

Instructions

Instructions form the final building block for the survey questionnaire. Instructions can be part of the question itself, or they can serve to introduce or close the questionnaire or make meaningful transitions between different topics or sections within it. The principal criterion to use in evaluating instructions is their utility in ensuring that the question or questionnaire is answered in the way it should be. For example, sometimes the instruction, "Record verbatim," is used with open-ended questions to encourage the interviewer to capture the respondents' answers in their own words to the maximum extent possible. Instructions are also used alongside response categories to tell the interviewer or respondent the next question to skip to, depending on the answer to that question. Instructions are also useful in guiding the interviewer through the steps for selecting the respondent to interview or in showing the respondent to a mail questionnaire how to fill it out. Instructions are often designated by using parentheses, all capital letters, or some other typeface to set them apart from the questions.

Questionnaire

The survey questions and accompanying response formats and instructions are then ordered and integrated into the survey questionnaire itself. The order and context in which the items are placed has an impact on the meaning of certain questions and how respondents answer them. "Context effect refers to differences in responses to a given question that depend on aspects of the items preceding or following that question" (Steinberg, 2001, p. 340). Some of these context effects may be a result of how the respondent responds to the way in which the questions are presented, in terms of both the sequence of questions and the types of information requested (internal to the structure of the questionnaire). Order and context effects in surveys have been an important focus in the applications of cognitive psychology to questionnaire design (Lavine, Huff, Wagner, & Sweeney, 1998; National Center for Health Statistics, 2004b; Rockwood, Sangster, & Dillman, 1997; Schwarz & Hippler, 1995b; Schwarz & Sudman, 1992; Steinberg, 2001). Specific design principles for understanding and addressing order and context effects in survey questionnaires are detailed in Chapters Nine through Twelve.

Questionnaire Administration

The various elements that can give rise to response effects or errors in the answers actually obtained in a survey include (1) the structure of the survey task itself, especially the questionnaire; (2) the characteristics and performance of the survey respondents; (3) the characteristics and performance of the interviewers charged with gathering the data; and (4) the mode (or method) of data collection (Biemer & Lyberg, 2003; Sudman & Bradburn, 1974).

With mail questionnaires, errors associated with the interviewer are eliminated. The characteristics of the task and the respondents do, however, take on even greater importance in deciding how to design and administer the questionnaire in order to maximize the quality of the data obtained in the survey. As discussed in Chapter Five, the mode of data collection (in-person, telephone, mail), as well as whether paper-and-pencil or computer-assisted methods are used, can affect how certain types of questions are answered. Instrument development and pretesting procedures should ultimately employ the procedures to be used in the final study.

Special Considerations for Special Populations

Research on conducting surveys of special populations, such as ethnic minorities, intravenous drug users, teenagers or the elderly, or low literacy populations, document that the approaches to answering questions may well differ for these groups (Morales, Weidmer, & Hays, 2001; Owens, Johnson, & O'Rourke, 2001; Scott, Sarfati, Tobias, & Haslett, 2001; Weech-Maldonado, Weidmer, Morales, & Hays, 2001).

Implementing "warm" procedures (such as ethnographic interviews, focus groups, and consumer-based or participatory action research) that involve informal and more intimate contacts with individuals like those to be included in the final study in the early stages of developing the questions before proceeding with more formal ("cold") procedures for evaluating them (think-aloud protocols, structured experiments, behavior coding, or larger-scale pretesting), may be particularly useful for designing culturally sensitive and relevant questionnaires (Brown, 2004; Call et al., 2004; Cassidy, 1994; Cornelius et al., 2004; Israel et al., 1998).

Surveys that involve contacts with large numbers of non-English-speaking respondents should have fully translated versions of the questionnaire, especially in the light of earlier comments made about how bilingual subjects may respond to questions. At a minimum, any translation of the original questionnaire should be back-translated by someone other than the first translator. In this way, questions that arise about different interpretations of the survey's words or concepts by different subgroups that purportedly speak the same language can be addressed. If possible, it would also be helpful to use a team of translators to scrutinize the translation of the questionnaire to capture both the cultural equivalence of the terms and the assurance that the translations represent the technical aspects of the subject area being examined in this study. A team is emphasized here because one translator may not possess sufficient technical knowledge regarding all the topics in the survey. Alternative language versions of the questionnaire should also be fully pretested with respondents similar to those who will be included in the final study before it goes to the field (Harkness, 2004; Harkness, van de Vijver, & Mohler, 2003; Marín & Marín, 1991).

Selected Examples

In the UNICEF Multiple Indicator Cluster Survey study, a core set of questions as well as site-specific questions were developed for implementation in this multinational study (UNICEF, n.d.). These questions were obtained from a model questionnaire that was developed by the World Summit for Children (WSC) to enable countries to determine whether they were reaching twenty-seven WSC goals. Although the questions were provided in English, administrators were advised to translate the questions into the local language, using two translators before conducting the study. They were also advised to pretest the questionnaire to identify any potential misinterpretations of the questions, sensitivity to the questions, difficulties the respondents might have in answering the questions, or problems the interviewers encountered in administering the questionnaire.

The instruments used in the California Health Interview Survey (CHIS) have undergone extensive testing, using many of the question development and review procedures detailed here: pretests that focused on the length of the questionnaire and the ability of the respondent to answer the questions as worded, the use of behavior coding to monitor the respondent during the interview, and the completion of a full dress rehearsal pilot test (UCLA Center for Health Policy Research, 2002b). The questionnaire was translated into Spanish, Chinese, Khmer, Korean, and Vietnamese using a team of translators for each language that was translated. Given that 12 percent of the households sampled in the CHIS 2001 survey completed the screener in a language other than English, translating and conducting the interviews in the language of the respondent became an important part of enhancing the survey response rate (UCLA Center for Health Policy Research, 2002d).

In the National Dentist Malpractice Survey, several existing questionnaires and scales were combined to form a survey that focused on dentist-patient communications, practice characteristics, practice finances, malpractice insurance and claims experience, and demographic characteristics. Survey developers used questions that came from a pilot study where they validated providers' responses regarding malpractice insurance and claims experience against claims data provided by a malpractice carrier (Milgrom et al., 1994; Milgrom, Whitney, Conrad, Fiset, & O'Hara, 1995).

Guidelines for Minimizing Survey Errors and Maximizing Survey Quality

The principles and procedures highlighted here are intended to minimize the inaccuracies or inconsistencies in the answers to survey questions—as a function of how the question is posed, who asks it *and* who responds, as well as the method used to ask it (telephone or personal interview or self-administered). These are referred to as "response effects" introduced by the questionnaire, interviewer, respondent, or mode of data collection, respectively (see Figure 8.1). These various types of effects are highlighted and the chapters with the approaches to addressing them are provided in Table 8.1.

**TABLE 8.1. SURVEY ERRORS: SOURCES AND SOLUTIONS—
GENERAL PRINCIPLES FOR FORMULATING QUESTIONS.**

	Systematic Errors			*Variable Errors*		
	Questionnaire Effects: Under- or Over-reporting	Respondent Effects: Yea-Saying	Mode Effects: Systematic	Questionnaire Effects: Order and Context	Interviewer Effects: Interviewer Variability	Mode Effects: Variable
Solutions to Errors	See Chapters Ten and Twelve.	See Chapters Ten, Eleven, and Twelve.	See Chapters Five and Ten.	See Chapters Ten, Eleven, and Twelve.	See Chapter Thirteen.	See Chapter Five.

A good offense is the best defense in minimizing these types of errors. That is, survey developers should consult previous research regarding the factors that are most likely to give rise to these errors, as well as plan plenty of "preseason practice" by implementing some or a combination of the pretest procedures outlined earlier for designing and evaluating survey questions.

The chapters that follow build on the principles and criteria introduced here to suggest guidelines for reducing the response errors in health surveys depending on *how* the survey questions are asked, as well as on *what* they are asked about.

Supplementary Sources

Sources that provide straightforward guidance on how to compose survey questions to minimize the kinds of errors discussed in this chapter include Biemer and Lyberg (2003); Bradburn, Sudman, and Wansink (2004); Dillman (2000); Foddy (1993); Fowler (1995); National Center for Health Statistics (1999); Salant and Dillman (1994); and Tourangeau, Rips, and Rasinski (2000).

CHAPTER NINE

FORMULATING QUESTIONS ABOUT HEALTH

Chapter Highlights

1. The selection of questions about health for health surveys should be guided by the principles of total survey design and survey quality.
2. The specific steps for selecting questions about health or other topics for health surveys are (1) decide how to measure the concepts, (2) relate the concepts to the survey design and objectives, (3) match the scale for the measures chosen to the analysis plan, (4) evaluate the reliability of the measures, (5) evaluate the validity of the measures, (6) choose the most appropriate method of data collection, (7) tailor the measures to the study sample, and (8) decide how best to ask the actual questions.

Deciding how best to measure health may summon much of the same perplexity and diversity of perspective as when the blind people were asked to take the measure of the proverbial elephant. Health surveys have traditionally served a variety of purposes and objectives, and the array of applications in both the public and private sectors continues to multiply. Correspondingly, different disciplines or fields of study or practice dictate different approaches to defining and measuring health as well as variant criteria for critiquing them.

Five major applications of health surveys can be identified, each of which illuminates contrasting perspectives in measuring health. First, health surveys have been widely used in community needs and asset assessment activities or as a basis for planning health programs in a given market or service area. This perspective takes a broad look at the population's health, its determinants, and the various risks for poor health that exist for different members of the community. International and national health agencies, local public health providers, and public and private strategic planners are most likely to design and implement these types of studies (Aday, 2001; Drukker & van Os, 2003; Evans, Barer, & Marmor, 1994; Evans & Stoddart, 1990; Fremont et al., 2005; Wallace, 1994).

Surveys may also be used to evaluate the impact of experimental or quasi-experimental interventions on the health of affected groups. These studies dictate consideration of indicators of health that are sensitive to change over time or differences between groups to capture meaningfully any effects the programs yield. The RAND Health Insurance Experiment, an experimental study to evaluate the impact of different types of coverage and associated out-of-pocket costs on use and health (Brook et al., 1979), and the Medical Outcomes Study (MOS), an observational study of the health outcomes of patients with selected illnesses in different practice settings, and related International Quality of Life Assessment Project initiatives (Alonso et al., 2004; Stewart & Ware, 1992), have made substantial contributions to research on the measurement of health status and health-related quality of life. These studies have also contributed to informing national health care debates about the appropriateness of different models of financing and delivering services.

A third application of health surveys is for the purpose of gathering data on health plan patients or enrollees regarding their health status, satisfaction, and access to care, as components of "report cards" that are made available to current and prospective enrollees to assist them in evaluating the performance of health plans. These report cards are also used by plan administrators to compare their plan's performance against others, as well as to make improvements in the management of the plan. An example of a report card used to evaluate the quality of care delivered by providers is the Health Plan Employer Data and Information System, developed by the National Committee for Quality Assurance (NCQA), an independent nonprofit organization formed to assess the quality of managed care organizations (National Committee for Quality Assurance, 2005, June 13). Patient access and satisfaction surveys are an increasingly important component of report cards for evaluating the quality of care delivered in both inpatient and ambulatory settings (Agency for Healthcare Research and Quality, 2003; "Characteristics of Community Report Cards," 1997; Schauffler & Mordavsky, 2001).

A fourth application of health surveys is epidemiological and clinical research to investigate the determinants or course of disease (based on case-control or cohort designs) and test the effectiveness of alternative treatments (using randomized clinical trials). The proliferation of managed care in the private sector and the large role the federal government plays in providing coverage (especially for the elderly through Medicare, and the corollary concerns of these payers with the efficiency and effectiveness of services) have generated a burgeoning interest in health and medical care outcomes assessment and accountability. For example, the Agency for Healthcare Research and Quality (1999, 2000) assumed a role in funding research examining treatment effectiveness, the cost and economics of health care, and patient management.

Finally, a fifth application is the use of health status assessment instruments in direct clinical practice to select treatments and monitor patient outcomes. The impetus for this application has been encouraged by the growing interest in evaluating and reporting the performance of health care plans and providers. It also surfaces a unique set of concerns from the perspective of providers regarding the utility, cost, and feasibility of implementing such procedures in the real world of clinical practice (Crawford, Caputo & Littlejohn, 2000; Wu et al., 2000).

Criteria for Developing and Evaluating Measures of Health

A variety of criteria may be applied in developing and choosing measures of health, including theoretical, psychometric, economic, clinimetric, and pragmatic norms.

Theoretical considerations surface fundamental differences in the definition or conceptualization of health. Those who assume a perspective on the health of a community and the array of factors that influence it, for example, are likely to argue for the importance of gathering data on a broad set of subjective and objective indicators of quality of life (employment, school quality, crime, social support, and so on), based on the implicit assumption that an array of (medical and nonmedical) sectors and interventions is ultimately needed to improve the health of a community (Kindig & Stoddart, 2003). A contrasting perspective on the part of those principally concerned with measuring the effectiveness of medical care makes a strong case for distinguishing health-related quality-of-life measures, arguing that medical care should be held accountable only for those outcomes that it can most directly influence (Kane, 2004). This discussion is similar to that regarding the need to distinguish between short-term (proximal) and long-term outcomes (distal) in examining the social determinants of population health. Proximal factors represent immediate psychosocial causes of illness (for example, smoking), while distal factors represent macro social-structural factors reflecting underlying socioeconomic conditions or resources (for example, income) and their distribution across populations and subgroups (Link & Phelan, 1995). These contrasting perspectives may dictate an emphasis on the inclusion of a different complex of measures in designing surveys to evaluate the success of programs in improving the health of communities.

A related theoretical contrast is reflected in the distinctions drawn by critics of standardized approaches to questionnaire design and administration between the voice of the research world and the voice of the community (the experiences of everyday life) and their respective influences on how health is ultimately defined and measured (Cornelius, Booker, Arthur, Reeves, & Morgan, 2004; Israel, Schulz, Parker, & Becker, 1998). The research world seeks to elicit the truth about an underlying physiological state through standardized, scientifically validated language and research procedures that are designed and administered by the scientific community, while the community seeks to capture the reality of individuals' experiences of health and function as lived in their respective environments through seeking and hearing the stories the patients have to tell in their own words.

Psychometric criteria for evaluating health items, indexes, and scales refer primarily to assessments of the validity and reliability of the measures discussed in Chapter Three. The fields of psychophysics, psychology, and psychometrics provide the theoretical and empirical foundation for this approach. Psychophysics, a field of study that began in the late nineteenth century, explored the application of the measurement procedures relating physical intensities (such as the magnitude of light) to internal sensations (individuals' perceptions of varying intensities of light). It formed the conceptual basis for category scaling techniques, which entail placing a line on a page with clearly defined end points or anchors (perfect health versus death) and asking respondents to rate the desirability of various (health) states in relationship to these anchor points (Froberg & Kane, 1989b).

Economic norms refer to the preferences that individuals have for different health states (levels of functioning) that are likely to influence their choice of treatment alternatives. Economists in particular are concerned with measuring the values (utilities) consumers assign to different options when making purchasing decisions or choices regarding health care interventions. The conceptual foundation for quantifying these values is rooted in the axioms of utility theory developed by von Neumann and Morgenstern regarding the process of decision making under conditions of uncertainty (Froberg & Kane, 1989b). Preference-based approaches to medical decision making based on economic theory include measures of quality-adjusted life year measures, visual analog scales, and the standard gamble and time trade-off approaches to assessing the value of selected health states (Petrou & Henderson, 2003). (These approaches are discussed in detail later in this chapter.)

Clinometric norms are those raised by practicing physicians as they survey patients in their own practices to assess the effectiveness of the care delivered in general and for individual patients in particular (Ersser, Surridge, & Wiles, 2002; Feinstein, 1987). Clinometric criteria may, in fact, conflict with or contradict norms grounded in other schools of thought. Standards of clinical judgment or measures of the pain or distress that patients experience do not have gold standard points of reference for formally assessing criterion validity but may nonetheless be viewed by clinicians to have a high amount of implicit (face) validity. Some of the most useful clinical indicators of health status, such as the Apgar score assigned to newborns, include a consciously heterogeneous, rather than homogeneous, set of items. Clinicians may therefore be more interested in parsimony than redundancy (and hence reliability) in measuring the health of the patients seen in their busy practice.

A final set of norms are pragmatic ones. These include considerations of the cost and complexity of data collection and the ease of interpretation of the profiles or scores used to measure health concepts. These pragmatic concerns take on increasing importance as those who are not necessarily experts in the design and construction of such measures (patients, providers, and policymakers) are called on either to take the survey, administer it, or interpret the results as a foundation for deciding a course of action (choosing a health plan, deciding on a type of treatment, or defining the benefits that should be covered in a publicly sponsored health plan).

The relative weight or emphasis assigned to these respective criteria in developing or choosing measures of health is likely to mirror the disciplinary interests and points of view represented by the audiences and purposes motivating the conduct of a given survey. Survey designers must, however, be prepared to shed their disciplinary blinders and consider the applicability of this array of norms in order to maximize the clarity and precision of their own look at health.

Utility-Related Scaling Methods

The fields of psychometrics and economics have most influenced the development of health status measures. The focus of the psychometric approach is to generate descriptions of individuals' health states or outcomes, while the economic approach focuses on measuring individuals' preferences for these alternative states or outcomes. The Likert scaling methods and, to an increasing extent, Rasch models and item response theory have been used in developing psychometric-based summary measures of health status. These approaches to scale development were discussed in Chapter Three with particular reference to their application in developing a major psychometric-based measure of health status, the MOS 36-Item Short-Form Health Survey (SF-36) and related adaptations of it (SF-12, SF-8).

The principal utility-related approaches to health status measurement are described in this chapter and highlighted in Figure 9.1. Selected examples of major generic health status measures from both traditions, the concepts measured by each, as well as the mode of administration, extent to which they have been adapted or translated into multiple languages, scaling method, number of questions, and scoring procedures are summarized in Table 9.1 (Andresen & Meyers, 2000; Coons, Rao, Keininger, & Hays, 2000; Ware, 1995).

Both types of measures have been employed to measure the health-related quality of life (HRQOL), although this construct has been a particular focus of the utility-related measurement approaches (Bardwell et al., 2004; Bosch et al., 2004; Cella, 1995; Neudert, Wasner, & Borasio, 2004; Shafazand, Goldstein, Doyle, Hlatky, & Gould, 2004; Sharma, 2004). Coons et al. (2000, p. 14) indicate that HRQOL "refers to how health impacts an individual's ability to function and his or her perceived well-being in physical, mental and social domains of life." Two classes of HRQOL instruments are currently being used: generic HRQOL instruments and disease specific. Generic HRQOL instruments are designed to be used across the full range of medical conditions, populations, or interventions, while disease-specific HRQOL measures are meant to be used in examining a particular condition or disease state (Coons et al., 2000).

Within these two classes of instrument, two types of HRQOL scales are currently in use: HRQOL scales that provide a profile according to a series of dimensions or domains that can be also averaged together into a summary score (for example, the SF-36, the Nottingham Health Profile, the Sickness Impact Profile, and the Dartmouth Coop Charts), and utility-related HRQOL scales that provide a single number summary ranging from 0 to 1—for example, the Quality of Well-Being Scale (QWB), the Health Utilities Index (HUI), and the EuroQol Instrument (EQ-5D) (Bartman et al., 1998; Coons et al., 2000).

The basic metric in quantifying quality of life, based on utility-related preference scales such as the QWB, the HUI, and the EQ-5D, is an interval or ratio scale that ranges from 0 to 1, with 1 being a perfect state of health and 0 being death, with varying states of health represented by the points in between. Raters are then asked to evaluate their preference for alternative states of health compared with others or with death. For example, being able to eat, dress, bathe, and go to the toilet without help, and have no limitations in normal work, school, or play activities might be assigned a value of 1.00. Comparatively, having some limitation in these latter role activities may receive a score of .94. Needing help with all the personal care activities and not being able to engage in one's normal social roles may lower the rating considerably to .50, reflecting that it is much less preferable than being able to function fully in these activities (1.00) but nonetheless still preferred to death (0) (Patrick & Erickson, 1993). It is also possible that some states (such as being in a coma on life support systems) may be deemed worse

FIGURE 9.1. SELECTED UTILITY-RELATED SCALES.

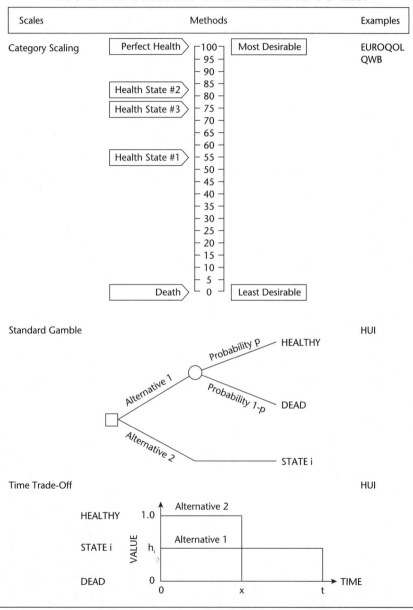

Scales	Methods	Examples

Category Scaling — Perfect Health — 100 — Most Desirable — EUROQOL QWB

Health State #2, Health State #3, Health State #1 ... Death — Least Desirable

Standard Gamble — HUI

Alternative 1 — Probability p — HEALTHY
Probability 1-p — DEAD
Alternative 2 — STATE i

Time Trade-Off — HUI

HEALTHY 1.0 — Alternative 2
STATE i h_i — Alternative 1
DEAD 0

VALUE, TIME, 0, x, t

TABLE 9.1. SELECTED GENERAL HEALTH STATUS MEASURES.

Concepts and Characteristics	Psychometric					Utility Related		
	SIP	NHP	COOP	DUKE	MOS SF-36	QWB	EUROQOL	HUI2, HUI3
Concepts								
Physical functioning	*	*	*	*	*	*	*	*
Social functioning	*	*	*	*	*	*	*	
Role functioning	*	*	*	*	*	*	*	
Psychological distress	*	*	*	*	*		*	
Health perceptions (general)		*	*	*	*		*	
Pain (bodily)	*	*	*	*	*		*	*
Energy/fatigue		*		*	*	*		
Psychological well-being				*	*			*
Sleep	*	*						
Cognitive functioning	*			*				*
Quality of life			*					
Reported health transition			*		*			
Characteristics								
Administration method (S = Self, I = Interview, P = Proxy)	S, I, P	S, I	S, I	S, I	S, I, P	S, I, P	S	S, I, P
Scaling method (L = Likert, R = Rasch, T = Thurstone, U = Utility)	T	T	L	L	L, R	U	U	U
Number of questions	136	38	9	17	36	107	9	31
Scoring options (P = Profile, SS = Summary Scores, SI = Single Index)	P, SS, SI	P	P	P, SI	P, SS	SI	SI	SI
Number of non-English multiple language/cultural adaptations	7	10	9+	NA	6	5+	16+	12+

Note: SIP = Sickness Impact Profile (1976); NHP = Nottingham Health Profile (1980); COOP = Dartmouth Function Charts (1987); DUKE = Duke Health Profile (1990); MOS SF-36 = MOS 36-Item Short Form Health Survey (1992); QWB = Quality of Well-Being Scale (1992); EUROQOL = European Quality of Life Index (1990); HUI = Health Utilities Index-Mark III (1993). NA = This characteristic was not available for the scale.

Bibliography: SIP: Bergner, Bobbitt, Carter, & Gilson, 1981; Bergner, Bobbitt, Kressel, Pollard, Gilson, & Morris, 1976; Medical Outcomes Trust, 2001, July.

NHP: Hunt & McEwen, 1980; Hunt, McEwen, & McKenna, 1992; Hunt, McKenna, McEwen, Williams, & Papp, 1981.

COOP: Beaufait et al., 1992; Nelson et al., 1987; Nelson, Wasson, Johnson, & Hays, 1996.

DUKE: Medical Outcomes Trust, 2001, July; Parkerson, Broadhead, & Tse, 1990; Parkerson, Gehlbach, Wagner, James, Clapp, & Muhlbaier, 1981.

MOS SF-36: McHorney, Ware, Lu, & Sherbourne, 1994; McHorney, Ware, & Raczek, 1993; Medical Outcomes Trust, 2001, July; Ware, Kosinski, & Keller, 1994; Ware & Sherbourne, 1992; Ware, Snow, Kosinski, & Gandek, 1993.

QWB: Bush, 1984; Kaplan, 1989; Kaplan & Anderson, 1988; Medical Outcomes Trust, 2001, July; Patrick, Bush, & Chen, 1973.

EUROQOL: EuroQol Group, 1990; EuroQol Group, n.d.

HUI: Boyle, Furlong, Feeny, Torrance, & Hatcher, 1995; Health Utilities Group, 2005, Jan. 12.

Source: Adapted from Table 1 (p. 330) in Ware, 1995. Reprinted, with permission, from the *Annual Review of Public Health,* volume 16, copyright © 1995 by Annual Reviews (www.annualreviews.org). Information on language/cultural adaptations drawn from Coons, Rao, Keininger, & Hays, 2000.

than death and would then be assigned negative values. The scores derived for each state can then be used as weights applied to the actual or anticipated years of life to compute quality-adjusted life years, an operational indicator of health-related quality of life incorporating both the quality and quantity of years lived (Highland, Strange, Mazur, & Simpson, 2003; Morrow & Bryant, 1995; Petrou & Henderson, 2003; Robine, Mathers, & Bucquet, 1993; Torrance & Feeny, 1989).

Although a number of utility-related measures have been developed, three have been most widely used and evaluated in measuring HRQOL: category scaling, standard gamble, and time trade-off (Feeny & Torrance, 1989; Froberg & Kane, 1989a, 1989b, 1989c, 1989d; Patrick & Erickson, 1993; Petrou & Hendersen, 2003; Torrance, 1986, 1987). The first has its roots in psychophysics and the latter two in economics. The response format and examples of each are portrayed in Figure 9.1.

In general, raters are asked to assign health states to a point on a scale that ranges between 0 (death) and 100 (perfect health), assuming that the points on the scale can be considered equal intervals. Those assigned closer to the perfect or most desirable state (100) would be preferred to those that are not. Thermometers or comparable metrics are used as devices for registering the relative rating of different health states, levels of function, or pain (Szende, Svensson, Ståhl, Mészáros, & Berta, 2004; van Exel, Reimer, & Koopmanschap, 2004).

The standard gamble approach involves making two types of choices: the certainty of one choice (for example, death from not having a needed kidney transplant) and a gamble with two possible outcomes, each of which is assigned a probability between 0 and 1. In this case, the individual estimates the probability of two outcomes from having a kidney transplant: one results in living in good health for a period of time, and the other is dying as a result of a postsurgical complication. The first choice is assigned a probability of (p), while the second choice is assigned a probability of $1 - p$.

The concept of probability underlying the standard gamble approach is complex and may not be readily understandable by some respondents. For example, it may be difficult to summarize the complex array of scenarios that can be produced under such an approach (Dobrez & Calhoun, 2004; Sjöberg, 2000). The time trade-off method was developed as an alternative that would be simpler to implement and interpret. Under the time trade-off option, the respondent is asked to consider the amount of time he or she is willing to trade to live in a particular state of health. Thus, under this approach, the person who was deciding whether to have a kidney transplant would be offered an alternative of having the transplant and living a certain number of years ($x = 5$) of the estimated remaining years of life ($t = 20$) in a relatively healthy state, compared with living out his or her life (twenty years) on dialysis. The preference for living in this state (h) can be computed (x/t) based on these trade-offs ($5/20 = .25$). A score of .25 reflects a low evaluation of the transplant compared with not having it given the few years of healthy life gained (Torrance, 1986).

Preferences and valuations, based on these approaches, provide the foundation for utility-related scales of health-related quality of life. Respondents can be asked their current state of health or level of functioning, and the ratings (or weights) derived from these respective approaches can then be used in assigning overall HRQOL scores.

The reliability and validity of these and other approaches to constructing the preferences for treatment alternatives and associated health outcomes are unresolved issues in health services research. As noted earlier, it may be difficult for respondents to calculate the options under each utility scenario, or there may be a tendency for survey respondents to give systematically higher or lower scores using one method versus another. Factors such as poor health, depression, or anxiety could also affect ratings (Dobrez & Calhoun, 2004). It is important in studies where they are used to employ relevant methods for evaluating the reliability and validity of these complex but important utility-based measures of health.

Intra- and inter-rater reliability (the consistency within and between raters), as well as test-retest reliability, are the most relevant forms of reliability analyses for these measures. There is no expectation that the varying stimuli (states) presented to respondents will have high intercorrelations (internal consistency reliability). In general, the intra- and inter-rater and test-retest reliability of these approaches has been found to be variable but acceptable (.70 or higher), although as might be expected, the test-retest reliability diminishes the longer the time is between measurements (Froberg & Kane, 1989b).

Content and construct validity are most applicable to these types of measures. There is no gold standard against which these judgments can be compared to evaluate their criterion validity. Studies of health-state preferences differ widely in the format and content of health states that are presented to raters, and the content validity of these scenarios is rarely discussed. The convergent validity among the different methods and the hypothetical associations of these preferences with other variables have been neither extensively examined nor supported in the literature. The category rating scales appear to be the easiest for raters to understand and yield the most valid scale values (Froberg & Kane, 1989b).

Methodological concerns with these approaches relate to who is asked to do these ratings (general population, patients, health professionals) and the extent to which the ratings might differ for different groups; the impact of how the question is framed, the content of the descriptions of the health states, and the risk aversiveness of respondents on responses provided; and the paucity of comprehensive validity analyses (using the multitrait multimethod approach, for example) comparing the various methods (Bartman et al., 1998; Cella, 1995; Gill & Feinstein,

1994; Froberg & Kane, 1989a, 1989b, 1989c, 1989d; Rutten-van Mölken, Bakker, van Doorslaer, & van der Linden, 1995; Torrance, 1986, 1987). As these types of measures are increasingly used in making critical policy and clinical choices, the need for collaborative and effective partnerships between and among researchers from the disciplines of psychometrics, economics, and cognitive psychology in resolving these controversies takes on a heightened importance.

Steps in Developing and Evaluating Measures of Health

The discussion that follows applies the principles of survey design discussed in other chapters to illustrate the total survey design approach for deciding which questions on health and other topics to include in a health survey.

Deciding How to Measure the Concepts

A primary consideration in deciding which questions to ask in a health survey is the conceptualization of health that best operationalizes the research questions to be addressed in the study (see Table 3.1 in Chapter Three). If there is an interest in profiling a population's overall health status, then general health status measures such as the MOS-SF-36 may be most appropriate. If the focus is on eliciting patient preferences for the health states that might result from alternative treatment choices, then utility-based scales such as the Health Utilities Index (HUI) may be the health status measure of choice.

A number of overviews of health status measures are available (Andresen & Meyers, 2000; Bowling, 2005; Brook et al., 1979; Cella, 1995; Coons et al., 2000; Keith, 1994; Larson, 1991; McDowell & Newell, 1996; Patrick & Bergner, 1990; Patrick & Deyo, 1989; Patrick & Erickson, 1993; Scientific Advisory Committee of the Medical Outcomes Trust, 2002; Stewart & Ware, 1992; Streiner & Norman, 2003; Szende et al., 2003; Ware, 1987, 1995; Wilkin, Hallam, & Doggett, 1992; Wu et al., 2000).

Multidimensional Concept of Health. Health is a complex and multidimensional concept. The World Health Organization (WHO) has defined *health* as a "state of complete physical, mental, and social well-being and not merely the absence of disease or infirmity" (World Health Organization, 1948, p. 1). Comprehensive efforts to conceptualize health and develop empirical definitions of the concept have tended to distinguish the physical, mental, and social dimensions of health reflected in the WHO definition (Ware, 1987, 1995). Efforts have been made to highlight the interrelatedness of physical and mental health (U.S. Public Health Service, Office of the Surgeon General, 1999). Instead of using the term *physical* health, *somatic* health is used to note the nonmental functions of the body. This notion shifts the focus to the brain as the center of both mental and nonmental activities in the body (Cox, Donohue, Brown, Kataria, & Judson, 2004; Taft, Karlsson, & Sullivan, 2001).

Although physical and mental health indicators clearly "end at the skin," to use Ware's phrase, indicators of social well-being extend beyond the individual to include the quantity and quality of his or her social contacts with other individuals (Orth-Gomer & Unden, 1987; Ware, 1986). There is evidence that the number and nature of such contacts influence individuals' physical and mental health. Also, whether individuals can perform appropriate social roles and thereby be productive members of society is the bottom line in evaluating the impact of their physical and mental health on their overall social well-being. Social capital theory, for example, focuses on examining the type and intensity of interrelationships among families, neighborhoods, and communities and their effect on health and well-being (DeGraaf & Jordan, 2003; Drukker & van Os, 2003; Steury, Spencer, & Parkinson, 2004).

In arriving at the kinds of health questions to ask in health surveys, researchers need to decide which dimensions of health—physical, mental, or social—they want to study. If they want to focus on more than one dimension, they must determine what the various dimensions convey, separately or together, about the target population's health.

Positive Versus Negative Concepts of Health.

Positive Versus Negative Concepts of Health. Another conceptual consideration that influences how health might be measured is that health status can be defined in positive or negative terms. Examples of positive indicators of health include criteria such as norms for age- and sex-specific measures of height or weight, measures of individual or family coping strengths, and scales of positive mental health. As for negative indicators, death may be said to reflect the total absence of health, measured by total or disease-specific mortality (death) rates (Doornbos, 1996; Hatfield, 1997; Jones, 1996; Schene, 1990; Schirmer & Lopez, 2001).

Concepts of morbidity serve to define the middle range of a continuum defined by theoretical positive and negative end points that mark the total presence or absence of health. Health providers and patients may, of course, apply different criteria in defining morbidity and associated health status. Some of these conceptualizations of morbidity are culturally bound (U.S. Public Health Service, Office of the Surgeon General, 2001). For example, in some cultures, a patient experiencing emotional stress may choose to somatize it—that is, say he or she has a physical problem rather than say he or she is feeling anxious or depressed. At the same time, some cultures may lack the words to express concepts like death (as an end state) because death and life are viewed as being part of a single continuum.

Provider Versus Patient Concepts of Health. The assessment of the presence or absence of disease relies on clinical or diagnostic judgments of the underlying medical condition. Efforts to identify diseases in the target population of a survey would be obtained by administering physical exams or tests, such as taking participants' blood pressure or administering a glucose-tolerance test, as is done in the NCHS–Health and Nutrition Examination Survey. Another approach would be to ask respondents or their physicians to report diagnosed conditions, as in the NCHS–National Health Interview Survey and the NCHS–National Ambulatory Medical Care Survey, respectively. Comparable mental health diagnoses can be obtained by sampling clinic records or asking mental health professionals to provide this information for the clients they see in their practices.

An approach to defining morbidity based on conceptualizing it as illness tends to rely more on the individuals' own perceptions of their physical or mental health than on provider or medical record sources or respondents' reports of clinically diagnosed conditions. The emphasis here, then, is on the person's perceptions rather than on provider judgments. Questions about symptoms that people experienced during the year or their perceptions of their health—whether they consider it to be excellent, good, fair, or poor and how much they worry about their health—are questions that respondents, not providers, can best answer. These questions tap the person's subjective experience of the illness.

Different individuals' perceptions of the same underlying medical condition may vary as a result of cultural or subgroup differences in how illness is defined or because of individual variations in the thresholds of pain or discomfort felt to be experienced. There is also evidence that providers' perceptions of cultural issues related to end-of-life decisions may influence their diagnoses of certain types of diseases, such as chronic and severe morbidities (Becker, Gates, & Newsom, 2004; Searight & Gafford, 2005).

Asking questions to get at people's perceptions of their mental or physical health may tap something different from what providers would say about their health. The choice of approach should be guided by conceptual considerations of which ways of measuring health make the most sense given the aspects of health the investigator wants to learn about from the study and from whose point of view.

A third approach to estimating morbidity is in terms of the individual's ability to perform certain functions or activities. Examples of measures of functioning include activities of daily living or instrumental activities of daily living. These indicators are based largely on behavioral but may also include perceptual or clinical criteria (Adler, Clark, DeMaio, Miller, & Saluter, 1999; Andresen, Fitch, McLendon, & Meyers, 2000). For example, WHO developed a measure of functioning that encompassed both behavioral and perceptual criteria. Under the International Classification of Impairment, Disability and Handicap (ICIDH), functioning represents the cognitive, emotional, and motivational status of the individual and is influenced by the person's health condition, body functions, and interaction with their environment. The measurement of functioning under this scenario entails measuring not only disability but also coping strengths. It may, however, be difficult to fully reconcile the behavioral and perceptual criteria in measuring health-related quality of life. Study subjects with high limitations may report a score of zero or near perfect health. The same condition may also have a different impact on different people's level of functioning. A broken arm may represent a limited disability for a lawyer but a major handicap for a professional baseball player (Andresen & Meyers, 2000; Ueda, 2002).

Researchers need to decide whether behavioral indicators of health are important for their purposes and, if so, what level of functioning it is most appropriate to capture with these measures and for whom.

Generic Versus Disease-Specific Concepts of Health.

Another important distinction to consider in selecting relevant measures of health status is generic versus disease-specific indicators. As highlighted in the earlier discussion regarding the generic HRQOL scales and the disease-specific HRQOLs, generic measures encompass an array of relevant dimensions of health and quality of life (such as general perceptions of health, psychological function, physical and role function, and social function) that are relevant across disease or illness categories. Disease-specific measures are those that are most relevant to measuring the health impact of specific conditions, such as cancer, arthritis, or chronic back pain. Disease-specific measures may be particularly useful in measuring the responsiveness of patients to interventions in a clinical practice setting and generic measures for profiling the needs of a population in a program's service area.

One example of such a measure is the WHOQOL-HIV instrument, which examines the quality of life of persons who are HIV positive (O'Connell et al., 2003). It is an expansion of a generic QOL instrument, the WHOQOL-100, which focuses on the specific needs of persons who are living with HIV or AIDS. Whereas the WHOQOL-100 focuses on physical facets, psychological facets, level of independence, social relationships, the environment, spirituality, religion, and personal beliefs, the WHOQOL-HIV includes questions regarding the symptoms of HIV, attitudes and feelings regarding living with AIDS, body image, social inclusion, death and dying, and forgiveness. Thus, one may want to assess whether a generic or a disease-specific instrument is more appropriate to use in planning a study.

Relating the Concepts to the Survey Design and Objectives

Next, researchers should consider the particular study design being used in their survey (Table 2.1 in Chapter Two) and the types of research questions that can be addressed with the design (Table 2.2 and Figure 2.1 in Chapter Two). Different methodological criteria should be emphasized in choosing health indexes for different types of study designs (Kirshner & Guyatt, 1985).

Cross-Sectional Designs. Cross-sectional survey designs are often used to estimate the prevalence of disease or the need for certain health services or programs in the target population. Researchers must decide, for example, whether disease-specific or generic health status measures are appropriate in gathering data on the target population. Disease-specific measures are appropriate for assessing the health of a patient population that has a particular disease or condition and generic measures for assessing health across a variety of populations or patients. Designers of needs assessment surveys must clearly define the needs they are trying to assess in deciding which health questions to ask in their study.

Group-Comparison Designs. Kirshner and Guyatt (1985) point out the importance of discriminative criteria in selecting health indexes for group comparison designs. This type of design allows researchers to detect real differences between groups. Researchers then need to ask which groups are the focus of the survey and if the instrument is sufficiently discriminating to detect meaningful degrees of difference on the relevant health dimensions between these groups.

For example, one type of functional status indicator would be required if the study focuses on comparisons between different age and sex groups in a general population survey, while another type would be required for a study comparing the same groups in a survey of the institutionalized elderly. The indicators chosen would need to have very different scales for measuring physical functioning for these different groups. Health indexes that measure the ability to feed or dress oneself or walk, such as Katz's Index of Independence in Activities of Daily Living (Katz, Ford, Moskowitz, Jackson, & Jaffe, 1963), would be appropriate for the institutionalized elderly sample but not for the general population sample, because the majority of those in the latter sample would be able to perform these tasks.

The use of general health status measures such as the MOS Trust SF-36 scale may, for example, result in floor or ceiling effects for selected populations. A group that is largely in good health would concentrate at the top of the scale (ceiling effect) and those with poor health at the bottom (floor effect). Using the overall score (rather than the physical and mental health subscores) on this scale also may not fully distinguish key differences in mental versus physical health within and across groups (Bardwell, Ancoli-Israel, & Dimsdale, 2001; Cox et al., 2004; Taft et al., 2001).

In comparing the major subgroups of interest and particularly within the general population sample, researchers may need to consider the appropriate roles (working, going to school, for example) for different groups in collecting information that can be meaningfully compared between them.

Longitudinal Designs. With longitudinal designs, Kirshner and Guyatt (1985) point out the importance of considering predictive criteria. That is, the individual items and the summary scales developed from them should predict changes in certain criterion measures over time. One would, for example, expect health questions in surveys inquiring about the numbers and types of medical conditions to be associated with subsequent mortality rates for a cohort of individuals being followed over time in epidemiological surveys.

In conducting longitudinal studies of this kind, survey researchers need to be particularly sensitive to the extent to which variations in the health indicators could be affected by other external factors in the environment, as well as to the fact that changes in the questions in successive waves of the study could introduce errors in detecting true changes in these indicators over time. Improved diagnostic and treatment techniques for a selected illness can lead to a higher survival rate of people with the disease and, hence, a higher, rather than lower, prevalence of the disease over time. Increased access to medical care can result in more "prescribed" days of disability (limiting one's usual routine because of illness) or to the diagnosis of previously undiagnosed conditions. Changing the survey methodology to increase the reporting of health events will also reduce the comparability of survey results with data from previous years.

Measuring changes in health indicators requires that investigators be aware of the factors to which those indicators are sensitive and whether they are the "true" changes that the investigators are interested in measuring or simply noise that confounds the interpretation of any differences that are observed over time.

Experimental Designs. Evaluative criteria should be applied in the development or choice of health indexes for surveys used in experimental studies. These criteria determine whether the indicator is sensitive to detecting the changes hypothesized to result from some clinical or programmatic intervention.

The researcher should consider what changes in an individual's health, such as specific levels or types of physical functioning for people with rheumatoid arthritis, are predicted to result from the intervention—the use of a new drug or physical therapy regimen, for example. Furthermore, health promotion interventions that focus on producing "good health" may require indicators that define the positive end of a continuum conceptualized as the presence or magnitude of health or well-being, while more treatment-oriented interventions may require that the negative end of the continuum—the presence or magnitude of "illness"—be defined.

Health measures in experimental or quasi-experimental designs should be scaled to be responsive to different levels or types of interventions and at the same time should not be subject to large random variation between questionnaire administrations.

Matching the Scale for the Measures Chosen to the Analysis Plan

The third major set of considerations in deciding the types of health questions to ask in surveys is the level of measurement and type of summary scale that would be most appropriate to use in asking or analyzing the questions. As discussed in Chapter Three, variables can be nominal, ordinal, interval, or ratio levels of measurement (Table 3.1). There are also a variety of devices for condensing the information from several different questions into a single summary or scale score (Figure 3.3 and Table 3.4). Ultimately, and perhaps most important, the kinds of analysis that can be conducted with the data are a function of how the variables are measured (see Chapter Fifteen). In deciding how to ask the questions, then, the researcher should give considerable thought to what he or she wants to do with the data once they are collected.

Level of Measurement. Researchers might decide that a simple classification of individuals into categories—those who can climb stairs or dress themselves versus those who cannot—is adequate for their purposes. If so, asking questions that rely on nominal dichotomous responses (yes or no) would be sufficient. Typologies can also be constructed on the basis of cross-classifications of these variables: "can climb stairs and dress oneself; can climb stairs but not dress oneself; can dress oneself but not climb stairs; or can do neither."

If finer discrimination is required to detect varying levels of functioning for different individuals, then a question or scale with an ordinal level of measurement would be more appropriate. For example, the study subjects could be rank-ordered according to whether they can perform more or fewer functions or seem to be more or less happy with their lives. Different ordinal summary devices could be used if this type of discrimination is desired, including simple indexes that add up the number of tasks the subjects can accomplish or Likert-type scales that summarize scale scores reflecting the extent to which they can perform these tasks.

Ratio or interval measures or summary scales provide more information for the researcher to use in order to estimate not just whether the "health" of certain individuals is better than that of others but also how much better. Building in this level of discrimination in choosing questions to include in the study could be particularly important in experimental or quasi-experimental designs in which the investigator is interested in determining the magnitude of improvement that results from different levels (or dosages) of an experimental treatment applied to study subjects. Utility-related measures generally assume a cardinal (interval or ratio) level of measurement (Torrance, 1986, 1987).

Number of Items. A related measurement issue in choosing the questions to include in a health survey is whether the survey designer wants to use a single-item or a multi-item scale to measure the health concept of interest. There are advantages and disadvantages to each approach. Single items are easier and cheaper to administer and are less of a burden for the respondents to answer. Health variables based on one or only a few questions may, however, be less reliable than multi-item scales that more consistently capture a larger part of the concept. It may be advantageous in such cases to compare shorter versions of scales with longer versions to evaluate the trade-offs between reducing respondent burden by administering a shorter scale versus a losing validity or reliability. For example, Hurst, Ruta, and Kind (1998) compared the MOS SF-12 with the SF-36 in a sample of rheumatoid arthritic patients to examine the comparability of the scales. They found only a slight decrease in the reliability of the scale as a result of eliminating some of the questions from the longer scale. They concluded that the slight decrease in reliability was acceptable, however, given the lower respondent burden in answering the shorter form.

However, there are some disadvantages in asking a number of different questions. For example, a single score summarizing across a variety of dimensions can be hard to interpret substantively and may not adequately capture differing patterns of responses to different dimensions or indicators of the concept.

Both single-item and multi-item approaches to asking questions about people's health are used in health surveys. One question used with considerable frequency as an indicator of overall health status asks whether a respondent thinks his or her health is excellent, good, fair, or poor. The precise wording of this question has varied in different surveys. The California Health Interview Survey (CHIS) survey asks, "In general, would you say your health is excellent, very good, good, fair or poor?" (CHIS 2001, section B, question AB1). This is similar to the question asked in the National Health Interview Survey. In the 2004 NCHS–NHIS study, the question was, "Would you say your health, in general, was excellent, very good, good, fair, or poor?" (National Center for Health Statistics, n.d.). This question captures the point of view of the person's own experiences and perceptions. It also tends to be a particularly sensitive indicator of the presence of chronic and serious but manageable conditions, such as hypertension, diabetes, thyroid problems, anemia, hemophilia, and ulcers and to be correlated with individuals' overall utilization of physicians' services (Burgos, Schetzina, Dixon, & Mendoza, 2005; Ivanov, 2000; Preville, Herbert, Boyer, & Bravo, 2001).

Many of the individual questions from the CHIS that ask whether people were unable to perform age-appropriate roles because of health limitations (CHIS, 2001, section B) are used quite often as single-item indicators of health status.

Many health status indicators, however, are based on a number of questions and may capture various dimensions of health (physical, mental, and social) as well as provide a summative evaluation of health as a whole.

Evaluating the Reliability of the Measures

An important methodological criterion to consider in evaluating any empirical indicator of a concept is its reliability. Methods for evaluating the test-retest, inter-rater, and internal consistency reliability of survey measures were described in Chapter Three (see Figure 3.1).

Survey designers should review information of this kind when deciding whether the measures they are considering are reliable enough for their purposes. More precise (reliable) measures are required when the focus is on estimates for particular individuals—such as changes in physical functioning of individual patients as a result of a clinical intervention—than when looking at differences between groups, especially groups for which substantial differences are expected to exist. An example of the latter would be the degree of social functioning for disabled versus nondisabled children.

As mentioned earlier, reliability will probably be lower for single-item than for multi-item indicators of health. The reliability of certain measures may be less for socioeconomically disadvantaged groups (those with less income or lower levels of education) or individuals whose impairments (such as poor sight or hearing) limit their ability to respond adequately to certain types of survey forms or questions.

If information is not available on measures that others have formulated or for new items or scales developed for a survey, then survey designers can assess the reliability of those questions through pilot studies or split-ballot experiments before fielding their study questionnaire if time and resources permit.

Evaluating the Validity of the Measures

Validity—the accuracy of empirical measures in reflecting a concept—is another important methodological criterion to consider in evaluating survey questions. Approaches for assessing the content, criterion, and construct validity of survey measures were summarized in Chapter Three (see Figure 3.2). Often, however, data on the validity of survey questions are limited.

The place to start in examining the validity of health status measures is their content: Do the items seem to capture the domain or subdimension of health (physical, mental, or social health or health in general) that is the focus of the study? Researchers should systematically scrutinize the items being considered and try to determine whether the items seem to capture adequately and accurately the major concept or subdimension of health that they are interested in measuring. Factor analysis and multitrait, multimethod analyses are also useful in making more sophisticated quantitative judgments about whether the items adequately discriminate one concept from another (see the discussion in Chapter Three). In general, valid measures are those that accurately translate the concept they are supposed to measure into the empirically oriented language of surveys.

Choosing the Most Appropriate Method of Data Collection

Once researchers have clearly delineated the major questions they want to address with a study, the ways in which the questions will be conceptualized and measured, and the probable validity and reliability of the measures they will use to summarize the data, they should give thought to practical implementation decisions, such as how they will go about collecting their data.

Certain indicators require certain forms of administration (by expert raters, interviewers, or self-administered formats) (McDowell & Newell, 1996). If researchers are thinking about one of these measures, they need to consider whether it is appropriate to use the method used originally in designing and administering the scale or to adapt it to their study. They also need to consider the implications that a change will have for the overall reliability and validity of the resulting data.

The burden (time, effort, and stress) on respondents in participating should always be taken into account when deciding on the numbers and kinds of questions to ask in health surveys. Researchers also need to consider both the personal and pecuniary costs and benefits of different data collection approaches (such as those outlined in Table 5.1 in Chapter Five) and whether certain methods of gathering the information are more appropriate than others, given who is the focus of the study.

Tailoring the Measures to the Study Sample

A related practical issue in deciding the kinds of questions to ask and how to ask them is the type of sample that will be drawn for the study. Generic health status questions may be more suitable for general surveys of the noninstitutionalized population, while disease-specific questions may be more appropriate for samples of hospitalized patients.

Furthermore, it may be necessary to design and test screening questions to ask of family or household informants so that people with certain types of medical conditions can be oversampled if they are a particular focus of the study. To be most efficient for this purpose, such questions should have good criterion validity, that is, high levels of specificity and sensitivity and, correspondingly, few false-positive or false-negative answers (see Figure 3.2 in Chapter Three).

Deciding How Best to Ask the Questions

In deciding exactly how to phrase the questions that will be in a survey, researchers should follow the principles outlined in the preceding chapter and in Chapters Ten and Eleven. They should consider the precise words, phrases, and resulting sentences to be used; the instructions to be provided with them; and the possible effect of the order and format in which they appear in the questionnaire on people's propensity to respond reliably and accurately.

Certain questions about physical, mental, or social health—such as whether respondents are incontinent or have had feelings that life was not worth living— may be highly sensitive and threatening. In asking these types of questions, survey designers should consider the principles outlined in Chapter Ten for asking threatening questions.

Special Considerations for Special Populations

Considerations that come into play in measuring the health of special populations are numerous. Different cultural, racial, or ethnic groups may experience and express illness in different ways (Becker et al., 2004; Institute of Medicine, 2003; Searight & Gafford, 2005; U.S. Public Health Service, 2001). It is therefore particularly important to employ culturally sensitive and relevant approaches to item and instrument development to capture these variant meanings. Translations of standardized health status questionnaires that an investigator would like to use or adapt may (or may not) be available. Even if they are, the reliability and validity of the scale should be assessed and compared with the estimates provided for the English and translated versions on other studies. The results may well differ.

Furthermore, one size does not fit all for certain health status questions across age groups, such as the functional impact of disability for children, adults, and the elderly. In addition, some types of questions or modes of administration will be particularly burdensome or problematical for those whose health one might be most interested in measuring—the elderly or people with low levels of literacy or cognitive, physical, hearing, or visual impairments, for example. Thought must then be given to strategies that are appropriate for facilitating obtaining information from these populations (amplified audio data collection techniques, the use of proxies, or observational rather than respondent report methods, for example).

Selected Examples

While the National Dental Malpractice Survey did not have the measurement of health status or health-related quality of life as a primary focus, this is a central component of the UNICEF Multiple Indicators Surveys and the California Health Interview Survey. Topics in the UNICEF survey include maternal mortality, child disability, tetanus toxoid, maternal and newborn child health, immunizations, care of illness, and malaria, for example (UNICEF, 2000). Topics in the 2001 and 2003 California Health Interview Surveys differed to some extent, but included a wide array of health topics, such as measures of health status, specific health conditions (such as asthma, arthritis, and heart disease), health behaviors (such as dietary intake and physical activity), women's health, cancer history and prevention, dental health, mental health, and injury and violence, among others. Extensive methodological reports are available on the methods used in the California Health Interview Survey and the resulting implications for the quality of the data gathered in the survey (UCLA Center for Health Policy Research, 2005).

Guidelines for Minimizing Survey Errors and Maximizing Survey Quality

This chapter identified a variety of norms that might be applied in selecting and evaluating measures of health status. The best advice to minimize both the systematic and variable errors in measuring health is to be aware of what a given perspective might either illuminate or fail to surface. Disciplinary or methodological parochialism may shed light on parts of the proverbial pachyderm, but the essence and magnitude of the beast as a whole may well be hidden or distorted in the viewing.

As suggested in Table 9.2 it may be possible to end up using questions that do not accurately capture the meaning of what they were intended to measure (poor or low validity) or evidence substantial instability (poor or low reliability). These errors can occur as a result of not determining whether the aspect of health being measured is understood by the respondent or because of differences in the

**TABLE 9.2. SURVEY ERRORS: SOURCES AND SOLUTIONS—
FORMULATING QUESTIONS ABOUT HEALTH.**

	Systematic Errors: Low or Poor Validity	Variable Errors: Low or Poor Reliability
Solutions to Errors	Use existing questions or scales that have been demonstrated to be valid, or evaluate validity during the pretest or final study, or both (see Chapter Three).	Use existing questions or scales that have been demonstrated to be reliable, or evaluate reliability during the pretest or final study, or both (see Chapter Three).

meanings of the linguistic interpretations of the terms across populations. These types of errors can be minimized by using questions or scales that have been validated with the population of interest or in the design and conduct of formal evaluations of the reliability and validity of the questions either prior to or in the course of the study.

Supplementary Sources

See the following sources for a more comprehensive treatment of health status measurement: Andresen and Meyers (2000); Bowling (2005); Coons, Rao, Keininger, and Hays (2000); McDowell and Newell (1996); Patrick and Erickson (1993); Revicki et al. (2000); Scientific Advisory Committee of the Medical Outcomes Trust (2002); and Streiner and Norman (2003).

CHAPTER TEN

FORMULATING QUESTIONS ABOUT DEMOGRAPHICS AND BEHAVIOR

Chapter Highlights

1. In selecting the sociodemographic and socioeconomic questions to ask people in health surveys, researchers can start with items comparable to those in the U.S. Census, federally sponsored health surveys, or related health surveys that have undergone extensive testing, and either adapt them or develop new ones as needed to enhance their relevance for a given study purpose or population.
2. In selecting and adapting demographic questions, researchers may want to consider carefully the analytical intent of the study, as recent research has reframed some of the ways that characteristics like gender, marital status, and race/ethnicity are defined.
3. In developing factual, nonthreatening questions about behaviors, researchers should try to reduce "telescoping" errors (overreporting) by using devices such as bounded recall and errors of omission (underreporting) by means of aided recall, diaries, or respondent record checks, as well as cognitive survey research techniques, to design and implement the survey questionnaire.

4. Rules for developing sensitive questions about health behaviors should focus on how to reduce the kind of underreporting that results from respondents' feeling threatened when acknowledging they engaged in those behaviors.

This chapter presents rules for writing questions to gather facts about the target populations of surveys. Three types of questions are considered: (1) questions about demographic characteristics, (2) nonthreatening questions, and (3) threatening questions about health and health care behaviors of survey respondents and their families. Different tasks and respondent burdens are associated with different types of questions. Questionnaire designers should take these differences into account in formulating their questions, as well as in evaluating items that others have developed.

Questions About Demographics

We are often interested in looking at demographic factors because of an interest in examining subgroup differences. Data on race/ethnicity, education, and income are, for example, relevant for identifying health or health care disparities between groups.

One does not have to start from scratch when developing questions about the basic sociodemographic and socioeconomic characteristics of study respondents and their families. The use of standardized items of this kind has several advantages. They (1) reduce the time and effort needed to develop and test such questions, (2) permit direct comparisons of the sample of a given survey with the results from a variety of other studies, and (3) in some instances, have documented evidence of their reliability or validity in previous studies.

In selecting the sociodemographic and socioeconomic questions to use in health surveys, those asked in the U.S. Census, federally sponsored surveys, or related health surveys that have undergone extensive testing provide a useful place to start (Bradburn, Sudman, & Wansink, 2004). Using items from these studies offers several advantages: these surveys follow the guidelines or requirements of the Office of Management and Budget and other federal statistical agencies such as the Bureau of the Census and have often undergone multiple stages of questionnaire design and testing before implementation. Nevertheless, the researcher should think about whether using questions identical to those in other surveys makes sense given the emphases of a particular survey. Modifying questions to operationalize fully a major concept of interest to the investigator or adapting questions to a particular mode of data collection or study population would certainly be appropriate.

Examples of the majority of the demographic questions to be discussed appear on the U.S. Census Bureau (2003) Web site; in the revised edition of *Asking Questions* (Bradburn et al., 2004), a classic guide for how to pose survey questions; and in the UNICEF Multiple Indicator Cluster Survey and California Health Interview Survey (see Resources A and B). When appropriate, relevant modifications, such as those used when data are collected over the telephone, are mentioned. Selected questions in the CHIS 2001 and UNICEF MICS End-Decade (MICS-2) Survey questionnaire are referenced as examples. See the Web sites for the CHIS and UNICEF surveys for revisions to how the questionnaires were modified in subsequent waves of data collection (UCLA Center for Health Policy Research, 2005; UNICEF, n.d.).

Household Composition

An important change has occurred in the procedures for identifying individuals who live in a sampled household and their relationships in the United States: national surveys now start with the "reference person" rather than with the "head of the household." The reference person is defined as "the person or one of the persons who owns or rents this home." Questions about the relationship of others in the household are then asked of this designated reference person. This convention was adopted by the U.S. Bureau of the Census for the Current Population Survey and other surveys to reflect better the nontraditional composition of many U.S. households and the emerging sensitivity on the part of many American families to identifying any one member as the head of the family.

The 2000 U.S. Census asked: "How many people were living or staying in this house, apartment, or mobile home on April 1, 2000?" (question 1); "Please print the names of all the people who you indicated in question 1 were living or staying here on April 1, 2000. Start with the person, or one of the people living here who owns, is buying, or rents this house, apartment, or mobile home. If there is no such person, start with any adult living or staying here" (question 2) (U.S. Census Bureau, 2003).

The UNICEF Multiple Indicator Cluster Survey (MICS) End-Decade Study Household Listing Form provides another example of how the members of the household might be listed (UNICEF, n.d.). It makes use of a matrix comprised of columns for each question regarding the characteristics of household members and rows (or lines) for each person in the household on which responses to the respective questions can be recorded. The MICS still uses the referent of "the head of the household," defined as "the person who is considered responsible for the household," with it being up to the respondent to define who is head (UNICEF, 2000, p. A1.6).

For most of the questions in the CHIS, an adult is asked to provide the responses to the survey. However, the respondent who is identified as the "Most Knowledgeable Adult" (MKA) is asked to answer the Child Questionnaire, while separate permission is solicited from teenage members in the household for questions relating to them.

Age and Sex

To accurately capture a person's age and minimize the chance of error, the U.S. Census Bureau asks two questions: "What is this person's age and what is this person's date of birth?" (U.S. Census Bureau, 2003). The answers can be checked against each other at the time of the interview and any discrepancies resolved at that time. If only a single question is asked, Bradburn et al. (2004) recommend asking year of birth, because it may be less threatening than asking directly about age.

The primary question used in the CHIS 2001 to find out ages is, "What is your date of birth?" (CHIS 2001, section A). If the respondent does not provide a date of birth, the interviewer proceeds with asking either, "What month and year were you born?" "What is your age now, please?" or "Are you between 18 and 29, between 30 and 39, between 40 and 44, between 45 and 49, between 50 and 64, or 65 or older?" respectively. These alternative forms are asked in an iterative computer-assisted telephone interviewing (CATI) interview to minimize the degree of item nonresponse to the age question. In the UNICEF MICS-2, the household respondent is asked either, "How old is (name)?" or "How old was (name) on his/her last birthday?" (UNICEF MICS-2, Household Listing Form, question 4).

In a study comparing methods that conform closely to the census and CHIS approaches with questions comparable to those used in the MICS, Peterson (1984) found that all the questions tended to yield fairly accurate responses. However, he found that asking, "How old are you?" resulted in the greatest number of refusals to answer (9.7 percent) and that asking people to put themselves into age categories—eighteen to twenty-four, twenty-five to thirty-four, and so on—resulted in the highest percentage of inaccurate responses (4.9 percent) among the methods that were compared. Based on these findings, asking the respondent's date of birth or month and year of birth would seem to be the best means of minimizing reporting errors when people are asked their age.

Gender is generally recorded on the basis of observation. However, the question may have to be asked for family members who are not present at the time of an in-person interview or directly of the household respondent in a telephone interview—"What is this person's sex?" (U.S. Census Bureau, 2003); "Are you male or female?" (CHIS); or "Is (name) male or female?" (MICS)—if not apparent from the person's name or other information provided during the interview. For studies of transgendered or transsexual populations, it may be helpful to distinguish between the respondent's gender at birth and current gender identity, since respondents may classify themselves as "transgender" or "transsexual" (Fikar & Keith, 2004; Kenagy, 2005; Lindley, Nicholson, Kerby, & Lu, 2003; Nemoto, Operario, Keatley, Han, & Soma, 2004; Shankle, Maxwell, Katzman, & Landers, 2003).

Marital Status

The U.S. Census asks, "What is this person's marital status?" The response categories provided are "now married, widowed, divorced, separated, or never married" (U.S. Census Bureau, 2003). For every person age fifteen or older in the UNICEF MICS-2, the respondent is asked, "What is the marital status of (*name*)?" The categories provided to respond are currently "married/in union, widowed, divorced, separated, and never married." For persons eighteen years of age or older, the CHIS 2001 asks, "Are you now married, living with a partner in a marriage-like relationship, widowed, divorced, separated or never married?" (CHIS 2001, section H, question AH43). It should be noted that the response categories like "in union" and "living with a partner in a marriage-like relationship" expand the definition of marital status to include individuals who are living as committed partners, even if they are not formally married, which may be important to consider, depending on the analytical intent and population that is the focus of the study.

Race and Ethnicity

A multitude of approaches have been used since the late eighteenth century in the United States to collect data on race and ethnicity, each reflecting trends in U.S. history relating to racial and ethnic populations. Included are the collection of data on "whites," "slaves," and "Indians" in the 1790 Census; data on ethnic immigrants in the nineteenth century to reflect the influx of immigrants into the United States; and data on racial and ethnicity in the 1960s to monitor the reinforcement of the 1964 Civil Rights Acts and the 1965 Voting Rights Act. In the 1990s, recommendations to gather data on a multitude of racial and ethnic groups reflect findings from methodological research, discussions regarding the effect of the U.S. Census undercount by race and ethnicity on research, and expressed preferences for multiracial classifications (Anderson & Fienberg, 2000; Johnson et al., 1997; Wallman, Evinger, & Schechter, 2000).

The 2000 U.S. Census first asked, "Is this person Spanish/Hispanic/Latino?" followed by the question, "What is this person's race?" with the instruction, "Mark one or more races to indicate what this person considers himself/herself to be." Response categories were "White," "Black, African American, or Negro," "American

Indian or Alaska Native," as well as a variety of Asian groups ("Asian Indian, Chinese, Filipino, Japanese, Korean, Vietnamese, Native Hawaiian, Guamanian or Chamorro, Samoan, Other Pacific Islander, Other Asian"), or some other race (U.S. Census Bureau, 2003).

The Office of Management and Budget (OMB) race and ethnicity standards call for the use of self-reporting as the preferable means of identifying the race and ethnicity of the respondent (Office of Management and Budget, 1997; Wallman et al., 2000). Unlike earlier versions of these standards, it requires federal researchers to offer the respondents the option of selecting one or more racial or ethnic designations. The minimum racial categories required are "American Indian or Alaska Native, Asian, Black or African American, and Native Hawaiian or other Pacific Islander," and the minimum categories for ethnicity are "Hispanic or Latino" and "Not Hispanic or Latino." However, the 2000 U.S. Census questions on race and ethnicity provide considerable more detail than required by the minimum OMB standards.

Underlying the decision to modify the way that race and ethnicity were asked in surveys are responses to concerns raised by respondents regarding their preferences for how they wished to be identified (U.S. Department of Labor, Bureau of Labor Statistics and Bureau of the Census, 1996); the merits of forcing them to choose only one race or ethnicity category as well as the fact that the substitution of a category for mixed race persons increased the number of respondents who identified themselves as being of mixed race (Johnson et al., 1997); and findings that indicate that a higher response rate (an increase from 82 to 91 percent) was found for the Hispanic origin question when the question was asked before the one on race as opposed to asking it after asking about the respondent's race (Anderson & Fienberg, 2000).

The approaches used in the CHIS conform with the directives for asking these questions issued for federally supported surveys by the Office of Management and Budget (CHIS 2001, section A, questions AA4–AA5F) (Office of Management and Budget, 1997). In CHIS 2001 the interviewer asked two questions during the screening interview to identify racial or ethnic subpopulations: "Do any of these adults who live in your household consider themselves to be (ETHNICITY) or of (ETHNICITY) descent?" and, "Do any of these adults who live in your household consider their ancestry to be Pakistani, Indian, Bangladeshi, Sri Lankan or Bhutanese descent?" (UCLA Center for Health Policy Research, 2002b, p. 2-2). In the core interview, the respondents were first asked, "Are you of Latino or Hispanic origin?" (question AA4). If they answered yes, then questions were asked about their specific Latino or Hispanic ancestry or origin (question AA5). The question that follows on race asks, "Also, please tell me which one OR MORE of the following you would use to describe yourself. Would you describe yourself as Native Hawaiian, Other Pacific Islander, American Indian, Alaska Native, Asian, Black, African American, or White?" (question AA5A). Other questions ask about specific Asian and Native American groupings (questions AA5B-E).

One of the issues to consider in deciding which type of race/ethnicity question should be included in a survey is how important it is to be able to analyze findings by race/ethnicity. If in developing the objectives of the study, as noted in Chapter Two, the researcher determines that race/ethnicity is a central determining factor of the outcomes of interest or there is an interest in detailed racial/ethnic subgroup comparisons, then an expanded set of questions, as reflected in CHIS questionnaire, may be required. If not, a single question (for example, question AA5A in the CHIS 2001) might suffice.

Education

The 2000 U.S. Census asked, "What is the highest degree or level of school this person has COMPLETED?" (U.S. Census Bureau, 2003). The question used in the Current Population Survey (CPS) to determine the educational level of persons fifteen years of age and older is similar to that used in the census: "What is the highest level of school completed or highest degree completed?" (U.S. Census Bureau, 2002).

For everyone eighteen years of age older in the CHIS 2001, the following question is asked to elicit information about years of schooling: "What is the highest grade or year of education you have completed and received credit for?" The response categories differ somewhat from those used in the CPS and census, but generally include no formal education, grade school, high school or equivalent, four-year college or university, graduate or professional school, two-year junior or community college, and vocational, business, or trade school (see question AH47 in CHIS 2001).

Two questions were used in the UNICEF MICS-2 to ascertain the respondent's education. For persons five years of age or older, respondents were asked, "What is the highest level of school (*name*) attended?" as well as, "What is the highest grade (*name*) completed at this level?" For children ages five through seventeen, respondents are asked, "Which level and grade is/was (*name*) attending?" In the MICS, the respondent is given broad categories (preschool, primary, secondary or nonstandard curriculum) as response options for the level of school attended (UNICEF MICS-2, Education Module, questions 15–22).

Bradburn et al. (2004) suggest that to obtain the most accurate measure of educational level, one should ask separate questions regarding the highest degree received and the number of years of school completed because some individuals may have received a diploma (for example, GED) while having completed fewer years of formal schooling. It is also important, they argue, to clearly specify the level or number of years actually completed to reduce the upward bias likely from asking about the level or years simply attended.

Employment Status

The U.S. Census and Current Population Survey collect detailed data on employment status (Bradburn et al., 2004; U.S. Census Bureau, 2002, 2003; U.S. Department of Labor, Bureau of Labor Statistics, 2001, n.d.). The CHIS provides a useful example of a parallel but more circumscribed set of questions on employment status. In the CHIS 2001, the respondent is asked a core question regarding his or her employment status followed by a series of follow-up questions on employment (CHIS 2001, section K). In the first question on employment, the respondent is asked, "Which of the following were you doing last week?" Depending on whether the respondent indicated that he or she was "working at a job/business," "with a job/business but not at work," "looking for work," or "not working at a job/business," the respondent was asked a series of questions regarding the nature of his or her employment activity. A respondent who was not working was asked, "What is the main reason you did not work last week?" The person who was working was asked, "On your MAIN job, are you employed by a private company, a federal, state, or local government, OR are you self employed, OR are you working without pay in a family business or farm?" By distinguishing between individuals who are self-employed or working in a family business or farm, the interviewer is attempting to sort out those who work for themselves from those who work for others.

This series of questions regarding employment status is used to determine whether an individual is employed, and if not employed, whether he or she is actively seeking a job. This questioning is typically used to replicate the methods used to compute estimates of unemployment using a definition that is similar to how the Bureau of Labor Statistics defines unemployment. The survey designer will need to decide what level of detail is necessary, given the purposes to which the data will be put.

Occupation

Asking respondents to fit themselves into precoded categories of occupations designed by the researcher may result in considerable variability based on how different individuals think their job should be coded. Yet asking individuals an open-ended question about what their occupation is may yield insufficient detail to code accurately many responses.

The questions asked in the CHIS about the type of job and industry in which people are employed are used to code occupations according to guidelines developed by the U.S. Bureau of the Census (U.S. Census Bureau, 1992). A series of questions is asked, including "What is the MAIN kind of work YOU do?" and "What kind of business or industry is this?" (CHIS 2001, section K, questions AK5–6).

Occupation as well as education and income are traditionally used to construct measures of socioeconomic status (SES). The researcher choosing an approach for asking about occupation—or wondering whether to include such a question at all—must weigh the costs and benefits of asking it. This may include evaluating the burden of asking the questions, coding and processing the data, as well as the overall analytical merits of having comprehensive composite measures of SES that combine occupation, educational status and earnings, given the study objectives (Warren, Sheridan, & Hauser, 1998).

Income

Questions about income are some of the hardest to get good data on in surveys and generally result in the highest rates of refusals by survey respondents. There are potential problems that can occur as a result of item nonresponse, over- or underreporting amounts, sources of income and types of incomes, errors that can occur in the process of retrieving information (memory and recall problems), and problems relating to cognitive misunderstanding regarding what certain terms may mean, for example, "non-wage cash payments" (Moore, Stinson, & Welniak, 2000).

A "split-point" form of asking the question, in which the respondent is asked whether family income is above or below a certain amount, has been found to reduce the threat to the respondent and, hence, to make him or her more willing to answer (Locander & Burton, 1976). The CHIS makes use of this and other devices to maximize the quality and completeness of the information obtained on this question. The CHIS 2001 asks, "We don't need to know exactly, but could you tell me if your HOUSEHOLD'S ANNUAL income from all sources BEFORE TAXES is more than $20,000 per year or is it less?" Depending on whether the respondent reported a family income of more or less than $20,000, different computer screens with a number of income categories appear, which then allow the interviewer to ask the respondent, "Is it . . . ?" followed by a series of income groups (CHIS 2001, section K, questions AK11-AK16).

To increase the accuracy of reporting, it might have been helpful to incorporate a detailed list of items that should be included in this family income figure, as is done in the 2004 National Center for Health Statistics–Health Interview Survey (NCHS, n.d.), for example: "Now I am going to ask you about the total combined income in [year], including income from all sources we have just talked about such as wages, salaries, Social Security or retirement benefits, help from relatives and so forth. Can you tell me that amount before taxes?"

In developing income questions, one must consider how many questions to ask to get this information. The scope of questions asked in any given survey must be dictated by the perceived importance of a certain item for analysis of the data as well as by the cost and quality trade-offs that the researcher may find it necessary to make.

Nonthreatening Questions About Behaviors

Methodological research on survey question design has demonstrated that different cognitive processes come into play when people answer factual questions about their previous behaviors or experiences depending on how threatening they perceive the questions to be. Bradburn et al. (2004) suggest that one test for determining whether a question is potentially threatening is to consider whether the respondent might think there is a "right" or "wrong" answer in terms of what a socially acceptable response would be. Questions about alcohol consumption or sexual practices—as are the questions regarding alcohol consumption in the CHIS 2001 (CHIS 2001, section E, questions AE11-AE14) and the contraception and the HIV/AIDS modules in the MICS-2—could be considered threatening. Some respondents may feel that other people would frown on these activities. Questions about whether people went to a doctor or were hospitalized in the year may be seen as less threatening because they put the respondent at less risk of being criticized for behaving one way or the other.

Formulating answers to nonthreatening questions about past behaviors relates to the second stage of the question-answering process: the memory and recall of relevant events identified by Tourangeau and his colleagues (Tourangeau, 1984; Tourangeau, Rips, & Rasinski, 2000). The two major types of memory errors that occur in surveys are that the respondent reports too much (overreporting) or too little (underreporting) relative to his or her actual experiences based on comparisons with some external criterion source, such as provider medical records or third-party payer forms.

Overreporting and Underreporting Errors

The problems that may lead to overreporting or underreporting occur in situations where respondents (1) telescope, that is, include events from outside the time period being asked about in the question, or (2) omit events that should have been included within the reference period. A respondent's ability to recall events is a function of the time period over which the events are to be remembered (past two weeks, six months, or year, for example) and of the salience or significance of the event to the person (being hospitalized, for example, is a more salient event for respondents than the number of times they ate carrots in the past year). Manipulating the recall period for the target behaviors can result in opposite effects in terms of telescoping and omission errors. The shorter the recall period, the less likely it is that respondents will omit events but the more likely they are to telescope behaviors from the surrounding periods of time into this shorter reporting period. In contrast, the more salient an event is, the less likely it is to be omitted, but the more likely it is to be incorporated into the time period about which the question is asked even when it occurred outside that period.

In the CHIS 2001, respondents are asked, "During the past 12 months, how many times have you seen a medical doctor?" and for those who had not seen a doctor in the past twelve months, "About how long has it been since you last saw a medical doctor about your own health?" (CHIS 2001, section H, questions AH5-AH6).

The accurate recall of physician visits, as well as of hospitalizations, decays (diminishes) substantially for longer as opposed to shorter periods of recall. This would suggest that it is important to consider the frame of reference that respondents use when asked to recall events and the devices that can be applied in developing questions to minimize both underreporting and overreporting errors in survey reports of health events.

Cognitive Survey Research Procedures

Cognitive research on surveys in general and health surveys in particular has documented the importance of more fully understanding the thought processes in which respondents engage in answering factual questions, as well as the factors that constrain or enhance recall, as a basis for deciding how best to design such questions (Collins, 2003; Jobe, Tourangeau, & Smith, 1993; Lee et al., 1999; McCarthy & Safer, 2000; National Center for Health Statistics, 1994b; Rasinski, Willis, Baldwin, Yeh, & Lee, 1999; Schwarz, 1999; Schwarz & Oyserman, 2001; Schwarz & Sudman, 1994).

Respondents' memory and reporting of events are influenced by both the structure of the task (questions or questionnaire) and the techniques (or schemata) they may call on in answering them. A basic assumption underlying cognitive survey research is that respondents are "cognitive misers," that is, they will try to minimize the thought and effort needed to complete a task (respond to a question) by looking for clues (or a frame of reference) from the stimulus (item) that is presented to them or from convenient and familiar rules of thumb based on their previous (specific and general) experiences.

One of the most important frames of reference derived from the question itself, for example, is the response categories that are provided to answer it. Methodological research has documented that the distributions of answers people give to questions about the number of times they engage in a particular behavior is influenced by the format and range of values provided in the response categories (Bless, Bohner, Hild, & Schwarz, 1992; Gaskell, O'Muircheartaigh, & Wright, 1994; Moxey & Sanford, 2000; O'Muircheartaigh, Gaskell, & Wright, 1993; Schwarz, 1990; Schwarz & Bienias, 1990; Waterman, Blades, & Spencer, 2001; Wright, Gaskell, & O'Muircheartaigh, 1997). For example, respondents who were given a high-frequency scale regarding the number of times they watch television on average each week (ranging from up to ten hours to more than twenty-five hours) were more likely to report a higher rate of television watching than those provided a low-frequency scale (up to two and a half to more than ten hours). This tendency is greater for relatively frequently occurring (or mundane) behaviors (eating certain foods regularly) than for rare (or salient) events. A questionnaire design alternative to deal with this problem is to use an open-ended rather than a closed-end response format, especially when it is unclear what frequency range for a question may be most fitting for a given study population.

Cognitive survey researchers have also helped to surface the internal schemata or approaches respondents use in answering questions. Respondents may try to recall and count the specific events (episodes) that occurred relatively infrequently during the reference period (three or fewer times), but they are much more likely to use various estimation strategies for events that occurred more often. An array of hypotheses have been explored in both laboratory and field settings to attempt to identify these strategies.

For example, respondents may set limits to (or bound) their answers based on previous experiences or an implicit or implied comparison with others; they may round their estimates to prototypical values (such as seven, fourteen, or thirty days); they may think of a kind of autobiographical time line or landmark public or private event (a presidential election or the birth of their first child) as a point of reference; disaggregate (break down) the task into a series of simpler tasks (the different reasons for their child's going to see a doctor) and then sum or impute a summary (total visits to the doctor) based on these discrete computations; or they may consider what they typically do or what they know they "should" do (get a Pap smear or mammogram) (Blair & Burton, 1987; Burton & Blair, 1991; Crawford, Huttenlocher, & Engebretson, 2000; Huttenlocher, Hedges, & Bradburn, 1990; Jobe et al., 1993).

Trying to recall accurately specific episodes, especially frequently appearing events, may lead to the underreporting of these events, whereas employing estimation strategies can result in overreporting. Research has suggested that when the approach to asking questions attempts to take into account the heuristic or devices that respondents use in trying to answer a question, then more accurate reporting can result (Czaja, Blair, Bickart, & Eastman, 1994; Gwyer & Clifford, 1997; Kurbat, Shevell, & Rips, 1998; Mooney & Gramling, 1991; National Center for Health Statistics, 1989a, 1989b, 1991, 1992a, 1992b, 1994a; Waterman et al., 2001).

Employing cognitive interviewing and think-aloud strategies during the instrument development stage is a good way of surfacing the ways respondents go about answering a question (see Chapter Eight). There is also evidence from research on the recall of visits to a physician (Jobe et al., 1990; Means & Loftus, 1991; National Center for Health Statistics, 1989a), the use of preventive procedures (Bowman, Redman, Dickinson, Gibberd, & Sanson-Fisher, 1991; National Center for Health Statistics, 1994a; Warnecke et al., 1997), stressful events (Shrimpton, Oates, & Hayes, 1998), and diet (Armstrong et al., 2000; Buzzard & Sievert, 1994; Kohlmeier, 1994) that when respondents are provided greater opportunity for free recall of relevant events, use explicit cognitive techniques (think-aloud, time line, or the decomposition of their answer into parts) in choosing how they come up with an estimate, or are given more time for responding, they provide more accurate answers.

Bounded Recall Procedures

The primary device used to reduce overreporting of health events as a result of telescoping events from other time periods—especially those that took place before the date specified in the interview—is the bounded recall procedure. This procedure was developed for continuous panel surveys, where respondents could be interviewed at the beginning and end of the time periods referenced in the survey questionnaire. The first interview would serve to identify events that occurred before the interview period so that they could clearly be eliminated if the respondent later reported that they occurred during the period between the first and second interviews. This bounded recall device was used in panel surveys conducted in connection with the 1977 National Medical Care Expenditure Survey (NMCES) and the 1987 National Medical Expenditure Survey (NMES), and more recent Medical Expenditure Panel Survey (MEPS) in which summary reports of what respondents said during the previous interview were provided to interviewers. Interviewers could then use these reports to make sure that events were not reported a second time as well as to complete certain questions through information that had become available since the previous interview (such as hospital or doctor bills) (see Resource E).

Sudman, Finn, and Lannom (1984) developed and tested an adaptation of the bounded recall procedure for a cross-sectional survey using several of the questions asked in the National Health Interview Survey. This study involved an adaptation of the survey questions about disability days, days spent in bed, physician visits, and nights spent in a hospital for a personal interview survey of a probability sample of Illinois residents. Respondents were administered questions about their health behaviors in the previous month (the inclusion dates being referenced were specified) and were then asked about corresponding events in the current calendar month. After adjustments for the numbers of days on which reporting was based, the results showed that the events reported in the current (bounded) month were less than the previous (unbounded) month and that comparable National Center for Health Statistics–National Health Interview Survey (NCHS–NHIS) estimates fell in between these two estimates. The authors concluded that "the use of bounded recall procedures in a single interview reduces telescoping" (p. 524) and that if the comparable NCHS–NHIS questions were explicitly bounded they might produce lower estimates as well. Subsequent research has documented that asking people about the same procedure twice, first in connection with a given reference period (physical exam within the last six months) and then in connection with the reference period of interest (within the last two months), can also reduce overreporting (Loftus, Klinger, Smith, & Fiedler, 1990).

Memory Aid Procedures

The main question design devices used to reduce errors of omission help jog the respondent's memory or recall of relevant events. They include using aided recall techniques, records, and diaries.

Aided Recall Techniques. These methods are the simplest of the three memory aid devices and place the least burden on respondents. They basically provide explicit cues to aid respondents in recalling all the events they should recall in thinking about the question. Clues are included in the questions about physician visits to make sure respondents explicitly consider visits that they may have made to a number of different physician specialists as well as those with a nurse or someone else working for the doctor: "During the past 12 months, did you delay or not get any other medical care you felt you needed—such as seeing a doctor, a specialist, or other health professional?" (CHIS 2001, section H, question AH22).

Methodological studies comparing these versions of the questions with those in which memory aids were not provided showed that larger numbers of visits were reported in general and for the types of providers listed in the version in which aids were used (National Center for Health Statistics, 1985). Other research has shown that the use of memory aids led to a lower rate of overreporting of the number of weeks of missing work because of illness, reports of one's own income, the number of weeks unemployed, and health behaviors, such as self-reports of estimated minutes of walking (Belli, Shay, & Stafford, 2001; Johnson, Sallis, & Hovell, 2000).

Records. A second memory aid recommended to reduce the underreporting of health events is to ask respondents to consult personal records, such as checkbooks, doctor or hospital bills, appointment books, or other sources during or in advance of the interview to aid them in answering certain questions. Large-scale national surveys carried out by NCHS and the Agency for Healthcare Research and Quality (see Resource E) have employed this technique, generally by sending a letter in advance of a personal interview to inform respondents about the study and encourage them to have relevant records handy when the interviewer came.

This device is less useful for telephone surveys, especially those that are based on random digit dialing techniques. These techniques provide no advance warning to the interviewer or the respondent about who will fall into the study and therefore no opportunity to encourage them to get relevant information together beforehand. There is also a much greater opportunity for the respondents to terminate the interview or refuse to cooperate when called back a second time after being asked to check their records. As mentioned in Chapter Six, computerized databases linking telephone numbers to addresses are commercially available, however. Although it would add to the time and cost of doing the survey, such databases can be used to identify mailing addresses for sending an advance letter, if it is particularly useful to do so.

Finally, using records as a means of collecting data may also be a useful approach to consider when collecting data about specific testing procedures such as childhood immunizations when respondents may not have cognitively encoded the information initially or have very poor recall of the specifics of the events (Lee et al., 1999).

Diaries. A third technique to aid respondents' reporting of events is the use of a diary in which they can record these events on a regular basis, as they occur (Garry, Sharman, Feldman, Marlatt, & Loftus, 2002; Graham, Catania, Brand, Duong, & Canchola, 2003). In the NMCES, NMES, and MEPS surveys described earlier, respondents were asked to use calendars provided by the researchers to record certain relevant health events when they occurred (they took a day off work due to illness, had an appointment with the doctor, had a prescription filled, and so on). The respondent then consulted the diary when interviewed about these events.

Log diaries have been used in the National Ambulatory Medical Care Survey and other physician surveys in which doctors and their staffs are asked to record selected information about a sample of patients who come into their office during a particular period of time. In these instances, diaries were the major data collection devices. Diaries are useful for recording information on events that occur frequently but may not have a high salience to respondents (such as recalling what one ate). Two of the biggest problems in identifying the nutritional content of the foods people eat relate to the accuracy of recall in what was eaten even twenty-four hours prior to an interview and to the representativeness of this one day for eating habits in general. Asking respondents to record what they eat over a several-day period can help reduce errors of this kind.

Study participants often perceive keeping diaries to be burdensome and time-consuming, and this may result in inaccurate or incomplete information being provided. In addition, monitoring and processing diaries can be expensive. For some types of studies, as in the food-intake example, it may be the best or even the only way to gather the required information. In this case, the researcher will need to consider the trade-offs in terms of the cost and quality of gathering data in this way and if incentives to study participants to maximize cooperation might be helpful.

Threatening Questions About Behaviors

Different rules need to be considered when formulating threatening questions about health and health care behaviors. Tourangeau (1984) suggested that at the final or response stage of answering a question, considerations other than the facts come into play as respondents contemplate the answers they will provide.

Respondents may feel less inclined to provide responses to threatening questions if they feel that they are being treated like "objects" as opposed to being treated like "subjects." For example, Ross and Reynolds (1996, p. 901) indicate that when survey respondents are treated as objects, the focus is on using question wording, order, or other aspects of questionnaire design, as well as using interviewer characteristics and appearance or payments to "convince or manipulate the respondent into participating." In the process of treating the respondents as subjects, researchers focus on examining the internal rational decision-making processes respondents use when answering a question as well as their possession of the knowledge needed to respond to a question.

It is understandable then that in the face of threatening questions, respondents may decide to provide a less-than-honest response if they think their answer will cause them to be viewed as "deviant" or, at a minimum, as behaving in a socially "undesirable" way. Various researchers have suggested a number of devices in designing threatening questions for reducing these tendencies on the part of respondents (Bradburn & Danis, 1984; Bradburn et al., 1979, 2004; Lee, 1993; Tourangeau, 1984; Tourangeau et al., 2000). Their suggestions are presented in terms of each of the building blocks that were outlined in Chapter Eight for constructing survey questions: examining words, phrases, sentences, responses, instructions, questions, and questionnaire design, as well as understanding the cognitive processes respondents use to answer survey questions.

Words

The words used in phrasing threatening questions should be familiar to the respondent, especially because words may not mean the same thing to all respondents (Amaya-Jackson, Socolar, Hunter, Runyan, & Colindres, 2000; Binson & Catania, 1998; Michaels & Giami, 1999; Schwartz, 2000; Smith, 1999). For example, Schwartz (2000, p. 817) notes that there is extensive debate around the use of specific words and phrases such as "force," "held down," "gave you alcohol," and "you could not give consent" in studies of violence against women because of disagreements regarding their meaning and the impact of the way they are asked in surveys.

The approach employed in the UNICEF MICS-2 to determine the types of birth control methods the women in the survey used is to ask them to indicate which method they have used in their own words, without prompting them in terms of a specific response. This allows them to answer the question with terms that they understand and are comfortable in using (UNICEF MICS-2, Contraceptive Use Module, question 4).

Phrases

Concerning the balance of the phrasing to use with threatening questions, Bradburn et al. (2004) suggest that it may in fact be better to load the questions to reduce a tendency for respondents to underreport socially undesirable behavior when answering such questions. One approach to loading a question deliberately is to suggest that others also engage in the behavior. For example, a statement of this kind is provided in the UNICEF MICS (UNICEF MICS-2, Contraceptive Use Module, question 3): "Some couples use various ways or methods to delay or avoid a pregnancy. Are you currently doing something or using any method to delay or avoid getting pregnant?"

A second approach to loading a question to reduce the underreporting of what may be perceived to be undesirable behaviors is to suggest that people in authority support these behaviors. An example of this technique is used in a

Chicago area general population survey on AIDS knowledge and attitudes: "Some government health officials say that giving clean needles to users of illegal drugs would greatly reduce the spread of AIDS. Do you favor or oppose making clean needles available to people who use illegal drugs as a way to reduce the spread of AIDS?" (Aday, 1996, p. 411).

A third approach is to ask the question so as to imply that the person does engage in the behavior by asking how often he or she engages in it, not if he or she does. For example, a question to elicit the consumption of alcoholic beverages could be posed, "In the past two weeks, on how many days did you drink any alcoholic beverages such as beer, wine, or liquor?" rather than asking, "Did you? [drink any of these beverages]?" A response category could be provided for those who said none. A risk in asking questions in this way is that people who do not engage in these behaviors might be offended by what seems to be a built-in assumption that they did engage in what they believed would be perceived to be socially unacceptable practices.

Sentences

Another way to reduce the underreporting of what are thought to be socially undesirable practices is to make the sentences used in asking them longer rather than shorter. There are several examples of this approach in the UNICEF MICS (UNICEF MICS-2, HIV/AIDS Module, question 3, Contraceptive Use Module, question 2). In these instances, several sentences of explanation about the question are read to respondents before they are asked to respond directly themselves. Longer questions tend to increase the reported frequencies of socially sensitive behavior compared with shorter questions. A longer question gives the respondent more time to think about the question, provides a fuller explanation of what is being asked and why, and is generally thought to underline the importance of answering it (Bradburn et al., 1979, 2004).

Responses

Another technique recommended to increase the reporting of behaviors that are traditionally underreported is to use open-ended rather than closed-end response formats. With closed-end formats, respondents may assume there is a ceiling on what they should report or perceive based on the ranges provided and that they must be odd people if the frequency with which they engage in the behaviors meets or exceeds that limit. For example, the question in the CHIS 2001 about the number of cigarettes smoked each day over the past thirty days (CHIS 2001, section E, question AE16) is open-ended in format. It asks the respondent "how many" without providing categories in responding.

Instructions

Another useful device in designing questionnaires is to build in transition sentences or introductions at points when the topic being addressed changes. This may be particularly important when introducing threatening topics so that the respondent is forewarned about what is coming next and given an opportunity to decide how he or she wants to respond. Both the UNICEF MICS and CHIS surveys make frequent use of this device. For example, in the UNICEF survey, when the interviewers introduce a series of questions about perceptions regarding the transmission of HIV, they are told to say, "Your answers are very important to help understand the needs of people in (*country name*). Again this information is completely private and anonymous. Please answer yes or no to each question" (UNICEF MICS-2, HIV/AIDS Module, question 3).

Questionnaire

Other suggestions about asking threatening questions relate to the order and context in which they appear in the questionnaire. For example, Bradburn et al. (2004) suggest that when asking about undesirable behaviors, it is better to ask whether the person had ever engaged in the behavior before asking about his or her current practices. For behaviors that are perceived to be socially desirable, they advise asking about current practices first. They argue that respondents will also be more willing to report something in the distant past first because past events are less threatening. Interviewers should then progress toward asking them about current behavior.

This device was used in the CHIS 2001 in asking a series of questions on the topic of smoking. Respondents were asked, "Have you smoked at least 100 cigarettes in your ENTIRE LIFE?" Then they were asked, "Do you now smoke cigarettes every day, some days or not at all?" followed by, "In the past 30 days, when you smoked, how many cigarettes did you smoke per day (on the days you smoked)?" (CHIS 2001, section E, questions AE15-AE16).

Survey designers may thus need to consider a combination of strategies to reduce the threat perceived by respondents in answering questions about socially undesirable events and to increase the reporting of these events—asking them how often they engage in some behavior now after moving them through a somewhat less threatening sequence of questions about whether they ever engaged in it.

It is also desirable for threatening questions to appear at the end of the questionnaire, after respondents have a clearer idea of what the study is about and the interviewer has had an opportunity to build a rapport with them. Such questions could also be embedded among others that are somewhat threatening or sensitive so that they do not stick out like sore thumbs. For example, one of the most sensitive questions in the CHIS 2001 questionnaire—"Are you gay, (lesbian,) or bisexual?"—appears near the end of the survey after questions that deal with citizenship status and whether they felt that they have ever been discriminated against in receiving health care (CHIS 2001, section H, question AH45). All of these questions may, to some extent, be considered sensitive ones. But placing the question about sexual orientation in this context and at this point in the questionnaire may reduce the threat some may feel in answering it. This is an example of the art of thinking through the placement of such questions; the science of how to do it is far from well developed.

Questionnaire Administration

Field procedures that can help reduce the threat of sensitive questions include relatively anonymous methods, such as using self-administered questionnaires rather than personal or telephone interviews, using a combination of telephone interviewing and interactive voice response technology, having questions read aloud to the respondents through earphones using computer-assisted personal interviewing surveys, or asking a knowledgeable informant rather than the individuals themselves to provide the information. Respondents may be more inclined to report threatening behaviors for others than about themselves. Under certain circumstances (such as administering an interview in a private setting way from home), the interviewer administration of sensitive questions may produce data that are more accurate than self-administered surveys. What is central is that the respondent feels that confidentiality and anonymity are assured (Corkrey & Parkinson, 2002; Hay, 1990; Fowler & Stringfellow, 2001; Martin, Anderson, Romans, Mullen, & O'Shea, 1993; Rasinski, Willis, Baldwin, Yeh, & Lee, 1999; Schwartz, 2000; Tourangeau & Smith, 1996).

A device to maximize the anonymity of respondents' reporting of threatening events is the randomized response technique (Fox & Tracy, 1986; Warner, 1965). This technique involves giving the respondent a choice of answering either a threatening or a nonthreatening question: "In the past five years, have you used a needle to inject illegal drugs?" or "Is your birthday in August?" The respondent is then told to use a randomization device, such as flipping a coin, to decide which question to answer—if "heads," to answer the first question, and if "tails," the second. The interviewer or test administrator will neither see nor be told the results of the coin toss and, hence, which question the respondent was supposed to answer. Researchers, however, would be able to compute the probability of a particular (yes) response to the nonthreatening question. Any departure from this probability in the actual responses can be used to estimate the proportion of responses to the threatening item.

The randomized response technique does not enable responses to be linked to individual respondents, which limits the explanatory analyses that can be conducted with other respondent characteristics. There are few studies validating the technique, and evidence exists that some respondents are still likely to lie, but it is difficult to determine how many and who they are. Furthermore, the procedure may seem like a complex one to respondents, many of whom may be suspicious and therefore reluctant or unwilling to cooperate in answering the question (Beldt, Daniel, & Garcha, 1982; Biemer & Lyberg, 2003; Bradburn et al., 2004; Fox & Tracy, 1986; Landsheer, van der Heijden, & van Gils, 1999; Umesh & Peterson, 1991).

Health surveys have always dealt with sensitive topics. This focus has become even more pronounced in recent years, with morbidities such as HIV/AIDS, mental illness, and drug and alcohol abuse coming increasingly to the public's attention. More research needs to be conducted to examine the reliability and validity of the variety of mechanisms for asking questions about threatening topics.

In general, however, the best advice is to (1) try devices that seem to have worked in other studies; (2) attempt to validate aggregate estimates on the behaviors for which data are gathered against other data—if available; (3) conduct pilot studies using split-ballot alternatives of the questions to see if they agree—when time and money permit; and (4) ask respondents directly at the end of the interview which questions they thought were particularly threatening. This last step makes it possible to determine if respondents' perceptions of threat are associated with different rates of reporting behaviors and, if so, to take this into account when analyzing and interpreting the findings.

Special Considerations for Special Populations

Asking people of color or ethnic minorities to indicate their race, ethnicity, or ancestry or to respond to questions about whether they engage in what are thought to be "socially undesirable" practices (substance abuse, physically disciplining a child, high-risk sexual behaviors) does in fact place them in a kind of double jeopardy. Such questions are often difficult or troublesome to answer in general because of the categories that are presented for responding or the fear of either informal (social rejection) or formal (legal recourse) sanctions if answered honestly. The historical and contemporary realities of racism and xenophobia further confound both the message and the meaning of asking such questions of minority groups (Jones, LaVeist, & Lillie-Blanton, 1991; Kluegel, 1990; Mays & Jackson, 1991; Williams, 1994). Methodological research suggests that racial and ethnic minorities tend to underreport sensitive behaviors and respond differently to vague quantifiers (such as "very often") when answering questions about the frequency with which they have engaged in these or other behaviors (Aquilino & Lo Sciuto, 1990; Fendrich & Vaughn, 1994; Ford & Norris, 1991; Schaeffer, 1991).

In addition, questions regarding race and ethnicity, income, occupation, or socioeconomic status may lead to suspicion regarding how the data will be used or concerns about what the question is really measuring. For example, some have argued that race/ethnicity is in fact an imperfect concept since it is not clear whether the question represents a genetic or biological designation or a sociocultural designation. If the former is the case, then interventions would focus on individual biology or behavior; if the latter, activities would focus on social, economic, and environmental policies to problems facing ethnic populations (Nazroo, 2003). In the same vein, asking indigent respondents about their income may evoke feelings regarding perceived powerlessness since income is used as a means of determining status in society (Ross & Reynolds, 1996). These findings argue for greater cultural sensitivity and the implementation of cognitive survey development strategies in designing and evaluating such questions in general and for minority subpopulations in particular.

Selected Examples

The California Health Interview Survey and UNICEF MICS studies provide helpful examples of standardized questions to use in asking basic demographic information. The CHIS used questions that had been subjected to cognitive testing or extensive analysis and were then pretested prior to being fielded. The UNICEF surveys have been widely adopted, tested, and implemented in many countries. As has been pointed out in this chapter, questions from these studies and the National Dental Malpractice Survey provide good examples of how to ask questions to maximize the recall of nonthreatening behaviors or maximize the willingness to respond to questions addressing sensitive topics.

Guidelines for Minimizing Survey Errors and Maximizing Survey Quality

The simple and useful proverb "Square pegs do not fit well into round holes" has merit and meaning in designing survey questions that ask people to fit themselves into categories describing who they are or how often they do things that they may not readily reveal even to those closest to them. As amply documented in this chapter, respondents will try to place themselves into the categories that survey designers construct. These categories may, however, be ill-fitting ones and the survey respondents' presentation of themselves and their experiences may be distorted as a result. It is useful, then, to encourage respondents like those to be included in the survey to define the contours of their thinking about the topics to be covered in the study before developing the questions that are presumably intended to reveal them.

The use of poorly written or untested questions can lead to inaccurate responses from respondents. Likewise, the use of outdated questions that do not account for the nuances of new living situations (marital status), sexual orientation, racial or ethnic differences, or related issues can result in inaccurate and incomplete reflections of the lives of the respondents. The application of state-of-the-art principles of questionnaire design serves as a first step in avoiding or minimizing these problems. This can be supplemented by conducting pilot studies (for example, cognitive testing of questions or split-ballot tests of questions) to examine variations of questions before beginning a study (Table 10.1).

Supplementary Sources

For additional information and examples in developing demographic and threatening and nonthreatening behavioral questions, see Fowler (1995), Lee (1993), and Bradburn, Sudman, and Wansink (2004). Also see the Web sites for the U.S. Census Bureau, the National Center for Health Statistics, and the Agency for Health Care Research and Quality (see Resource D).

TABLE 10.1. SURVEY ERRORS: SOURCES AND SOLUTIONS— FORMULATING QUESTIONS ABOUT DEMOGRAPHICS AND BEHAVIOR.

	Systematic Errors			*Variable Errors*
	Questionnaire Effects: Under- or Over-reporting	**Respondent Effects: Social Desirability Bias**	**Mode Effects: Social Desirability Bias**	**Questionnaire Effects: Order and Context**
Solutions to Errors	Employ cognitive question and questionnaire design and evaluation procedures, and use bounded recall and memory aids to improve the accuracy in answering non-threatening questions about behavior.	Employ cognitive question and questionnaire design and evaluation procedures to enhance the honesty in answering threatening questions about behavior.	Consider using more anonymous modes of data collection.	Conduct split-ballot experiments to evaluate how answers to questions vary when they appear in a different order in the questionnaire.

CHAPTER ELEVEN

FORMULATING QUESTIONS ABOUT KNOWLEDGE AND ATTITUDES

Chapter Highlights

1. Rules for formulating questions about people's knowledge of different health or health care topics should focus on how to minimize the threat that these questions may pose and the tendency of respondents to guess when they are not sure of the "right" answer.
2. In formulating attitude questions, it is particularly important to be aware of any previous research on the specific items being considered and of general methodological research on the response effects associated with alternative ways of asking or answering this type of question.

This chapter presents guidelines for formulating questions about knowledge of and attitudes toward health topics. These types of questions are more subjective than the ones discussed in Chapter Ten because they ask for judgments or opinions about—rather than simple recall of—facts.

Important assumptions underlying cognitive survey research on knowledge and attitude questions are that they are systematically stored in long-term memory and that answering them is a product of the four-stage process identified for answering survey questions in general: interpreting the question, retrieving relevant beliefs and feelings, applying them in making appropriate judgments, and selecting a response. Respondents' decisions regarding how to respond are related to their perception regarding whether their opinion would be supported as well as their willingness to speak out (Glynn, Hayes, & Shanahan, 1997; Tourangeau & Rasinski, 1988; Tourangeau, Rasinski, & D'Andrade, 1991; Tourangeau, Rips, & Rasinski, 2000).

Bradburn, Sudman, and Wansink (2004, p. 121) note, "In general, opinion is most often used to refer to views about a particular object such as a person or a policy, and attitude is more often used to refer to a bundle of opinions that are more or less coherent and are about some complex object." For opinion or attitude questions, the third stage of replying to the question (the judgment stage) may be particularly relevant. At that stage, respondents evaluate the information retrieved from memory and its relevance to answering the question and then make subjective judgments about what items of information should be combined, and how, to answer it (Bradburn et al., 2004; Tourangeau, 1984). Guidelines for formulating such questions focus on the means for accurately capturing and describing these judgments.

Knowledge questions have a somewhat more objective grounding than attitude or opinion questions because some standard or criterion for what constitutes a "right" answer is presumed to exist. Researchers should, however, think through the "correct" or "most nearly correct" answer to such questions and how they will be scored before asking them. If it turns out that more than one answer is correct or that the correctness of a given answer is open to question, then the respondents' answers may be more appropriately considered their opinions or attitudes on the matter than an indication of their knowledge relative to some standard of accuracy.

Questions About Knowledge

Questions concerning knowledge about the risk factors for certain diseases or methods to prevent or treat them have long been important components of health surveys. With the emphasis in the public health and medical care community on the impact of individual beliefs, knowledge, and behavioral change on reducing the risks of certain diseases, such as cancer, hypertension, and HIV/AIDS, questions of this kind have been asked with growing frequency in health surveys. For example, many of the Year 2010 Health Objectives for the Nation are concerned with health promotion and disease prevention activities related to smoking, alcohol consumption, obesity, lack of exercise, poor diet, and so on. Programs for effecting changes in these and other behaviors that put people's health at risk require information about the general knowledge of the risks associated with the practices, attitudes toward them, and current or anticipated behaviors in those areas.

Surveys used to gather information for developing or assessing the performance of these programs are sometimes referred to as knowledge, attitude, and behavior (KAB) surveys. The 2004 National Center for Health Statistics–National Health Interview Survey (NCHS–NHIS) is an example of a KAB study of the American public to find out about health practices related to achieving the Year 2010 Health Objectives for the Nation (National Center for Health Statistics, 2005h, n.d.)

KAB surveys have been used extensively to examine HIV/AIDS knowledge, attitudes, and behavior. Since 1990 the Centers for Disease Control and Prevention has asked respondents in the Behavioral Risk Factor Surveillance System survey a series of questions about their knowledge of and attitudes toward HIV/AIDS. These data have been used directly for planning and evaluating HIV/AIDS prevention programs (Centers for Disease Control and Prevention, National Center for Chronic Disease Prevention and Health Promotion, 2005).

KAB surveys have also been used to assess the knowledge and attitudes of needle exchange participants regarding HIV/AIDS transmission, condom use, and HIV/AIDS-related risk factors (Ksobiech et al., 2004), and to obtain information from physicians in or near such areas regarding their knowledge of the disease, their attitudes toward homosexuals in general and treating HIV/AIDS patients in particular, and their technical and clinical management of HIV/AIDS patients (Lewis, Freeman, & Corey, 1987; Richardson, Lochner, McGuigan, & Levine, 1987).

Another example of an application of KAB surveys is the use of such surveys to examine knowledge, attitudes, and responsiveness to smoking cessation interventions. For example, Ganley, Young, Denny, and Wood (1998) developed and evaluated the validity and reliability of an instrument to examine KABs relating to chewing tobacco and smoking among fourth graders. They found that students who had a negative attitude toward tobacco were far less likely to use tobacco than those with a positive attitude toward it. In another study, Ma, Yajia, Edwards, Shive, and Chau (2004) found, based on analyses of the pre- and postintervention scores related to tobacco and tobacco use of Asian American youth who participated in a culturally tailored smoking prevention program, that more than 90 percent of the respondents were able to identify the link between smoking and tobacco-related illnesses. They also found a significant change in attitude toward tobacco and smoking as a result of participating in this intervention. Studies like these have been useful in helping practitioners understand the effectiveness of smoking cessation programs.

Smoking cessation has gained substantial attention in the implementation of health programs that emanated from the multistate tobacco settlement with several U.S. tobacco companies. In 1998, the nation's largest tobacco companies signed the Master Settlement Agreement (MSA) with the attorney generals of forty-six U.S. states where they agreed to pay approximately $206 billion over a twenty-five-year period as reimbursement for tobacco-related health costs, such as Medicaid expenditures. Four other states (Florida, Mississippi, Texas, and Minnesota) had signed an earlier agreement for $40 billion in payments over a twenty-five-year period. As of 2001, 54 percent of the MSA payments had been used for health interventions (including smoking cessation), tobacco control, or economic development programs for tobacco growers (U.S. General Accounting Office, 2001). KAB surveys can be helpful in evaluating the consequences of smoking cessation and other initiatives funded under the auspices of this settlement.

Questions

In considering the specific questions to ask to find out about people's knowledge of a health topic, survey designers should first screen for whether respondents are likely to have any knowledge of the topic. At a minimum, knowledge questions are useful for finding out who has heard of the disease or diseases that are the focus of a health survey. In the UNICEF Multiple Indicator Cluster Survey (MICS)-2, for example, a key screening question asked early in the questionnaire is, "Now I would like to talk to you about what you know about serious illness, in particular, about HIV and AIDS. Have you ever heard of the virus HIV or an illness called AIDS?" (UNICEF MICS-2, HIV/AIDS Module, question 1). Those who answered no to this question were skipped out of the subsequent detailed questions that asked about respondents' KABs with respect to the disease.

Hernandez, Keys, and Balcazar (2003) found that out of twelve studies that examined knowledge of the Americans with Disabilities Act (ADA) among employees, adults with disabilities, and students of rehabilitation counseling, nine studies asked, "Have you ever heard of the ADA?" and, "How knowledgeable are you about the ADA?" to assess respondents' knowledge about the ADA. Such questions could be a likely starting point for a series of questions regarding the ADA, but these authors noted that only three of the twelve studies administered a test to examine knowledge of the specific provisions of the ADA. They suggest that future research should focus on the development of psychometrically sound measures of the knowledge of specific ADA provisions.

In general, it is advisable to ask more than one question to capture people's knowledge or understanding of the issue. Simply asking, "Do you know what causes (*disease*)?" will tell you very little about the state of awareness of those who say yes. Also, as in any other test-like situation, when people are asked to answer questions on what they "know" about an issue, those who are not sure of the right answer are likely to guess. If only one question is asked, there is a 50 percent chance that the person will get the right answer by guessing. People's summary performance on a number of items is thus a better indication of their overall knowledge of the topic. For example, in the UNICEF MICS-2, respondents are asked a number of questions regarding their knowledge about the risk factors and modes of transmission for HIV/AIDS (UNICEF MICS-2, HIV/AIDS Module, questions 2–12). (See the discussion in Chapter Three of how a knowledge index could be created from these questions.)

The main reason people claim to know more than they actually do when asked such questions is to prevent them from being viewed as ignorant on the topic. To reduce this threat, Bradburn et al. (2004, p. 205) suggest phrasing knowledge questions as though they were intended to elicit the respondents' opinions about, rather than their knowledge of, the issue or using phrases such as, "Do you think . . . . ?" "Do you happen to know . . . . ?" or "Can you recall offhand . . . . ?" The device of phrasing knowledge questions regarding HIV/AIDS so that they sound more like opinion questions is used in the UNICEF MICS, such as, "Do you think a person can get infected with the AIDS virus through supernatural means?" (UNICEF MICS-2, HIV/AIDS Module, question 4).

While an initial step in the question development process for knowledge questions would be to see what questions may have already been developed that could be drawn on, consideration should also be given to whether (1) methodological studies are available that document the internal consistency or test-retest reliability of such questions; (2) items asked of one population group are relevant and appropriate to ask in a survey of a different group; (3) using the items in a different order or context in a different questionnaire might affect how people respond to them; and (4) new items will have to be developed to capture more sophisticated knowledge of the disease and the risk factors associated with it as the scientific and clinical understanding of the illness itself advances.

Responses

When numerical responses are required to answer knowledge questions, Bradburn et al. (2004) also recommend that the question be asked in an open-ended fashion so as not to provide clues about the right answer and make it harder for respondents to guess if they are not sure of the answer. If a "don't know" option is provided, respondents are quite likely to use it if they are unsure of the answer. These responses could, however, be scored accordingly in constructing a knowledge scale—assigning a score of 1 for a correct answer, −1 for a wrong answer, and 0 for a "don't know" response (Mondak, 2001; Mondak & Davis, 2001).

Questionnaire Administration

Another way to reduce the threat of knowledge questions is to use nonverbal procedures, such as self-administered questionnaires. In this case, explicit "don't know" responses can be provided for the respondents to check if they are not sure of the right answer. However, using self-administered forms of asking such questions is more appropriate in supervised group-administered data-gathering sessions than in unsupervised situations or in mailed questionnaires where respondents might cheat by looking up or asking someone else the answer.

A method for estimating whether respondents are overreporting their knowledge of certain topics is to use "sleepers"—fictional options—when asking respondents whether they are knowledgeable about various aspects of a topic (Bishop, Tuchfarber, & Oldendick, 1986; Bradburn et al., 2004). For example, when conducting a marketing study about the brand names of different headache remedies or the penetration of a new advertising campaign, this device can be used when asking respondents if they have heard of various health care plans or medical delivery organizations. When the respondents who say they "know" about the fictitious or nonexistent alternatives are identified, their records can be excluded from the analyses or their responses to the sleeper questions coded as "wrong answers" when scores of their knowledge of the topic are constructed.

Questions About Attitudes

As indicated earlier (Chapter Three), considerable developmental effort is often required to design reliable scales for summarizing individuals' attitudes on an issue. Therefore, researchers should begin with items that others have developed and used, particularly those for which reliability and validity have already been tested. Different types of scaling methods, such as Likert scales and item response theory, also make different assumptions about how attitude items should be phrased and about the criteria to use in selecting the final items to incorporate in the scale. Researchers should determine which of these approaches they want to use in summarizing the data for the attitude items relating to a particular topic before making a final decision about the questions to ask in their survey. As with factual questions, if respondents perceive a large burden in assembling or evaluating the evidence to use in answering attitudinal items, they are likely to engage in satisficing behavior; that is, they fail to draw on all the relevant input or engage in the cognitive work to process and integrate the information required to provide a complete or unbiased response (Krosnick, 1991; Krosnick, 2002).

Rules of thumb presented here to mitigate the satisficing tendency when asking attitude questions once again follow the outline for formulating survey questions described in Chapter Eight: words, phrases, sentences, responses, questionnaire, and questionnaire administration (see Figure 8.1).

Words

Bradburn et al. (2004) point out, "Attitudes do not exist in the abstract. They are about or toward something. That something is often called the attitude object" (p. 119). It is important, then, in choosing the words for attitude questions to be clear about the object or focus of the evaluations sought from respondents. For example, if researchers have an interest in learning about respondents' attitudes or opinions toward smoking, they should clarify whether the focus is on cigarette, cigar, or pipe smoking; smoking anywhere or in the workplace or restaurants; the direct or passive effects of smoking; and so on. Perhaps all of these dimensions are of interest to the investigator, in which case a series of attitude items could be asked about the topic. The point is that researchers should clarify what they want to learn before presenting a question to respondents.

The impact of the choice of words on the way in which people respond to attitude questions has been documented by split-half experiments, in which minor changes in wording have resulted in varying distributions on what are thought to be comparable questions. One example is the use of the words *forbid* and *allow* in public opinion polls that ask whether respondents think the government should "forbid" or "allow" certain practices: "Do you think the government should forbid cigarette advertisements on television?" versus "Do you think the government should allow cigarette advertisements on television?" There is some indication that because *forbid* sounds harsher than *allow*, respondents are more likely to say no to allowing the practice than yes to forbidding it. The impact of this change in wording may be greater for more abstract issues or attitude objects (such as free speech or antiterrorism activities) than for concrete ones (such as X-rated movies or cigarette advertising) (Hippler & Schwarz, 1986; Narayan & Krosnick, 1996; Schuman & Presser, 1981).

Phrases

Another important issue in designing attitude items is the phrasing used in those items. Some evidence suggests that formal balancing of the alternatives for responding to attitude or opinion items, such as asking respondents whether they agree or disagree with or support or oppose an issue, is warranted so that both alternatives for answering the questions are provided and it is clear to the respondent that either answer is appropriate.

However, it is more difficult to choose a clearly distinct and balanced substantive counterargument or alternative in asking respondents' attitudes toward an issue: "Do you feel a woman should be allowed to have an abortion in the early months of pregnancy if she wants one, or do you feel a woman should not be allowed to end the life of an unborn child?" (Schuman & Presser, 1981, p. 186). Some people, for example, may feel that having an abortion "later" in the pregnancy would be acceptable. For those individuals, the alternative in the second half of the questions is not the balanced or equivalent alternative to the option described in the first half.

Similarly, problems can emerge with double-barreled or "one-and-a-half-barreled" questions, in which more than one question is introduced or implied in what questionnaire designers present as a single question. In this situation, it is not clear to respondents which question they should be answering or how they should register what they see as different answers to different questions. Bradburn et al. (2004) therefore suggest using unipolar items (with one substantive alternative) if there is a possibility that bipolar items (with two alternatives) do not really capture independent (and clearly balanced) dimensions.

For example, in a survey in Washington State of dentists' preferences in prescribing dental therapy (Aday, 1996, Resource C, question 17; Grembowski, Milgrom, & Fiset, 1990), some dentists may have had trouble deciding the extent to which they agreed or disagreed with the statement, "The primary focus of dentistry should be directed at controlling active disease rather than developing better preventive service." For some dentists, both approaches may be important, while for others, other aspects of dental therapy may be more important. However, if respondents said they disagreed or strongly disagreed with the statement, it would not be clear whether they thought neither approach was important—that both should be the "primary focus of dentistry"—or that, as the survey designers intended, they thought "better preventive service" was a more appropriate focus than "controlling active disease." Interestingly, this item was eliminated in a factor analysis of this and other items in the dentists' survey to identify the major dimensions of practice beliefs (Grembowski et al., 1990).

Sentences

The length of the question or series of items used in attitude questions can also affect the quality of individuals' responses. There is evidence that a medium-length introduction to a question (sixteen to sixty-four words), followed by a medium-length question (sixteen to twenty-four words) or a long question (twenty-five or more words), yields higher-quality data than either short introductions followed by short questions or long introductions followed by long questions. Also, the quality of responses to batteries of items—those that contain a list of questions to be answered using the same response categories (such as yes or no; agree, disagree, uncertain; and so on)—also tends to decline as the number of items increases. The "production line" nature of such questions may lead to carelessness on the part of the interviewer or respondent in asking or answering them (Andrews, 1984; Bradburn et al., 2004).

Responses

Considerable research has been conducted on the appropriate response formats to use in asking attitude questions. In general, the use of open-ended response formats is discouraged except during the preliminary or developmental stages of designing new questions. It is difficult to code and classify open-ended verbatim answers to nonfactual, attitudinal questions. The results will therefore be less consistent and reliable across respondents—and interviewers—than when standardized, closed-end categories are used.

Sometimes open-ended questions are designed for the interviewer to "field-code." With field-coded questions, the respondents are asked the question by means of an open-ended format. However, precoded categories are provided for the interviewer to classify the response into closed-end codes. This technique reduces the time and expense associated with the coding and processing of open-ended answers and also makes it possible to check the reliability of interviewers' coding. This approach is not recommended for use with subjective, attitudinal questions because of the errors and inconsistencies that can result when interviewers try to fit what respondents say into such categories (Bradburn et al., 2004; Schuman & Presser, 1981).

Avoiding "Yea-Saying." A related methodological issue that has been raised with some frequency when considering appropriate closed-end response formats for attitude items is the problem of yea-saying. This refers to the tendency of respondents to agree rather than disagree with statements as a whole or with what are perceived to be socially desirable responses to the question (Bachman & O'Malley, 1984; Bishop, Oldendick, & Tuchfarber, 1982; Schuman & Presser, 1981).

As noted in Chapter Ten, there are a number of techniques for minimizing yea-saying and the problem of social desirability in surveys, including using a self-administered questionnaire to obtain responses to potentially threatening questions, placing threatening questions near the end of the questionnaire, and allowing respondents the opportunity to provide open-ended responses regarding the frequency of behaviors. (Also see Bradburn, Sudman, & Wansink, 2004, for other suggestions.)

Given the possibility that these problems may occur during the course of an interview, researchers should work diligently to design attitude questions that deal with yea-saying, social desirability, and other factors that can influence responses to attitude questions. It may be useful to analyze data from pilot tests for systematic patterns of responses by age, race/ethnicity, and educational level to pick up potential variations in the validity of these questions by sociodemographic characteristics (Dijkstra, Smit, & Comijs, 2001; Knäuper, 1999).

A number of solutions have been suggested for identifying and dealing with this tendency toward yea-saying in attitude questions that can result in social desirability bias. One method is to include both positive and negative statements about the same issue in a battery of items—for example, "People with HIV/AIDS deserve to have the disease," as well as, "People with HIV/AIDS do not deserve to have the disease." If respondents say they agree with both items or comparable alternatives for other items, this obviously suggests a tendency toward yea-saying.

One solution to mitigating this response tendency is to use a forced choice rather than an agree-disagree format in asking such questions (Bishop et al., 1982; Schuman & Presser, 1981; Sensibaugh & Yarab, 1997). The latter format involves asking respondents whether they agree or disagree with statements such as, "How much a baby weighs at birth is more likely to be influenced by the mother's eating habits during pregnancy than by her genetic background." With a forced-choice format, respondents would be asked instead, "Which, in your opinion, is more likely to account for how much a baby weighs at birth—the mother's eating habits during pregnancy or her genetic background?"

Other devices for reducing the yea-saying tendency relate to the order and form of response categories provided to respondents. Bradburn et al. (2004, p. 152), for example, suggest that rather than asking respondents to "circle all that apply" in a series of statements about various attitudes toward a topic, they should be asked to say yes or no (does it apply to them or not) for each item. They are then forced to think about every item separately and not just go down the list and check those that "look good." This is good advice for other types of questions as well, because if the respondent or interviewer is asked to circle or check only those that apply, it is not always clear whether those that were not checked did not apply, were skipped over by the respondent or interviewer when reviewing the list, or were missed simply because the respondent did not give much thought to the items.

Bradburn et al. (2004) also recommend that when survey designers provide a list of alternatives for individuals to use in answering a question, the "least socially desirable" alternative should appear first in the list—for example, "In terms of your own risk of getting AIDS, do you think you are at great risk, at some risk, or at no risk for getting AIDS?" (Aday, 1996, Resource B, question 29; Albrecht, Levy, Sugrue, Prohaska, & Ostrow, 1989). Otherwise the respondent may choose the more desirable response right away without waiting to hear the other possible responses. The precise effect that the order of the response categories has on how respondents answer questions is far from clear, however. Some studies suggest that people tend to choose the first category mentioned (primacy effect), others the last category mentioned (recency effect), and still others the categories toward the middle of the list. Though not consistent across studies, there is a tendency in self-administered surveys for respondents to choose the first option, while in personal or telephone interviews, they are more likely to pick the last one (Bradburn et al., 2004; Dillman, 2000; Krosnick & Alwin, 1987; Narayan & Krosnick, 1996; Payne, 1951; Salant & Dillman, 1994; Schuman & Presser, 1981).

Incorporating positively and negatively worded items or using a forced-choice format does not necessarily ensure that acquiescence will be reduced. In fact, it may produce other response effects (such as tending to choose the first or last option in a forced choice question). If there is concern about the effect that phrasing or ordering the responses in a certain way may have on respondents' answers to certain questions and if no methodological research has been done on these items, researchers may consider conducting their own split-half experiments during the piloting or pretesting stages of their study if time and resources permit.

The Marlowe-Crowne Social Desirability Scale is also used to identify respondents who may be distorting their answers to survey questions in a socially desirable direction; it asks a series of questions thought to reflect this tendency. Attitudinal items that are found to have a high correlation with this measure can then be eliminated. The Marlowe-Crowne scale has been criticized, however, in that it may not reflect social desirability bias but a real tendency toward social conformity on the part of survey respondents (Bradburn et al., 1979; Crowne & Marlowe, 1960). Loo and Thorpe (2000) found in a confirmatory factor analysis of a full version and several shorter versions of the scale that the shorter versions were actually better measures of response bias and social desirability bias than the long version of the scale.

Measuring Attitude Strength. An important issue in measuring people's attitudes is determining the strength with which the attitudes are held. This is measured through scales for rating or ranking the order of people's preferences for different attitudinal statements about a topic.

With *rating* scales, respondents are asked to indicate the level of intensity they feel about the statements along the dimensions provided by the researcher. For example, the first question in the National Dental Malpractice Survey asks respondents, "All in all, on a daily basis how satisfied are you with your practice in general?" Responses provided are "extremely satisfied, very satisfied, somewhat satisfied, somewhat dissatisfied, very dissatisfied, and extremely satisfied" (Resource C, question 1).

With *ranking* formats, respondents are asked to rank-order their preferences for different alternatives. For example, a major component of a study conducted of dentists in Washington State was to ask the dentists to rank-order the top three (most, second, third most important) patient, technical, and cost factors they considered in choosing among alternative dental therapies (Aday, 1996, Resource C, questions 1–16; Grembowski et al., 1990). Such rankings can occur, however, only when respondents can see or remember all the alternatives. Bradburn et al. (2004) suggest that respondents can handle no more than two to three alternatives at a time over the telephone. Even with self-administered or in-person interviews, in which visual devices or cards can be used to rank-order the options, they recommend that no more than four or five alternatives be provided.

An important issue to address in designing rating scales is how many categories or points should be provided in such scales. A large number of points (seven to ten) may, for example, permit the greatest discrimination in terms of attitude strength or intensity. But increasing the numbers of categories will make it harder for the respondent to keep all the responses in mind, particularly if verbal labels (such as strongly agree, agree, and so on) rather than numerical labels ("On a scale from 1 to 5 . . . ") are used to identify the respective points along the scale. Research suggests that scales with five to seven points are more valid and reliable than those with only two to three categories, although the gradations of opinion reflected in the verbal labels used with these formats may be difficult for certain groups (those for whom English is a secondary language or the elderly, for example). For detailed discrimination (along a ten-point scale, for example) numerical scale categories are recommended.

Research has suggested that verbally labeling only the end points of the scale and allowing the intermediate points to take their meaning from their relative position between the end points results in higher-quality data than labeling every point of such scales for those with seven or fewer categories (Alwin & Krosnick, 1985; Andrews, 1984; Bradburn et al., 2004). However, more respondents are likely to endorse the lower (less positive) range of an eleven-point scale that ranges from 0 to 10 compared with a scale that ranges from –5 to +5 even though the end points have the same verbal labels—"not at all satisfied" and "very satisfied." The explanation for this finding is that the 0 to 10 scale is implicitly viewed by respondents as unipolar—the extent to which the feeling is present—and the –5 to +5 scale as bipolar—the extent to which it is present (+1 to +5) or absent (–1 to –5). Respondents are therefore more reluctant to register the absence of any positive feelings invited by the negative (less positive) end of the bipolar rating scale

(Schwarz, Knäuper, Hippler, Noelle-Neumann, & Clark, 1991; Schwarz & Hippler, 1995b).

Verbal scales used in personal interview surveys (such as "completely, mostly, somewhat satisfied") are often converted to numerical scales in telephone interviews ("On a scale of 1 to 5, where 5 is completely satisfied, and 1 is not at all satisfied, how satisfied are you with . . . "). It may be easier for respondents to keep the numerical scale, rather than the complex-sounding verbal labels ("strongly agree, agree, uncertain, disagree, strongly disagree"), in their heads in answering questions over the telephone. Another device that is frequently used in telephone interviews is to ask whether the person agrees with, disagrees with, or is uncertain about a statement, and then, if the person agrees or disagrees, to ask whether he or she agrees or strongly agrees (or disagrees or strongly disagrees). In personal interviews, cards with the response categories printed on them can be handed to the respondents to facilitate the use of even a large number of verbal response categories. Other numerical devices that have been used to get respondents to register their opinion on an issue include providing pictures of thermometers or ladders for them to use in indicating how "warm" they feel about the issue or where they "stand" on it (Bradburn et al., 2004).

A related issue in designing rating formats is whether a neutral or middle alternative or "don't know" or "no opinion" option should be explicitly provided for respondents who do not have a strong attitude, one way or the other, on the topic. Research suggests that when such alternatives are explicitly provided, the proportions of those who say they don't know or don't have an opinion is naturally higher (Bishop, 1987; Presser & Schuman, 1980; Schuman & Presser, 1981).

In terms of the merits of using no opinion responses in attitude surveys, Krosnick (2002) found no difference in the reliability and validity of the responses provided by those who were attracted to a no opinion category than those who were not. At the same time, they found that respondents with a lower level of educational attainment, as well as those who devoted little time to responding to the question or those who were exposed to opinion questions later in the survey, were more likely than others to use the no opinion option. These findings support the results of an earlier study by Narayan and Krosnick (1996) that found a relationship between educational attainment and a variety of response order effects, including the preference for the use of the no opinion category, and a tendency toward yea-saying.

In a review of a series of studies on "no response" patterns, Krosnick (2002, p. 99) concluded that the choice to provide no response to attitude questions may reflect a decision not to reveal a potentially embarrassing attitude, ambivalence, question ambiguity, or the lack of willingness of a respondent to "do the cognitive work necessary to report it."

Beatty, Herrmann, Puskar, and Kerwin (1998) caution researchers to examine, whenever possible, the motivations respondents have for providing a response of "don't know." In particular, they suggest that researchers should determine whether respondents are indicating that they do not know because they honestly do not know (a truthful response) or indicating that they do not know because they either choose not to provide the information (an error of omission) or choose to provide untruthful information (an error of commission). There is also research suggesting that when one uses either a divider line or a space to separate options for registering "don't know" and "no opinion" from the other options there is a higher rate of item nonresponse (Tourangeau, Couper, & Conrad, 2004).

People who express an opinion when the neutral or no opinion options are not provided but opt for these categories when they are available are called "floaters." They are more likely to have lower levels of involvement in the issue, that is, assign it less importance or have less interest in it (Bishop, 1990; Gilljam & Granberg, 1993; Hippler & Schwarz, 1989).

Research indicates that the relative percentages (or proportions) of respondents who choose the other categories are not affected by explicitly adding these options. Although the addition of such alternatives may not affect the overall distribution of positive and negative responses, it is recommended that they be provided so that respondents do not feel forced to choose a category. Instead they are allowed to indicate that they have no opinion or no strongly felt opinion—one way or the other—on the topic, if that is the way they feel about it (Andrews, 1984; Bradburn et al., 2004).

Paired comparisons of different alternatives have been widely used in studies that ask respondents to choose among competing options. This approach is, for example, implicit in the utility-related approaches to estimating the preferences for different treatment alternatives, such as having a kidney transplant to be restored to normal health but confronting a three in ten chance of dying from the transplant versus not having it and continuing in a less desirable health state on dialysis (see the discussion in Chapter Nine).

However, if respondents are asked to make a large number of comparisons, this method can lead to considerable fatigue on their part and a resultant failure to concentrate on the choices they are making. Even when fully participating in the process, people may not always make entirely consistent choices across items.

In a comparison of rating versus ranking methods for eliciting people's value preferences for the characteristics children should have, Alwin and Krosnick (1985) concluded that neither method was necessarily superior to the other for that purpose. However, they did point out that the ranking method clearly forced the respondent to compare and contrast alternatives and choose between them, whereas the rating technique did not. Researchers thus need to decide whether explicitly asking respondents to make such choices is necessary given what they want to learn about their attitudes on a topic.

Questionnaire

A final issue to consider in asking attitudinal questions in surveys is the order in which such questions should appear. There is evidence that people respond differently to questions about their general attitudes on a topic (such as abortion), depending on whether they are placed before or after a series of questions that tap more specific attitudes on the issue (whether abortion is warranted in the instances of rape, incest, a deformed fetus, risk to the mother's health if she carries the baby to term, and so on). In general, it is recommended that the more general attitude items be asked before the specific ones. Otherwise respondents tend to feel that they have already answered the question or to assume that the general question refers to other (or residual) aspects of the issue that they were not asked about in detail earlier (Bradburn et al., 2004; Mason, Carlson, & Tourangeau, 1994; Schuman & Presser, 1981; Schwarz & Bless, 1992; Schwarz, Strack, & Mai, 1991; Tourangeau, Rasinski, & Bradburn, 1991).

Previous questions can influence respondents' answers, especially if they are on a related topic and the respondents view the issue as important but do not have a well-formed opinion about it. Survey developers should consciously consider the context in which such questions are asked when designing the survey questionnaire. There might be an interest in prompting respondents' recall of specific events (problems in getting medical care) before answering certain attitudinal questions (satisfaction with their regular provider) but not others (their opinion of pending national health care reform legislation). If there is not a clear rationale for ordering the questions, then it might be useful to conduct a split-ballot experiment to examine the impact of changing the order in which they appear in the questionnaire on survey responses.

Questionnaire Administration

Although proxy interviews may be sought for demographic or factual questions, it is not generally advisable to do so for knowledge or attitude items because they are uniquely intended to reflect the respondent's subjective, internal states or feelings, and not necessarily an objective, external reality readily observable by others (Lavizzo-Mourey, Zinn, & Taylor, 1992).

There are also other potential mode effects as they relate to responses to questions. Holbrook, Green, and Krosnick (2003) found that respondents in long telephone interviews provided a higher level of no opinion and socially desirable responses than respondents in long face-to-face interviews. They suggest that the length of the telephone interview may have an effect on the response patterns. It may also be the case that the length of the study in general can contribute to response bias. In general, there tends to be smaller social desirability bias in telephone surveys than face-to-face interviews, but telephone interviews also tend to be shorter than face-to-face interviews (Biemer & Lyberg, 2003).

As in the case of any other type of study, one may want to remain sensitive to the context under which attitude questions are presented (Schwarz & Hippler, 1995a). For example, Dillman (2000) suggests that because of the interviewer interaction process, respondents may provide more socially desirable responses in a face-to-face interview than some other mode to questions regarding potentially embarrassing behavior, such as cheating on one's spouse or substance abuse. At the same time, patients who are called by providers may also provide more socially desirable responses in a telephone interview regarding their satisfaction with services in comparison to an anonymous survey on the same topic.

Special Considerations for Special Populations

Yea-saying response tendencies are more likely to have been observed among Hispanics and other minorities and poorly educated respondents (Marín & Marín, 1991). This may be caused by a general tendency to give more socially desirable responses, but it may also reflect difficulty in discriminating among the fine gradations of opinion implied by the response categories provided or cultural or linguistic ambiguities in what is meant or intended by the question. The cognitive survey development techniques reviewed in Chapter Eight are useful in detecting these problems early on, and formal tests of the reliability and validity of the resulting summary scales (reviewed in Chapter Three), stratified (broken out) by major subgroups of interest, would document the extent to which these problems exist, once the data are gathered.

Selected Examples: Patient-Consumer Satisfaction

An array of knowledge and attitude questions illustrating the principles detailed in this chapter is reflected in the three major survey examples used in this book (Resources A through C). Selected knowledge and attitude summary scales based on these studies were highlighted in Chapter Three.

Although not a focus of these three surveys, questionnaires to tap patient and consumer satisfaction are increasingly being used to assess the performance and quality of health care services delivery. Patient satisfaction is viewed as a unique and patient-centered indicator of success in attending to the nontechnical as well as technical aspects of care (Agency for Healthcare Research and Quality, 2005; Goldstein, Elliott, & Guccione, 2000; Harpole et al., 2003; Lewis, 1994; O'Connell, Young, & Twigg, 1999; Quinn et al. 2004; Thomas & Bond, 1996; Tyson et al., 2001).

Furthermore, many of the principles for designing attitudinal questions in general come into play in developing these measures. A balanced response scale in which both positively and negatively worded items are used is recommended to minimize an acquiescent response set. Item response formats may take one of several forms of a Likert-type scale to tap satisfaction with different dimensions of care: direct ("very satisfied, satisfied, neither satisfied nor dissatisfied, dissatisfied, very dissatisfied"), indirect ("strongly agree, agree, uncertain, disagree, strongly disagree"), or evaluative response formats ("excellent, very good, good, fair, or poor"). Research has suggested that the evaluative rating scale may in fact be superior to the direct scaling method in measuring patient satisfaction because the resulting scores tend to be less skewed (toward higher levels of satisfaction), have greater variability, and be more likely to reflect the patient's intentions regarding seeking care (Sherbourne, Hays, & Burton, 1995; Ware & Hays, 1988).

The content, number of items, and response format used for selected scales of general satisfaction with medical care, physicians, and hospitals that have been employed extensively in developing report cards or other reports on provider performance are highlighted in Table 11.1. A number of sources provide a review and synthesis of the major conceptual and empirical approaches to measuring patient satisfaction (Agency for Healthcare Research and Quality, 2005; Coyle & Williams, 1999; Davies, Ware, & Kosinski, 1995; Di Palo, 1997; Gold & Wooldridge, 1995; Hudak & Wright, 2000; Jackson & Kroenke, 1997; Kirsner & Federman, 1997; van Campen, Sixma, Friele, Kerssens, & Peters, 1995; Williams, Weinman, & Dale, 1998).

The impetus for the first generation of satisfaction measures came primarily from a desire within the health services research and policy communities for valid and reliable methodologies for assessing the performance of the U.S. health care delivery system. The Medical Care Satisfaction Questionnaire, developed by Barbara Hulka and her colleagues (Hulka, Zyzanski, Cassel, & Thompson, 1970), and John Ware and associates' Patient Satisfaction Questionnaire (Ware & Snyder, 1975) have been used extensively in soliciting both patients' and the general population's satisfaction with medical care in national, state, and local surveys. The Visit Satisfaction Questionnaire (Ware & Hays, 1988), used in the Medical Outcomes Study (described in Chapter Three), measured patient satisfaction with specific visits to providers across the array of delivery settings that were the focus of that quasi-experimental health services evaluation.

TABLE 11.1. SELECTED PATIENT SATISFACTION MEASURES.

Concepts and Characteristics	Physician		Hospital	Services
	PSQ III	VSQ	PJS	SERVQUAL
Concepts	Interpersonal manner Communication Technical quality Financial security Time spent with physician Access to care General satisfaction	Physician access Telephone access Office wait Appointment wait Time spent with physician Communication Interpersonal aspects Technical quality Overall care	Admissions Daily care Information Nursing care Doctor care Auxiliary staff Living arrangements Discharge Billing Total process	Tangibles Reliability Responsiveness Assurance Empathy
Characteristics Number of questions	50	9	46	21
Response scale	Strongly Agree, Agree, Uncertain, Disagree, Strongly Disagree	Strongly Agree, Agree, Not Sure, Disagree, Strongly Disagree	Excellent, Very Good, Good, Fair, Poor, Don't Know	Two dimensions: Perception (low = 1 to high = 9); Expectation (low = 1 to high = 9)

Note: PSQ III = Patient Satisfaction Questionnaire, III (1984); VSQ = Visit-Specific Satisfaction Questionnaire (1985); PJS = Patient Judgment System (1987); SERVQUAL = Service Quality (1985).

Bibliography: PSQ III: Marshall, Hays, Sherbourne, & Wells, 1993; Rand Health, n.d.; Safran, Tarlov, & Rogers, 1994. VSQ: Measurement Excellence and Training Resource Information Center, n.d.; Peck et al., 2001; Rubin et al., 1993; Ware & Hays, 1988; Yancy et al., 2001. PJS: Hays, Larson, Nelson, & Batalden, 1991; Measurement Excellence and Training Resource Information Center, n.d.; Meterko, Nelson, & Rubin, 1990; Nelson, Hays, Larson, & Batalden, 1989; Nelson & Larson, 1993; Rubin, 1990. SERVQUAL: O'Connor, Trinh, & Shewchuk, 2000; Parasuraman, Zeithaml, & Berry, 1988.

Also see reviews by Gold & Wooldridge (1995) and van Campen, Sixma, Friele, Kerssens, & Peters (1995).

The impetus for the second generation of satisfaction measures (such as the Group Health Association of America Consumer Satisfaction and related National Committee for Quality Assurance Surveys) emanated from a growing interest on the part of the corporate provider community (particularly large-scale managed care organizations) in obtaining consumer assessments of the quality of care received from member providers (Davies & Ware, 1988, 1991; National Committee for Quality Assurance, 2004). The results of patient satisfaction surveys on plan performance were to be incorporated into report cards summarizing both clinical indicators and patient assessments of quality that could be used in marketing health plans to prospective consumers. Satisfaction surveys have also been incorporated into evaluations used in the private sector to examine the performance of health providers and organizations (Press Ganey Associates, 2005). The Picker/Commonwealth Program for Patient-Centered Care, supported by the Commonwealth Fund, provided support for the development of scales of hospital patients' satisfaction with care (Patient Judgment System) that could be used in assessing the quality of inpatient care from the perspective of those receiving the services (Nelson, Hays, Larson, & Batalden, 1989).

In addition to scales that focus on the hospital patients' assessment of services in general, Parasuraman and colleagues developed an instrument (SERVQUAL) for assessing the quality of services in general by calculating the difference between the consumer's perception of how services were delivered (a perception rating) and their expectation of how the services should have been delivered (an expectation rating). The perceived quality of care is determined by subtracting the perception rating from the expectation rating for different dimensions for evaluating services (Tangibles, Reliability, Responsiveness, Assurance, and Empathy) (O'Connor, Trinh, & Shewchuk, 2000; Parasuraman, Zeithaml, & Berry, 1988).

The literature is replete with scales to assess satisfaction with a variety of other health-related programs or services. The Agency for Healthcare Research and Quality (2005) sponsors the National Quality Measures Clearinghouse Web site that serves as a portal for measures of satisfaction of care. This site includes an archive of satisfaction measures and links to related resources.

Guidelines for Minimizing Survey Errors and Maximizing Survey Quality

A tendency toward yea-saying (or an acquiescent response set) may introduce systematic biases in responses to a series of attitude or knowledge questions (see Table 11.2). To reduce this tendency, the number of questions asked could be reduced in number or short-form equivalents of the scales employed. Variable errors re-

TABLE 11.2. SURVEY ERRORS: SOURCES AND SOLUTIONS— FORMULATING QUESTIONS ABOUT KNOWLEDGE AND ATTITUDES.

	Systematic Errors	*Variable Errors*
	Respondent Effects: Yea-Saying (Acquiescent Response Set)	**Questionnaire Effects: Order and Context**
Solutions to Errors	Reduce the length of a series of questions (or use a short form of scales) measuring knowledge or attitudes.	Conduct split-ballot experiments to evaluate how answers to questions vary when they appear in a different order in the questionnaire.

sulting from the order and context in which the questions are asked could also be explored through split-ballot experiments that systematically evaluate how answers to questions vary when placed in a different order or context in the survey questionnaire. Thought should be given in particular to the ordering of questions related to general versus more specific attitudes on a topic of interest.

Asking questions to find out deep-seated opinions and feelings is somewhat like digging for buried treasure. One must know where and how to look as well as what previous explorations might have surfaced. The objective of the undertaking (the concept to be measured) must be clearly defined, the tools (questions and response categories) for extracting it honed, and the environment (order and context) in which it is embedded taken into account. Both existing maps (previous research) and tailored scouting expeditions (pilot studies or split-ballot experiments) may be needed to surface the gems that are the object of the inquiry.

Supplementary Sources

Other sources to consult on attitude scale construction are DeVellis (2003), Nunnally and Bernstein (1994), and Oppenheim (1992).

CHAPTER TWELVE

GUIDELINES FOR FORMATTING THE QUESTIONNAIRE

Chapter Highlights

1. The format, order, and context in which questions are asked should all be considered in making final decisions about the form and content of the survey questionnaire.
2. Researchers should test and evaluate different approaches to formatting or ordering questions during the pilot and pretest stages of the study if they are not sure which approach will work best in their study.
3. In designing questionnaires for the Web, researchers should be sensitive to the ability of the users to navigate the questionnaire as well as the capacity of their Web browsers to handle complex graphics.

This chapter presents guidelines for formatting and ordering questions in a survey questionnaire. Three issues in particular are addressed: (1) the techniques for displaying the questions in mail, telephone, personal interview, and computerized questionnaires (format); (2) the order in which the questions appear; and (3) their relationship to other questions in the survey questionnaire (context). Each of these three factors affects the clarity and meaning of the questions and thus the respondent's ability or willingness to answer the questions reliably and accurately.

Format

Different modes of data gathering (mail, telephone, personal interview, or computerized) present somewhat different clues to the respondent about how to proceed with the survey questionnaire. Mail or self-administered questionnaires are often reliant solely on the clarity and appeal of the visual presentation of the questions, response categories, and accompanying instructions. With telephone interviews, auditory signals and the quality of the communication between the interviewer and respondent are central. In personal interview situations, visual and auditory stimuli as well as the norms of conversational and interpersonal interaction implicit in the exchange between the interviewer and respondent all come into play in encouraging or facilitating a response. As discussed in Chapter Five, computerized data collection methods, such as computer-assisted personal interviewing (CAPI), computer-assisted self-interviewing (CASI), computer-assisted telephone interviewing (CATI), and the Web, present unique challenges and opportunities in the questionnaire design and administration process.

With self-administered questionnaires, the principal criterion to consider in evaluating the instrument is whether the respondent can understand and answer the questions without having someone present to clarify or explain them. In telephone surveys, a key consideration is whether a question is likely to be understood if it were read exactly as it is written. In personal interview surveys, greater use can be made of visual aids, such as showing respondents a card with the response categories for a question listed on it or encouraging them to check relevant records before answering. Computer-assisted and Web-based data collection methods enhance the availability of an array of audio and visual cues to respondents and interviewers for understanding and answering questions. Advance letters are useful to provide prospective respondents information about a survey before they are actually contacted for the interview. (The content and format of these letters are discussed in Chapter Thirteen.) The introduction to a telephone survey is especially critical for enlisting respondents' cooperation. Salant and Dillman (1994) recommend a brief businesslike introduction that includes the interviewer's name, the organization and city from which he or she is calling, a one-sentence description of the survey, and a conservative estimate of how long the interview will take.

Exhibit 12.1 highlights the major do's and don'ts in formatting survey questionnaires in general. This chapter's discussion pinpoints their particular relevance and the adaptations required for different data-gathering methods. The examples in the exhibit are based primarily on conventions for developing survey questionnaires developed and recommended by Bradburn, Sudman, and Wansink (2004) and Dillman (2000).

EXHIBIT 12.1. DO'S AND DON'T'S OF QUESTIONNAIRE DESIGN.

Do	Don't

1a. Assign numbers to each question.
1b. Use letters to indicate subparts of a question when it has more than one part.
1a. If a center to treat people with AIDS was going to be set up in your neighborhood, would you *favor* or *oppose* it?
Favor **(Skip to Q. 2)**............1
Oppose.......................2
   (If "oppose"):
1b. Why is that? _____
	Don't leave off the question number.
	Don't leave off the letter for subparts of a question.
	If a center to treat people with AIDS was going to be set up in your neighborhood, would you *favor* or *oppose* it?
	Favor **(Skip to Q. 2)** 1
	Oppose...2
	   (If "oppose"):
	Why is that? _____

2. Use a vertical response format for closed-end responses. White.......................1 African American............2 Hispanic....................3	*Don't* list closed-end responses horizontally. White....1 African American....2 Hispanic....3
3. Use numerical codes for closed-end responses. In general, would you say that your health is . . . . **(Read categories and circle number for answer.)** Excellent....................1 Good........................2 Fair........................3 Poor?.......................4	*Don't* use alphabetical codes or blank lines to place X or check on, for closed-end responses. In general, would you say that your health is . . . Excellent _____ Good _____ Fair _____ Poor _____
4. Use consistent numerical codes and formats. Yes.........................1 No..........................2 *Don't know*.................8	*Don't* use different numerical codes and formats for comparable responses to different questions. 1 Yes 2 No 3 Don't know 1. Yes 2. No 8. Don't know

5. **Align response codes.**
   Yes.......................1
   No........................2
   Don't know..............8

   White.....................1
   African American..........2
   Hispanic..................3

6. **Provide clear instructions for open-ended items.**
   What was your blood pressure the last time you had it checked?
   RECORD HIGH VALUE: _____
   (systolic reading)
   RECORD LOW VALUE: _____
   (diastolic reading)

7. **Provide clear special instructions.**

   (Ask males only):
   Did you use a condom?

8. **Provide clear skip instructions.**
   8a. Do you smoke cigarettes?
       Yes **(Ask Q. 8b)**............1
       No **(Skip to Q. 9)**..........2
   8b. How many cigarettes do you smoke per day on average?
       RECORD NUMBER OF CIGARETTES: _____

9. **Phrase full and complete questions.**

   What is your age? or
   What is your date of birth?

Don't **vary alignment of response codes on a page.**
Yes...............1
No..................2
Don't know.........8

White.................1
African American......2
Hispanic..............3

Don't **just leave a space with no instructions for the answer.**
What was your blood pressure the last time you had it checked?
_____

Don't **have instructions about how to answer questions in same typeface and format as question.**
Ask males only:
Did you use a condom?

Don't **leave out explicit skip instructions.**
8a. Do you smoke cigarettes?
    Yes.........1
    No...........2
8b. How many cigarettes do you smoke per day on average?

Don't **simply use words or headings to elicit information from respondents.**
Age? _____

EXHIBIT 12.1. DO'S AND DON'T'S OF QUESTIONNAIRE DESIGN, *continued.*

Do	Don't

10. Use a forced-choice format for a list.

Should an employer be allowed to require job applicants to be medically tested for . . . (**Circle answer for yes or no to each.**)

	Yes	No
a. Sexually transmitted diseases (STDs)?	1	2
b. Using illegal drugs?	1	2
c. High blood pressure?	1	2
d. Having AIDS virus?	1	2

11. Use a column format for a series with the same response categories.

	Strongly agree	Agree	Disagree	Strongly disagree
a	1	2	3	4
b	1	2	3	4
c	1	2	3	4
d	1	2	3	4
e	1	2	3	4
f	1	2	3	4
g	1	2	3	4

12. Use a column format for a series with comparable skip patterns.

Don't ask respondent to indicate "all that apply" if he or she could indicate more than one response.

Should an employer be allowed to require applicants to be medically tested for . . . (**Circle all that apply.**)

a.	Sexually transmitted diseases (STDs)?	1
b.	Using illegal drugs?	2
c.	High blood pressure?	3
d.	Having AIDS virus?	4

Don't repeat a string of questions with the same response categories.

a. Male homosexuals are disgusting.

Strongly agree	1
Agree	2
Disagree	3
Strongly disagree	4

b. Male homosexuality is a natural expression of sexuality.

Strongly agree	1
Agree	2
Disagree	3
Strongly disagree	4

Don't fail to clearly link a series of questions to subsequent dependent items.

For each provider marked yes in Q. 1:

1. Did you go to see any of the following providers in the past twelve months, from **(date)** to **(date)**? (**Read list and circle number for yes or no.**)

	Yes	No
a. Dentist?	1	2
b. Chiropractor?	1	2
c. Psychotherapist?	1	2

2. How many times did you go see a **(provider)** during this period? (**Record number.**)

a.	_____ times
b.	_____ times
c.	_____ times

---

1. Did you go to see any of the following providers in the past twelve months, from **(date)** to **(date)**? (**Read list and circle number for yes or no.**)

	Yes	No
a. Dentist?	1	2
b. Chiropractor?	1	2
c. Psychotherapist?	1	2

2. How many times did you go see this type of provider during this period? (**Record number.**)

_____ times

---

13. Put all parts of a question on the same page. *Don't* split a question between pages, particularly when skip instructions are part of the question.

14. Allow plenty of space on the questionnaire. *Don't* crowd the questions and space for recording the answers.

15. Carefully consider the appearance of the questionnaire. *Don't* just start the questions on page 1 without introducing the study, identifying the sponsoring organization, and so on.

EXHIBIT 12.1. DO'S AND DON'T'S OF QUESTIONNAIRE DESIGN, *continued.*

Do	Don't

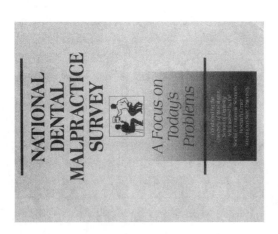

16. **End the questionnaire with a thank you.**

Your contribution to this effort is greatly appreciated. Please enclose the questionnaire in the stamped self-addressed envelope and mail to:

Don't forget to thank the respondent.

THE END.

17. **Consider how the data will be processed.**

Don't fail to anticipate how you will code and process the data as you design the questionnaire.

Adaptations for mail or self-administered surveys recommended by Don Dillman's tailored design method for mail questionnaires are highlighted in the discussion that follows (Dillman, 1978, 2000; Salant & Dillman, 1994). The tailored design method (TDM) refers to "the development of survey procedures that create respondent trust and perceptions of increased rewards and reduced costs for being a respondent, which take into account features of the survey situation and have as their goal the overall reduction of survey error" (Dillman, 2000, p. 27).

TDM is grounded in social exchange theory, which posits that human actions are motivated by the rewards, costs, and trust that are perceived to exist in a social situation. The tailored design approach to survey development attempts to identify the specific aspects of designing and implementing surveys that minimize the costs (for example, time, embarrassment) and maximize the rewards (for example, feeling appreciated, providing tangible incentives) and trust (for example, emphasizing the legitimacy of the study sponsorship) for survey respondents.

The National Dental Malpractice Survey in Resource C is based on Dillman's TDM guidelines for mail surveys. Proprietary Web and computer-assisted questionnaire design and data-gathering software packages have their own languages and protocols for designing and formatting a survey questionnaire, although many of the same basic principles apply when using these approaches (Couper et al., 1998; Dillman, 2000).

Assign Numbers to Each Question

All questions should be numbered in an easy-to-follow, straightforward sequence from the beginning of the question to the end of the document (as in the National Dental Malpractice Study, Resource C; also see Dillman, 2000, principle 3.9). Using an easy-to-follow, straightforward numbering system assists interviewers, respondents, data-processing staff, and analysts in locating the items on the questionnaire. Subparts of a question should also be clearly identified through indentation or assigning letters (for example, 1a, 1b). Some skip patterns or other instructions within the questionnaire may also require that particular questions be identified by number. Incorporating the question number into the names of analysis variables when constructing and documenting the data file for the study provides a clear road map to the source questions for those variables. Computerized data collection systems in particular require that each item on the questionnaire be identified through unique questions or code numbers.

Use a Vertical Response Format for Closed-End Responses

Another important rule of thumb for formatting closed-end response categories is to use a vertical format for the categories (Dillman, 2000, principle 3.19). In a vertical format, the categories and corresponding response codes are presented in list form, one right after the other (see UNICEF MICS-2, HIV/AIDS Module, question 3):

Yes 1

No 2

Don't know 9

This is in contrast to a horizontal format: "Yes: 1 No: 2." Dillman (2000) and Bradburn et al. (2004) point out that it is much easier for the respondent or interviewer to get confused and circle the wrong code for a response category when the horizontal format is used (for example, circling "1" for "No" in the horizontal format example). On a mail questionnaire, one may want to use a code of "3" rather than "9" for the "Don't know" response because some respondents may be confused by the jump from "2" to "9."

Use Numerical Codes for Closed-End Responses

Using numerical codes and circling them or putting an X through a box next to the category that best represents the respondent's answer are the recommended methods for closed-end response categories (Dillman, 2000, principle 3.21). Using an X rather than a check mark, and putting the X in a box rather than on a blank line, is likely to result in fewer errors because it is a somewhat more precise and constraining means of marking an answer to a question. The use of numerical response codes is likely to yield fewer problems in coding and processing the data than letters (a, b, c, d, and so on) because some statistical software packages present problems in handling these types of codes. They are also more limiting in terms of the number of unique codes (the twenty-six letters in the alphabet) that can be employed.

Use Consistent Numerical Codes and Formats

Follow a consistent pattern in assigning code numbers to comparable response categories for different questions. This recommendation is based on what is called the Law of Pragnanz, which states that "figures with simplicity, regularity, and symmetry are more easily perceived and remembered than are unusual or irregularly shaped figures" (Wallschlaeger & Busic-Snyder, 1992, as cited in Dillman,

2000, p. 109). This would suggest that being consistent in the development of response categories would lead to fewer errors in data processing. Assigning the same code numbers to comparable response categories for different questions throughout the questionnaire (for example, yes = 1; no = 2; respondent refused = 7; respondent doesn't know answer = 8) and using a consistent pattern for the placement of response codes for comparable types of questions (such as along the right margin in questions AB1 and AB2 in the Adult CHIS 2001 Survey) reduce the uncertainties for interviewers and respondents about which code to use in answering questions with similar response formats.

It has been argued that in mail surveys, respondents may answer in terms of the first categories on the list (primacy effect), while in telephone or personal interview surveys, they are more likely to respond in terms of the later categories (recency effect) (Ayidiya & McClendon, 1990; Salant & Dillman, 1994). However, subsequent research has suggested that these primacy and recent effects are far less predictable than what was previously thought to be the case (Dillman, 2000; Dillman et al., 1995). It is still important, though, to be aware of the possibility that this may occur in surveys. Procedures for minimizing these effects include reducing the number of categories presented to respondents, varying the order of presentation of the categories in interviewer-administered surveys, and (in personal interviews) showing cards to respondents with the response categories listed. Computer-assisted data collection methods offer particular advantages in addressing this issue, particularly in their ability to randomize the order in which options are presented to respondents.

Align Response Codes

A general rule of thumb is to align the response codes or the response boxes along the right margin for telephone or personal interviews (see questions 1 to 17 of the HIV/AIDS Module of the UNICEF MICS-2 survey), to the left of the response categories for mail questionnaires (see questions 1 and 2 of the National Dental Malpractice Survey, NDMS, Resource C), and in line with counterpart codes for questions that precede or follow (Dillman, 2000, principles 3.20 and 3.22).

Dillman (2000) notes that there are several considerations in deciding where to place the response categories. Placing response categories on the left in self-administered questionnaires may lead to respondents' overlooking skip pattern instructions that are placed on the right side of the response categories. Placing the codes along the right margin in interviewer-administered surveys is likely to result in fewer errors on the part of trained interviewers than might be the case with respondents who fill out the questionnaire themselves. In addition, it facilitates subsequent inputting of the data directly from the questionnaire. All things considered, with self-administered questionnaires, the ease and accuracy of respondents' recording their answers is primary, while with an interviewer-administered instrument, more weight can be given to formatting the questionnaire to facilitate data processing.

Provide Clear Instructions for Open-Ended Items

For open-ended items, clear instructions should be provided about how the information should be recorded (Dillman, 2000, Figure 3.16). It may be particularly important to specify the units to be used in responding, such as visits, patients, or procedures (see questions 28 and 29 of the NDMS questionnaire, Resource C).

Provide Clear Special Instructions

Any instructions relating to how the question should be answered or the skip patterns to be followed should appear next to the response category or question to which it refers (see question 18 of the HIV/AIDS module of the UNICEF MICS-2 survey). It is helpful to set off these instructions from the questions by presenting them in different type sizes (for example, fourteen-point type instead of twelve-point type) or using directional arrows to indicate where they should go next (Dillman, 2000, principle 3.27):

18. Is the woman a caretaker of any children under five years of age?

☐ Yes → GO TO QUESTIONNAIRE FOR CHILDREN UNDER FIVE and administer one questionnaire for each child under five for whom she is the caretaker.

☐ No → CONTINUE WITH Q.19.

Also, see question 35 in the NDMS (Resource C) for an example of the use of instructions to facilitate skip patterns.

Dillman's tailored design method for mail questionnaires recommends that the questions be set apart from the response categories by using dark type for questions and light type for answer choice (Dillman, 2000, principle 3.13 and Figure 3.12). (Note that the NDMS in Resource C, which was based primarily on Dillman's earlier total design method, used bold type for the response categories and regular type for the questions.) Any detailed instructions should be fully integrated in the question and not set apart in a separate instructional booklet for survey respondents (Dillman, 2000, principle 3.16 and Figure 10.4).

Provide Clear Skip Instructions

Both the respondent and the interviewer need to be instructed clearly with respect to where to go next when the answer to a particular question (as in question 18 from the MICS noted above) dictates the other questions they should answer. Dillman recommends that arrows (as in question 11 of the NDMS, Resource C) be used in self-administered questionnaires, although providing clear instructions in parentheses beside the response code to which it applies is also a useful strategy (see question 35 of the NDMS, Resource C). Another way this can be achieved is by presenting the instructions for the skip patterns in larger type sizes or in color (Redline & Dillman, 2002). Dillman (2000) cautions researchers against using multiple visual techniques in combination, as they may cause confusion or require cognitive adjustments on the part of the respondent.

In computer-assisted data collection, the relevant skip patterns or probes are programmed into the interview. As in paper-and-pencil questionnaires, these steps should be checked and double-checked before the questionnaire goes into the field to ensure that the instructions are directing the interviewer or respondent as they should.

Phrase Full and Complete Questions

Often single words or incomplete sentences are used in posing survey questions, such as "Age?" or "Occupation?" While respondents may understand what each of these terms mean, it may not be entirely clear who or what time period is being referenced (Dillman, 2000, principle 2.3). Thus, complete sentences should be used to clarify fully and precisely the information that is needed: "What is your age?" or "What is your date of birth?"

Use a Forced-Choice Format for a List

Questionnaires often ask respondents or interviewers to circle or mark all that apply among a series of categories provided. The danger of this approach is that it is not always entirely clear what *not* marking a response may mean. For example, it might mean (as intended) that it did not apply to the respondent. But it might also indicate that the respondent was not sure and left it blank or that it was inadvertently overlooked by either the respondent or the interviewer (Rasinski, Mingay, & Bradburn, 1994). This may also lead to a satisficing strategy on the part of respondents, in which they simply check the first few responses, but stop when they deem that they have checked "enough." This response pattern would result in a primacy effect, that is, a tendency toward the first rather than the latter items in the list being checked more frequently (Dillman, 2000, principle 2.10). It would better to pose questions as a series of options where the respondents have to make an explicit choice in favor of or against each statement (see, for example, question 39, NDMS, Resource C).

Use a Column Format for a Series with the Same Response Categories

Often a series of survey questions (especially those relating to respondents' attitudes toward a particular topic) have the same response categories (such as "strongly agree, agree, disagree, not sure, disagree, or strongly disagree"). To economize on the amount of space required for responding to these questions and facilitate the ease of recording the responses, a column format for arraying the questions and response categories is recommended. With interviewer-administered questionnaires, numbers (such as 1 through 5) can be assigned to the response codes or continuum (see question 3 in the National Dental Malpractice Survey, Resource C) and the interviewer can be instructed to circle the number that corresponds to the respondent's answer.

The labels for response codes can also be column headings for answers to a series of subparts to a question. These labels should be placed directly over the codes to which they apply (as in question 3 in the National Dental Malpractice Survey, Resource C):

Q-3. Please indicate the extent to which each of the following statements is typical of your ***unsatisfactory patient encounters***. (*Circle your responses*)

	Very Typical				Not at All Typical
	(*Circle one response for each item.*)				
1. The patient was trying to manipulate me.	1	2	3	4	5
2. The patient did not accept responsibility for his/her own dental health.	1	2	3	4	5

The Household Listing Form, Education Module, and Child Labour Module in the UNICEF MICS-2 (Resource A) illustrate the use of a matrix (or table) to gather information on all members of a household in an interviewer-administered survey. Each has questions in columns for which places to respond for each member of the household are provided in corresponding lines (or rows) of the matrix. Dillman (2000) cautions researchers against using such matrices in self-administered questionnaires, however. Matrices require complex skills in order to use them, and respondents may lose track of the basic navigational path through the matrix. Researchers are advised instead to separately break out and repeat the series of questions for each household member or event rather than consolidating them into a matrix (Dillman, 2000, principle 3.5). The use of such matrices is more feasible for interviewer-administered surveys, such as the UNICEF MICS-2, but interviewers would need to be carefully trained in the use of them.

Use a Column Format for a Series with Comparable Skip Patterns

Sometimes a series of questions may have a comparable skip pattern, such as asking how many times a particular type of health professional was seen after first asking questions about whether that type of provider was consulted or not (see item 12 in Exhibit 12.1). Once again, a column format, with the relevant questions and instructions serving as headings for the respective questions, is appropriate. This has many of the same advantages as noted for a series with the same response categories. It also ensures that the answers to any follow-up questions are clearly linked to the preceding (screener) questions. This is a relatively complex format, and it is not generally recommended for use in self-administered survey questionnaires.

Put All Parts of a Question on the Same Page

Questions and accompanying response categories should never be split between pages; the respondent or interviewer would have to flip back and forth to answer the question or might assume that the question ends on the first page and therefore fail to consider certain responses. Nor is it desirable to split subparts of a question, particularly if the same skip patterns or instructions apply to all parts of the question.

Allow Plenty of Space on the Questionnaire

There should be sufficient space provided in the questionnaire for responding to open-ended questions. A large and clear typeface should be used in printing the questionnaire or displaying the questionnaire on a computer screen. Also, the questions should not be crowded together on the printed page or the computer screen. Dillman recommends that blank spaces, rather than dividing lines, be used to separate questions in a self-administered survey and that space be provided at the end of a mail questionnaire for any additional comments respondents may wish to offer (see the last page of the NDMS, Resource C) (Dillman, 1978, 2000; Salant & Dillman, 1994).

Carefully Consider the Appearance of the Questionnaire

Dillman's TDM places considerable emphasis on the appearance of questionnaires, particularly that of mailed self-administered forms. It is generally desirable to put paper-and-pencil questionnaires into booklets to permit ease in reading and turning pages and also to prevent pages from being lost.

Dillman (2000) recommended that researchers consider one of the following three conventions when developing multipage questionnaires:

1. Use conventional legal-size paper (eight and a half by fourteen inches). Fold and staple it along the spine to create a booklet eight and a half by seven inches. This format can be used when printing one column or set of questions per page.
2. Use full-size pages (eleven by seventeen inches). Fold and staple along the spine to create a booklet eight and a half by eleven inches. This format can be used when dividing each page into two columns with sets of questions. When using this format, one should avoid printing items in smaller than twelve-point type.
3. Print pages of desired dimensions on one side only and staple them in the upper-left corner. If resources are constrained, this format can be used, but it is generally the least preferred of these options.

The front cover of the questionnaire should be a simple and neutral graphic design, complete with a title and the name and address of the survey sponsor (see Exhibit 12.1). The back cover of the questionnaire should merely consist of "an invitation to make additional comments, a thank you, and plenty of white space" (Dillman, 2000, p. 139). (See the back cover of the NDMS questionnaire, Resource C, and Dillman, 2000, Figure 3.24.)

It is helpful in interviewer-administered surveys to provide spaces for the interviewer to record the time that the interview began and ended, particularly during the pilot or pretest stages of the survey, so that the time it will take on average to do the interview can be estimated. With computer-assisted interviewing, the length of the interview can be logged automatically. The number of pages or amount of time for an interview will be influenced by the topic, the respondent's interest in it, the burden and complexity of the questionnaire itself, and the mode of data collection being used. As discussed in Chapter Five, interviewer-administered questionnaires can usually be longer than self-administered ones. Lengthy questionnaires may in particular affect the response rates to mail questionnaires. Dillman (1978) recommended that self-administered questionnaire booklets be no longer than twelve pages. For topics not especially salient to the respondents, the questionnaire should be much shorter.

End the Questionnaire with a Thank You

Questionnaires should always end with a thank you to respondents for their time and effort, as a way of demonstrating our appreciation for the time and effort the respondent took to complete the questionnaire (Dillman, 2000). Mail surveys should include instructions about where to mail the questionnaire.

Consider How the Data Will Be Processed

Thought should be given to how the data will be coded and computerized at the time the questionnaire is being designed. With computerized questionnaires, relevant coding and editing specifications can be built into the questionnaire. Deciding how data from paper-and-pencil questionnaires will be entered into a computer during the period the questionnaire itself is being designed is important for making sure that the data will be available in the form in which they will be needed. The trade-off in making all these decisions at the start is that it takes longer to get the questionnaire actually designed and tested. Procedures for coding and computerizing the data are discussed in more detail in Chapter Fourteen.

Order

The order in which questions are asked in the questionnaire affects respondents' willingness to participate in the study as well as the interpretation of the questions by those who do agree to be interviewed. We should view the questionnaire completion process in the same way we view a conversation: starting with an introduction and then moving from general questions to specific questions and sometimes to sensitive questions. Researchers also should think carefully about whether the order of questions or the way they are designed may affect the response. This includes examining some of the issues discussed in Chapter Eleven (such as yea-saying and the order of questions), as well as examining whether the respondent is inclined to perceive that a sequence of questions expects certain types of responses from them—termed "order effects."

Dillman (2000) describes five types of order effects that can influence responses to questions:

- *The norm of evenhandedness,* a value-based effect, where the respondent invokes norms of fairness or evenhandedness, based on his or her answer to a previous question, in responding to a subsequent question.
- *Anchoring,* a cognitive-based effect, where the respondent uses information from the answer to a previous question in responding to a subsequent question.

- *Addition (carryover) effect or subtraction effect,* where the respondent assumes that his or her answer to a previous question either carries over to the next question (addition effect) or that part of the next question has already been answered in the previous question (subtraction effect).
- *Increased positiveness of summary items when asked after specific items on the same subject,* due to respondents' having been asked to think about concrete aspects of their experience (for example, asking patients about their overall satisfaction with health care after asking them if they are satisfied with specific components of that care). This effect may occur because the specific questions may include information that the respondent may consider when answering the summary question or the respondent may think that he or she is being asked to provide an overall judgment when answering a general question following a series of specific questions on the same topic (Schwarz, Munkel, & Hippler, 1990; Sudman & Schwarz, 1989; Todorov, 2000; Wänke, Schwarz, & Noelle-Neumann, 1995).

The form and content of the study's introduction, which is read to respondents in interviewer-administered surveys or which respondents themselves read in self-administered questionnaires, should be carefully designed and pretested. Medium-length introductions (sixteen to sixty-four words), rather than very short or very long ones (fewer than sixteen words or more than sixty-four, respectively), are likely to elicit the best response. The introduction should state who is conducting the study and for what purpose, the topics that will be addressed in the interview, and the length of time it is expected to take (Andrews, 1984; Bradburn et al., 2004).

It is important that the first question be a relatively easy one for the respondent to answer, that it be on an interesting and nonthreatening topic that is salient to the respondent, and, ideally, that it relate to the focus of the study as set forth in the introduction. In fact, in the spirit of the survey as a conversation, these first questions should focus on issues that the respondent would find interesting to answer (Dillman, 2000). The first question asked in the NDMS, "All in all, on a daily basis how satisfied are you with your practice in general?" is related to the study topic, is about something that is likely to be of interest to the dentist, and should be relatively easy to answer (Resource C, question 1).

It is generally advisable to make the first question a closed-end one so that more structure is provided to the respondent for answering it. This question could, however, be followed by a related open-ended question if the topic is such that respondents are likely to be interested in elaborating on or explaining their answer to the previous question. Mail questionnaires, however, should never begin with open-ended questions because this would give respondents the impression that filling out the questionnaire will be a lot of work. As indicated in Chapter Five, the number of open-ended questions asked in self-administered questionnaires should be kept to a minimum.

Ideally, it is best to ask personal demographic questions—such as the respondent's or household member's age, sex, race, and income—at the end of the interview, after there has been an opportunity to convey clearly the purpose and content of the study and after the interviewer has established rapport with the respondents. Dillman (2000) particularly recommends this be done in mail questionnaires. But as in the California Health Interview Survey, it is often necessary to ask these as screening questions early in the interview in order to decide who to interview or to oversample certain population subgroups (CHIS 2001, section A). In that case, the rate of break-offs and refusals subsequent to asking these questions should be carefully evaluated during the pretest of the questionnaire, and the questions or other aspects of introducing the study to respondents should be redesigned to try to maximize cooperation.

For topics that have higher salience or when asking both general and specific questions about attitudes, it is advisable to ask general questions before specific ones. In contrast, for general questions about people's behaviors, particularly questions that might be less salient to respondents or rely on the recall of specific events, asking detailed questions about these experiences first might help them recall the details needed to answer the more general question. For example, in the CHIS 2001, questions about people's total number of visits to a physician in the year (CHIS 2001, section H, question AH5) follow a series of questions about the types of preventive exams and tests they have received, as well as questions regarding their usual source of care. This approach provides respondents with an opportunity to recall specific details about their experiences before they are asked to answer a more general question that summarizes them. It should be pointed out, however, that whenever individual items from other studies are used in a survey, the context for these items (the questions that precede and follow) may well differ, and this could affect the comparability in how respondents answer the questions.

Research applying the principles of cognitive psychology to questionnaire design has suggested that people tend to use autobiographical schemata in responding to survey questions, particularly those that require the recall of a series of events over time (Schwarz & Sudman, 1994; Tourangeau, Rips, & Rasinski, 2000). In designing such questions, researchers should phrase the question or series of questions in such a way that respondents are asked to respond in chronological order—either from the present backward in time or from some point in time in the past to the present. It may also be helpful to identify a salient autobiographical event of either a personal nature ("Since you were married . . . ") or a public nature ("Since the last presidential election . . .") that can serve as an anchor point for respondents to use in recalling these events.

In general, it is advisable to group together questions related to the same topic. Also, as mentioned in Chapter Eight, transitional phrases or instructions should be provided when new topics are introduced so that the shift does not seem abrupt to respondents and they have an opportunity to think about the topic before being called on to answer a question about it.

Consideration should also be given to arranging the order and format of questions so that respondents do not fall into an invariant pattern in responding to the items—referred to as a response set—because of boredom or the burden of providing discriminating answers to the questions. For example, a series of questions might ask respondents to report whether they saw certain providers in the year and, if so, how many times. If a great many questions in the questionnaire are of this kind, respondents may get wise and decide to start saying no when asked if they had certain types of experiences because they realize they can avoid answering many other questions if they do so. Varying the format and placement of such questions is thus important for enhancing the interest and variety of the questionnaire, as well as for reducing the chance of respondents' falling into these types of patterns in responding to the questionnaire.

In developing questionnaires, Dillman (2000) recommends that researchers carefully think through the navigational flow of the questionnaire as well as what devices would be used (for example, directional arrows, type sizes, skip patterns) to facilitate the movement through the questionnaire. In addition to developing and using navigational aids to steer respondents through the questionnaire, it is also helpful to design a flowchart that explicitly reflects the order in which questions are asked and the questions to which respondents are directed on the basis of answers to prior questions. Such flowcharts are imperative in designing computer-assisted data collection instruments and strongly advised in thinking through the arrangement of questions in paper-and-pencil questionnaires, especially those that have large numbers of items or complex skip patterns.

Context

The study of context effects in survey questionnaires is an area of methodological research that draws heavily on the concepts and theories of cognitive psychology (Hippler, Schwarz, & Sudman, 1987; Schwarz et al., 1990; Schwarz & Sudman, 1992; Sudman & Schwarz, 1989; Todorov, 2000; Tourangeau & Rasinski, 1988; Tourangeau, Singer, & Presser, 2003; Wänke et al., 1995).

Each of the stages in responding to a question (comprehension, retrieval, estimation or judgment, and response) can be affected by the questions that precede it. Earlier questions can provide information for the respondent to use in understanding the questions that follow. They can also prime respondents to consider particular types of beliefs that they might then call on later as they try to retrieve their opinion on a related issue. The earlier questions can provide some norm or standard of comparison for respondents to use in making a judgment about the right answer to the current question. Finally, in the response stage, respondents may feel that their answers should be consistent with attitudes or information they provided earlier in the questionnaire.

The context of survey questions becomes problematic when people answer what seems to be the same question differently depending on the content and order of other questions in the questionnaire. This would be a particular issue in using and comparing the same items between different surveys. It is advisable for survey designers to build in a split-ballot experiment or a think-aloud feedback strategy in evaluating different versions of the questionnaire during the pilot or pretest stages of the study if they think that context effects might be a problem in their study.

Special Considerations for Formatting Internet Surveys

In addition to the formatting recommendations provided above, when designing a survey that will be administered on the Web, survey designers will need to design questions that can be viewed on a variety of Web browsers since questionnaires that were designed using extensive computer programming may not load properly on some Web browsers. Dillman, Tortora, and Bowker (1999), for example, suggest the development of user-friendly designs such as a plain questionnaire without color and tables as a way to overcome this problem. In addition to examining the look and appearance of the actual questionnaire on the Web, survey designers need to think about the way that computer users use computer software when designing the survey (for example, tool bars, scroll bars, buttons). In particular, survey developers need to design a questionnaire that conforms to what users expect when they operate a computer. This is referred to as "usability testing," which is an important added dimension of developing and evaluating Web-based surveys (Murphy et al., 1999).

Dillman (2000) presents a series of principles for designing Web surveys—for example:

- Present each question in a manner that is similar to what is normally used in a paper self-administered survey.
- Restrain the use of color to encourage consistency in appearance and improving the navigational flow through the Web page.

- Provide specific instructions on how to execute the computer action (for example, "click the button on the bottom of the page") that is needed to flow through the form.
- Use drop-down boxes sparingly (drop-down boxes are boxes on a Web page that have a line with a triangle pointing to other hidden response options).
- Do not force a respondent to answer a question before going to another one.
- Develop skip patterns in a way that allows respondents to click on a link that takes them directly to the skip pattern.
- Exercise constraint in using question formats that have known measurement problems in paper questions (for example, "check all that apply").

Special Considerations for Special Populations

The form and format of survey questionnaires must acknowledge and take into account the capacities of potential respondents—aurally, visually, and cognitively. The respondent's familiarity with the norms and culture of survey research (that is, how to be a good survey respondent), the cultural norms of the target population regarding types of information individuals share with strangers, and the reluctance of respondents to admit they may have literacy or visual challenges may all influence the data that can be accurately obtained from survey respondents. Different modes of gathering data rely and call on different aptitudes on the part of survey respondents. The choice of method for formatting and presenting survey questions should therefore seek to optimize or match the unique strengths of a given method with the special capabilities of those of whom the questions are asked.

Selected Examples

The surveys in Resources A, B, and C drew heavily on many of the principles detailed here for designing and formatting survey questionnaires. The UNICEF MICS-2 presents special challenges because of the need to provide a core set of questions that can be answered across different countries while respecting the differences in culture across these countries. To strike a balance between the need to have a standardized protocol for administering the survey and the need to provide culturally sensitive instructions for completing the survey, the UNICEF MICS-2 instruction manual includes adaptation notes that indicate where in the questionnaire there may be variations in question wording, as well as when the survey coordinator needs to adapt the instructions to fit the need of the community being surveyed.

For example, in discussing the Child Labour Module, a notation in capital letters indicates, "THE UPPER AGE LIMIT FOR CHILDREN INCLUDED IN THE CHILD LABOUR MODULE MAY VARY FROM COUNTRY TO COUNTRY" (UNICEF, 2000, p. A1.1). In a second example, the survey coordinator in each country is advised to decide how to handle introducing the questions regarding contraceptive use. The coordinators are provided instructions regarding the types of interviewers who would be appropriate, as well as how the questions should be introduced to the respondent (UNICEF, 2000, pp. A1.19–A1.20).

The CHIS 2001 reflects adaptations required for computer-assisted telephone interviews, as in question AA5 of the Adult Questionnaire (Resource B), which instructs the interviewer to provide additional response choices ("IF NECESSARY, GIVE MORE EXAMPLES") for the respondent to choose from when answering the question, "And what is your Latino or Hispanic ancestry or origin? Such as Mexican, Chicano, Salvadorian—and if you have more than one, tell me all of them." Another adaptation in telephone interviews with questions that ask the extent to which a respondent agrees with a statement or was satisfied with aspects of their experience, for example, is to break the question into two parts: ask, "Do you agree or disagree?" or "Were you satisfied or dissatisfied?" and then ask, "Do you (dis)agree or strongly (dis)agree?"

Guidelines for Minimizing Survey Errors and Maximizing Survey Quality

Survey developers should employ the principles of questionnaire design highlighted in this and Chapters Eight through Eleven (see Table 12.1). Clarity, coherence, and consistency are sound principles to keep in mind in configuring the format, order, and context of survey questions, respectively. A lack of focus on how the visual flow of the questionnaire facilitates or hinders survey response can lead to item nonresponse. Solutions to this problem may need to be reflective of the different survey modes: face-to-face, mail questionnaires or Web-based surveys, for example. The content and format of the questions, response categories, and instructions must provide clear guidance to survey respondents and interviewers regarding how to answer them. Ideally the order in which questions are posed should reflect an underlying coherence in the concepts and the topics addressed in the questionnaire and their interrelationship. The context in which items

TABLE 12.1. SURVEY ERRORS: SOURCES AND SOLUTIONS—GUIDELINES FOR FORMATTING THE QUESTIONNAIRE.

	Systematic Errors: Questionnaire Effects: Under- and Overreporting, Yea-Saying	Variable Errors: Questionnaire Effects: Order and Context
Solutions to Errors	Employ the do's and don'ts of questionnaire design and related principles in general (Chapter Eight) and for specific types of questions (Chapters Nine, Ten, and Eleven).	Conduct split-ballot experiments to evaluate how answers to questions vary when they appear in a different order in the questionnaire.

are embedded should be governed by a self-conscious logic with respect to how preceding questions may influence those that follow.

Supplementary Sources

Dillman (1978, 2000), Salant and Dillman (1994), Fowler (1995), and Bradburn, Sudman, and Wansink (2004) provide guidance on the design and formatting of paper-and-pencil questionnaires. Couper et al. (1998) provides an overview of the issues in developing computer-assisted instruments, and Dillman (2000) offers guidance for Internet surveys.

CHAPTER THIRTEEN

MONITORING AND CARRYING OUT THE SURVEY

Chapter Highlights

1. Field procedures for carrying out a survey include deciding how to introduce the study to respondents, how to follow up with nonrespondents, when to schedule the initial and follow-up contacts, how to keep track of the results of those contacts, whether to provide cash incentives to respondents, whether to allow respondents to serve as proxies for other people, and what documentation to provide for these procedures.
2. The process of hiring interviewers for a personal or telephone interview should include a consideration of the applicants' physical, social, personal, and behavioral characteristics.
3. Interviewers should participate in a training session that provides a general introduction to survey interviewing and specific aspects of the study that interviewers will be carrying out.
4. Interviewer supervisors should monitor the following quality control tasks: (1) field editing, (2) interview validation, (3) interviewer observation, and (4) retrieval of missing data.
5. Survey management involves assuming responsibility for the overall conceptual development of the study, scheduling and

overseeing the tasks required to carry out the survey, monitoring
quality at each stage of the study's design and execution, and
monitoring expenditures relative to the project budget over the
course of the study.

6. Computer-assisted and Internet-based modes of data gathering
require a great deal of front-end planning but can greatly
expedite data collection, monitoring, and quality control.

This chapter presents the steps for testing and implementing the procedures
needed to carry out surveys designed according to the principles discussed in
the preceding chapters. In particular, it describes the steps in (1) specifying the field
procedures, (2) hiring interviewers, (3) training them, (4) supervising the fieldwork
for the survey, and (5) managing the survey as a whole. When applicable, specific
procedures used in the conduct of personal, telephone, and mail are discussed.
Special considerations in implementing computer-assisted and Internet-based surveys are highlighted at the end of the chapter.

Survey designers should consider the criteria discussed in this chapter whether
they are hiring or training their own interviewers or evaluating the quality of
the field operations of outside firms. If researchers decide to contract with an outside firm, they should request documentation on that firm's procedures for carrying out studies.

Specifying the Field Procedures

Before they begin to implement their survey, designers need to consider the nature of the first contact with respondents about the study.

Advance Notice

It is desirable to provide advance notice of a survey through the news media,
key informant and community contacts, or relevant professional or organizational
sponsors in the targeted communities. Interviews that are preceded by a letter or
other contact are called "warm contacts." Those in which no prior notice is given
to respondents are "cold contacts." Respondents tend to be more cooperative when
they are given advance notice that they will be contacted for an interview.

It should be noted that policies and trends regarding the protection of the privacy of respondents' information (such as the Health Insurance Portability and Accountability Act legislation in the United States, reviewed in Chapter One) may
influence how one can go about establishing the initial contact with the respon-

dent. For example, in conducting a study in a medical practice setting, in order to protect the privacy of the patient, it may be necessary for a member of the staff to first determine during a regular office visit whether the patient is interested in participating in a study before referring him or her to an interviewer. This would ensure that the subject recruitment process is kept separate from the interviewing process. By proceeding in this manner, one is able to ensure that the study does not take place without an explicit consent being obtained, before collecting any data.

Personal. In personal interview surveys, such as the National Center for Health Statistics–National Health Interview Survey (NCHS–NHIS), respondents are usually sent an advance letter that describes the study, intended to decrease the element of surprise when the household is contacted as well as lend legitimacy to the survey effort (National Center for Health Statistics, n.d.). It is also desirable for the interviewer to wear a printed project name tag and carry a signed original letter from the survey director that explains the purpose of the study and can be left with the respondents.

Telephone. Most telephone surveys, especially those based on a random digit dialing sampling approach, are cold contact surveys. However, with the exception of cell phones, databases in which the telephone numbers are linked to names and addresses can be used to identify potential respondents for the purpose of sending an advance letter to the addresses associated with targeted telephone numbers to increase the response rate to the survey.

In the California Health Interview Survey (CHIS), a short message was left on the answering machine the first time the interviewer encountered the machine when attempting an interview. The message described the purpose of the study and its sponsor and indicated that it was not a telemarketing call. This technique was used to perform the same function that an advance letter would serve in terms of helping respondents make an informed decision regarding whether to participate in the survey (UCLA Center for Health Policy Research, 2002b).

Mail. Mail surveys to special populations, such as groups of health professionals, can be preceded by a general announcement in professional newsletters or journals. Dillman's tailored design method recommends that a brief prenotice letter be sent a few days before mailing the actual survey (Dillman, 2000). The letter should notify respondents that an important survey will be forthcoming, briefly state why the study is being done, and convey that their participation would be greatly appreciated.

The tailored design method also points out the importance of the cover letter for eliciting respondent cooperation in mail surveys. Such letters should be addressed and sent to the specific individuals selected for the study (rather than to "Dear Dentist," for example), have the current date, and be signed with a blue ballpoint pen to convey a more personalized approach to the letter. It is particularly important to try to identify a specific individual to whom the questionnaire should be sent in conducting surveys of businesses or other organizations. An alternative to the hand-written signature is to preprint the signature in a color that is in contrast to the black type displayed on the letter. The letters should, at a minimum, explain the social usefulness of the study, why the recipients and their participation are important, the procedures that will be used to ensure the confidentiality of their responses, that their participation in the study is voluntary, the incentives or rewards for participating, and what to do or whom to contact if there are questions about the study. The cover letter should conclude with a thank you for participating (Dillman, 1978, 2000; Salant & Dillman, 1994).

Examples of advance letters and cover letters for personal, telephone, and mail surveys are provided in Chapter Four of *Mail and Internet Surveys: The Tailored Design Method* (Dillman, 2000). The cover letters and reminder postcard used in the National Dental Malpractice Survey appear in Resource C.

Schedule for Contacts

An important issue in designing the fieldwork for surveys is when to schedule contacts with the selected sample units. Launching a general population survey during major holiday periods, such as between Thanksgiving and New Year's Day, should generally be avoided because of the strong possibility that people will be away from home during those periods. The timing of data collection in relationship to specific study objectives should be carefully evaluated for surveys on topics that are likely to have large seasonal effects, such as surveys of allergy prevalence or colds and influenza during certain months of the year (Losch, Maitland, Lutz, Mariolis, & Gleason, 2002; Vigderhous, 1981).

Personal. Research to determine the times that yield the highest rates of interviews with respondents suggests that weekday evenings and weekends, especially Sundays, are the best times to contact households. Researchers may, however, encounter respondents who are too busy, unavailable, or physically or linguistically unable to participate whenever contacted. Special strategies may then be needed to encourage them to respond to the survey, especially in urban, high-density areas and in low-income communities (Couper & Groves, 1996; Stussman, Taylor, & Riddick, 2003; Weeks, Kulka, & Pierson, 1987). Providing interviewers with regular and positive feedback regarding the progression of the data collection activities and direct on-site supervision in the field led to an increase in the overall response rate of an evaluation of an antidrug initiative in four public housing projects, for example (Gwiasda, Taluc, & Popkin, 1997).

Telephone. Answering machines are increasingly in use in U.S. households either primarily to ensure that messages are received while the family is away ("connectors") or primarily to screen unwanted calls ("cocooners"). Call screening devices such as caller ID and call blocking are also increasingly being used to screen out unwanted calls. Urban households, those with higher family incomes, and younger adults are more likely to have answering machines, although once contacted, most are willing to grant the interview. Among users of call screening devices, households with younger adults and households with higher-income families may require more attempts to complete an interview than other households. The use of cell phones has also made reaching and identifying household respondents more difficult. Adults who have only wireless phone service are more likely to be young adults (age twenty-four or younger), male, living alone or with unrelated roommates, renting their home or apartment, and have household incomes below $10,000 (Blumberg, Luke, & Cynamon, 2004; Link & Oldendick, 1999; Oldendick & Link, 1994; Tuckel & Feinberg, 1991; Xu, Bates, & Schweitzer, 1993).

In the CHIS, the maximum number of calls was set at fifty each for the completion of the screener and the extended interviews. However, most screener interviews were completed after three calls, while most adult interviews were completed after two calls (UCLA Center for Health Policy Research, 2002b, 2002d).

Mail. In an analysis of factors contributing to nonresponse rates for 105 mail surveys focusing on natural resources, administered between 1971 and 2000, Connelly, Brown, and Decker (2003) found that administering a survey early in the year (the months of January through March) resulted in a 3 to 6 percent increase in the response rate compared to other times of the year. Dillman's tailored design method calls for a systematic series of timed contacts to elicit the fullest participation in a mail survey, which are described in detail in the discussion that follows (Dillman, 1978, 2000; Salant & Dillman, 1994).

Procedures for Follow-Up Contacts

An important aspect in carrying out a survey is following up with respondents who are not available or do not respond to the first contact. Different protocols for following up may be appropriate with different methods of data collection.

Personal. Returning to households to get a personal interview when respondents were not at home on the first visit can be expensive because of the time and travel. In the NCHS–NHIS, there is no specified upper limit of interviewer contacts at a household in order to obtain an interview, although most interviews were completed within three contacts (National Center for Health Statistics, n.d.). Many researchers or survey research firms have to limit the number of callbacks because of budgetary restraints. They must then consider the probable trade-offs in nonresponse rates relative to survey costs in deciding how many calls to allow interviewers to make. The location of interviewers' initial assignments and the protocols for recontacting households should be carefully designed so that the probable yield for each interviewer contact is maximized.

Telephone. Recontacts can be made more cost-effectively in telephone surveys than in personal interviews. With both personal and telephone interview surveys, all contacts and their outcomes should be recorded. A system of codes to record the disposition of each call, as well as forms on which interviewers can record this information, should be developed, so that a systematic accounting of the status of each case throughout the field period can be made. Different follow-up strategies may also be warranted for different outcomes. When respondents break off an interview or refuse to participate, it is often advisable to reassign the case to a different interviewer, a core group of interviewers whose principal job is to work with reluctant respondents, or an interviewing supervisor. For respondents who are not home at the time of the call or whose line is busy, specific call-scheduling protocols can be used to decide which interviewer should make the follow-up call and when. Most computer-assisted telephone interviewing (CATI) systems do in fact have computerized call scheduling and assignment procedures built into their basic data collection system.

Two approaches were used in the CHIS for determining the optimal time to contact the respondent. If the initial call resulted in no answer, a busy signal, or an answering machine, the automatic call scheduler would place the telephone number into a "time slice queue" (for example, Saturday, 10:00 A.M. to 6:00 P.M.) for a follow-up call. This method was used for up to fourteen attempts. Once the interviewer made contact with the respondent, all subsequent calls were made based on the respondent's assessment of the best time to call back.

Mail. Dillman's total survey design approach to mail surveys provides a systematic set of procedures to maximize the survey response rate (Dillman, 2000). It also argues for the value of multimodal approaches, such as following up with nonrespondents to mail surveys by telephone, to ensure a good response rate:

1. Send a personalized, advance letter to everyone selected for the study.
2. Within a week, mail a personalized cover letter with somewhat more detail about the study, a questionnaire, and stamped return envelope.

3. Four to eight days later, send a follow-up postcard to thank everyone who responded and to ask those who have not to do so.
4. Two to four weeks after the first questionnaire is mailed, send a new personalized cover letter to those who have not responded indicating that "we have
   not yet heard from you" and including a replacement questionnaire and
   stamped return envelope.
5. A final contact can be made by telephone, overnight express, special delivery,
   or priority mail (in contrast to using regular mail delivery for the previous mailings). This distinguishes the final contact from the other mailings.

Multimodal follow-up strategies, such as those proposed in the final stage of
the tailored design approach, are likely to be successful in enhancing survey response rates, though consideration does need to be given to possible mode effects for some questions (Fowler, Roman, & Di, 1998; Fowler et al., 2002).

The National Dentist Malpractice Survey employed Dillman's five steps for
implementing a mail survey. It also benefited from suggestions by Sudman on the
design of mail surveys of reluctant professionals: (1) point out the professional benefits given their time and effort involved in participating and (2) be sensitive to confidentiality issues. A five dollar bill was included in the initial mailing to dentists
as an incentive for them to participate. An overall response rate of 76.7 percent
was achieved in the study, which is quite a good rate of return for mail surveys
(Washington State University, 1993).

Incentives to Respondents

Survey designers may want to consider the cost-effectiveness of offering incentives
to respondents to participate in a study. Methodological research has borne out
the effectiveness of systematic follow-up strategies for achieving good response
rates, particularly in combination with sending even a modest monetary incentive
(one to two dollars) with an initial mailing or before an interview (Armstrong &
Lusk, 1987; Arzheimer & Klein, 1999; Church, 1993; de Leeuw & Hox, 1988;
Perneger, Etter, & Rougemont, 1993; Yammarino, Skinner, & Childers, 1991). Research also confirms that monetary incentives increase response rates without necessarily biasing study results (James & Bolstein, 1990; Shettle & Mooney, 1999;
Singer, van Hoewyk, Gebler, Raghunathan, & McGonagle, 1999; Singer, van
Hoewyk, & Maher, 1998, 2000; Willimack, Schuman, Pennel, & Lepkowski, 1995;
Yu & Cooper, 1983).

Nevertheless, criticisms may be made of such incentives, principally because
of concerns about setting unfortunate or unaffordable precedents for the field,
whether such incentives are warranted for well-paid health professionals, as well

as whether they may be viewed to be coercive for particularly vulnerable or at-risk respondents, such as patients in a selected medical practice or participants in a drug treatment program.

The U.S. Office of Management and Budget (OMB) forbids the offering of blanket financial incentives to respondents in federally sponsored surveys. The 1995 Paperwork Reduction Act required an explanation for a decision to provide any payment or gift. Requests must be submitted to OMB, and cases are decided on an individual basis. Compensation or remuneration is usually provided when particularly burdensome or time-consuming requests are made of study participants, who might not otherwise agree to participate in the study.

One type of nonmonetary incentive that some groups (such as members of a professional group being surveyed) may find appealing is the survey results. A return postage-paid postcard can be provided or respondents can be asked to indicate on the outside of the return envelope for the questionnaire if they would like to have a copy of the finished survey; in this way, they do not have to record their names and addresses on the questionnaire itself.

Another approach in mail, telephone, and personal interview surveys is the foot-in-the-door technique. This approach is a two-stage strategy in which respondents are asked to respond to relatively small initial request (such as being asked to answer a brief series of questions about health or exercise practices over the telephone) and then to participate in a larger data collection effort, which is the real focus of the study (for example, a more extensive series of questions on their use of health care facilities). Research on the effectiveness of this method has produced mixed results. Some studies have shown that it increases respondents' participation in the larger effort, and others have shown the opposite (Dillman, 2000; Hippler & Hippler, 1986; Hornik, Zaig, Shadmon, & Barbash, 1990).

Proxy Respondents

Another issue to consider when gathering survey data is whether respondents should be allowed to provide the interview or fill out the requested information (that is, act as proxies) for other individuals who were selected for inclusion in the study. Proxies are used, for example, when parents are interviewed about their children's health or health care practices.

Personal. It is not appropriate to ask proxies to answer subjective questions that seek to elicit the opinions, attitude, or knowledge of the sample person. Proxies may, however, be asked to provide verifiable factual information. The level of accuracy of reporting is likely to be greater, the greater is the level of communication between couples (that is, spouses or partners) regarding the issue. Proxies for patients with functional disabilities tend to report that the patients have greater limitations in instrumental activities of daily living (taking medication, using the telephone, shopping, preparing meals, doing housework, and so on) than do the patients themselves. Proxy respondents are generally better able to provide accurate responses for observable health conditions (for example, physical health and activities of daily living) than for nonobservable events (for example, symptoms) for elderly or disabled persons (Magaziner, Bassett, Hebel, & Gruber-Baldini, 1996; Magaziner, Simonsick, Kashner, & Hebel, 1988; Magaziner, Zimmerman, Gruber-Baldini, Hebel, & Fox, 1997; McGovern & Bushery, 1999; Menon, Bickart, Sudman, & Blair, 1995; Mosely & Wolinsky, 1986).

Telephone. Telephone surveys that gather information on everyone in the family from the person who happens to be at home at the time of the interview sometimes yield results that suggest that proxies tend to report more health problems for themselves than for others. Those who happen to be at home at the time may well be sicker than those who are not. In surveys in which healthy respondents are asked to respond for those who are too sick to respond for themselves, the opposite is likely to be true. Furthermore, as indicated in Chapter Ten, proxy respondents are less likely to underreport sensitive health behaviors for others than are those individuals themselves.

In the CHIS, the most knowledgeable adult was asked to answer the questions for children (under age twelve) and selected questions for adolescents (ages twelve to seventeen). Proxy reporting was also used when the sample respondents were over age sixty-five and unable to respond for themselves because of physical, mental, or emotional limitations (UCLA Center for Health Policy Research, 2002b).

Mail. Cognitive research on the level of agreement between self-reports and proxy reports suggests that the information processing strategy underlying how the questions are phrased (recalling specific episodes versus estimating the number of events), the order and context in which they are asked, and the extent to which the proxy and self-report respondent talk to each other about the activity or attitude being referenced all influence the convergence of proxy and self-reports (Bickart, Blair, Menon, & Sudman, 1990; Bickart, Menon, Sudman, & Blair, 1992; Menon et al., 1995; Moore, 1988).

In general, it is not advisable to ask someone to answer attitudinal, knowledge, or other perception-oriented questions for others. Proxy respondents who say they are knowledgeable about a selected individual's behaviors will probably do a good job of reporting this information for him or her, although it is advisable to ask additional questions in order to understand the extent to which the proxies have actually spent time with the sample persons or discussed the matters being referenced with them.

Documentation of Field Procedures

Survey designers should provide written documentation of the specific field procedures to be used in carrying out the survey. In personal and telephone interview surveys, these procedures can serve as resources for training interviewers as well as a reference for interviewers to consult in addressing problems or questions that arise in the course of the study.

Survey procedure manuals generally describe the purpose and sponsorship of the study and tell the respondents whom to contact and how if they want more information about the project. They describe the sample design and, when appropriate, give detailed instructions about how to carry it out. They include the project time schedule, the primary supervisor for the project and how to reach him or her, procedures for gaining the cooperation of and establishing rapport with respondents, and a sample of questions respondents might ask about the study and instructions on how to answer them. There is usually a description of the data collection forms and procedures to use in registering the status of cases that are in process, as well as those that did not result in completed interviews. These manuals give a brief overview of the screening and questionnaire materials, and include detailed question-by-question specifications that provide definitions for words or phrases used in the questionnaire.

Manuals of field procedures generally contain information similar to that found in the interviewer manuals of the California Health Interview Survey (UCLA Center for Health Policy Research, 2005) and the UNICEF MICS Study (UNICEF, 2000, n.d.). In addition, the CHIS publishes methodological reports describing survey procedures and resulting data quality (UCLA Center for Health Policy Research, 2002a, 2002b, 2002c, 2002d, 2002e).

Hiring Interviewers

In deciding to hire interviewers, consideration needs to be given to the types of interviewing that will be employed, that is, a standard interviewing approach versus a conversational interviewing approach, or a combination of the two. The primary distinction between standard and conversational interviewing is that in the former, the interviewer is expected to develop and use a protocol that provides a similar set of responses regarding how interviewers respond to questions from the respondent, how they should probe for responses, and so on. Conversational interviewing allows the interviewing to alter the wording of the question to fit the respondent's situation. These approaches may have an effect on the skills that are emphasized in hiring and training of interviewers (Biemer & Lyberg, 2003; Houtkoop-Steenstra, 2000).

The process of hiring interviewers for a personal or telephone interview survey should include consideration of applicants' physical, social, personal, and behavioral characteristics. Physical characteristics include age, sex, race, physical condition, physical appearance, and voice quality. Social, personal, and behavioral characteristics encompass experience and work history, education, intelligence, personality, attitude and motivation, adaptability, and accuracy.

Physical Characteristics

With respect to the desirable age for interviewers, some preference exists for mature individuals—those twenty-five to fifty-five years of age. Younger interviewers may, however, be appropriate for selected populations, such as adolescents (Berk & Bernstein, 1988; Hox & de Leeuw, 2002).

Most interviewers are women. There are assumptions in the survey research field that respondents are more likely to open their doors or continue with an interview over the telephone, as well as to respond to questions about sensitive or embarrassing issues, when contacted by a female interviewer. However, the choice of male or female interviewers should be guided primarily by the survey's subject matter and data collection design, and thought should thus be given to whether the gender of the interviewer is likely to be of any particular significance in the context of that study (Catania et al., 1996).

Another issue here is how respondents will respond to an interview conducted by someone who is not of their own race. This may be an issue in surveys dealing with explicitly racial topics, such as studies of attitudes about the effect of the sexual practices of different racial or ethnic groups on their risk of contracting HIV/AIDS or other sexually transmitted diseases. Minority respondents tend to provide more deferential or socially desirable responses to such questions when interviewed by a majority-race interviewer. If the subject matter of the survey deals directly with racially related topics, some thought should thus be given to matching interviewers and respondents along racial and ethnic lines. If a study is targeted to a particular racial or ethnic population subgroup, such as residents of an inner-city barrio, it would be important to talk with community leaders about these issues before hiring and assigning interviewers to such areas (Davis, 1997; Hurtado, 1994).

In personal interviews, it is important that an interviewer present a neat, pleasant, and professional appearance to respondents so that they feel comfortable admitting him or her to their home.

Research has been conducted on the impact of telephone interviewers' voice quality on refusal rates. Interviewers with the lowest refusal rates tended to have higher-pitched voices and greater ranges of variations of pitch, spoke more loudly and quickly, and had clearer and more distinct pronunciation. They were also rated as more competent overall and as taking a more positive approach to the respondent and the interview than those with higher refusal rates. Attention should thus be given to evaluating the overall quality of telephone interviewers' voices during hiring and training. The information and impression conveyed by the interviewers over the telephone are the only clues respondents have about whether the study is legitimate and, if they agree to cooperate, how they should approach answering the questions that are asked of them (Oksenberg, Coleman, & Cannell, 1986).

Social, Personal, and Behavioral Characteristics

Evidence of a responsible work history is generally a useful criterion to consider in hiring interviewers. Since many women use interviewing as a way of entering or reentering the workforce after a number of years as full-time homemakers, it is appropriate to inquire about relevant volunteer or nonsalaried work experience.

Previous experience as an interviewer or in seemingly related areas (sales or fundraising) does not necessarily indicate that a person will be a good interviewer in a given study. Different researchers or survey research firms may have different interviewer training protocols or data collection norms and procedures. Training for a new study or with a different organization may involve unlearning old habits, which might be hard for some people to do. Also, a sales or missionary zeal is not appropriate to surveys, which attempt to capture as accurately and objectively as possible what the respondent thinks or feels about a topic. Furthermore, respondents might refuse to cooperate if they feel that the interviewer is trying to sell them something. Training, commitment, and the accrual of relevant experience within a given study appear to be consequential correlates of interviewers' performance (Edwards et al., 1994; Groves, Cialdini, & Couper, 1992; Groves & Couper, 1998; Groves, Dillman, Eltinge, & Little, 2002; Groves et al., 1988; Parsons, Johnson, Warnecke, & Kaluzny, 1993; Snijkers, Hox, & de Leeuw, 1999).

Most interviewers have at least a high school education. It is sometimes desirable for interviewers to have some college education as well, particularly if the concepts or procedures used in a study are complex or require some degree of analytical or problem-solving ability. Too much education can be a liability, however, because highly educated individuals may feel overqualified for the job and become bored or careless as a result.

A related quality to look for in interviewers is native intelligence, although survey interviewing ordinarily does not call for exceptionally high levels of intellectual ability. The capacity to read and understand written materials, make sound and intelligent decisions, and express themselves clearly verbally and in writing sums up the qualities to look for when hiring interviewers. An interest in talking and listening to people is also a useful personality trait for an interviewer. In addition, interviewers should not be easily affected by others' lifestyles and attitudes.

Interviewing is demanding work; having people slam the door in your face or hang up the telephone when you call can be part of the daily experience. Furthermore, there is often the frustration of making repeated calls to a home and never finding the person there. Interviewers should therefore be highly motivated for the job and be adept at figuring out how to make the best use of their time to finish the required interviewing task and deal with difficult or frustrating situations in the field.

Another important prerequisite for a successful interviewer is adaptability and flexibility with respect to working hours. A survey of hospital executives might require interviewers to contact and interview them during a regular nine-to-five business day. In contrast, interviewing middle-class couples in a high-rise security complex might require trying to gain access through a security guard or answering machine or making calls during weekend or evening hours.

A willingness to try to enter or record accurately the answers provided by respondents is another important quality for an interviewer. Computer-assisted modes of data collection help to mitigate this issue.

Many of these qualities are hard to quantify on job applications or intake interviews. They are, however, the characteristics to look for in deciding who will probably make a good interviewer.

The task of ensuring that interviewers are qualified does not end with the hiring process. Interviewers must undergo a training period during which they are taught the general norms and guidelines of the particular firm or researcher in charge of the project, as well as the specific requirements of the survey in which they will be involved. In addition, their performance should be carefully evaluated before they conduct their first interview with an actual respondent, and the quality of their work should be monitored on a continuing or sample basis throughout the entire field period for the study.

Training Interviewers

Interviewer training usually encompasses both a general introduction to survey interviewing and fieldwork techniques and procedures and a review of the specific aspects of the study that the interviewer will be carrying out. General and study-specific interviewer manuals are important resources for the respective types of training. The following excerpt from Weinberg's chapter in the *Handbook of Survey Research* (1983, pp. 344–345) indicates that a typical study-specific interviewer training agenda addresses the following topics:

1. Presentation of the nature, purpose, and sponsorship of the survey
2. Discussion of the total survey process
3. Role of the professional survey interviewer (including a discussion of the ethics of interviewing—confidentiality, anonymity, and bias issues)
4. Role of the respondent (helping respondent learn how to be a respondent)
5. Profile of the questionnaire used (identification of types of questions and instructions, answer codes, precolumning numbers for data processing, and so on)
6. Importance and advantages of following instructions (examples of disadvantages to interviewer when instructions are not followed)
7. How to read questions (including correct pacing, reading exactly as printed and in order, conversational tone)
8. How to record answers (for each type of question)
9. How and when to probe (definition and uses of probes for each type of question)
10. Working in the field or on the phone (preparing materials, scheduling work, introduction at the door or on the phone, answering respondent's questions, setting the stage for the interview)
11. Sampling (overview of types of samples, detailed discussion of interviewer's responsibilities for implementation of last stage of sampling on specific survey)
12. Editing (reviewing completed questionnaires for legibility, missed questions, and so on)
13. Reporting to the supervisor (frequency and types of reports required)

The training sessions in the CHIS incorporated many of these elements.

Resources and techniques for interviewer training include (1) written resource materials, (2) lectures and demonstrations, (3) home study, (4) written exercises, (5) role playing, (6) practice interviews, and (7) coding of interviewer behavior. A study's interviewer manual contains the main written resource materials for a study. Interviewers are encouraged to read and study these materials at home before the training session and to refer to them during training and in the field as needed. Lectures and demonstrations are commonly used in interviewer training sessions. It is also helpful to demonstrate an actual interview so that interviewers can get a sense of how it should be carried out. Group discussions afford interviewers the opportunity to take an active role in raising questions or clarifying their understanding of aspects of the study. Written exercises on the more complex features of the questionnaire, such as the process of sampling within-household respondents, also help reinforce an interviewer's ability to handle those issues.

Round-robin interviewing and role playing are useful devices in training interviewers. An interviewer might administer the questionnaire to a supervisor or another interviewer who reads his or her answers from a script in which different aspects of an interviewing situation are presented. It may be desirable to have more than one script so that the interviewers can role-play different situations. This activity enables the supervisor to observe each interviewer's style of interviewing and provide feedback as appropriate.

The culminating—and perhaps most important—component of the interviewer training process is the opportunity to conduct a practice interview with an actual respondent. Interviewers may be asked to interview a friend or family member, for example, to get a sense of how an interview should go. The interviewer should then administer the interview to one or two other respondents who are recruited on a paid or voluntary basis. The supervisor can review the interviewers' performance during these trial runs. If the interview is satisfactory, the interviewers can be assigned to the field. If their performance is not acceptable, they can be retrained on those aspects of the study with which they seem to be having problems and asked to do one or two more practice interviews. If their performance is still not satisfactory, this could be grounds for dismissal from the project. Potential interviewers should, of course, be advised at the time they are recruited for the study that dismissal could be an outcome of training.

As mentioned in Chapter Eight, it may also be useful to observe and code systematically the behavior of interviewers to identify those who are having particular problems for the purposes of screening for hiring, devoting special attention to what are identified to be weak spots during training, or retraining or strengthening interviewer performance as the study proceeds (Edwards et al., 1994).

The length of the formal training period varies from study to study. The number of days of training should be based principally on the complexity of the questionnaire and associated field procedures and the level of interviewer experience with comparable studies. In most academic, professional survey organizations, training is generally two days at a minimum. Interviewers who receive less than one day of basic interviewer training are much more likely to display inadequate interviewing skills than those who received two or more days of training (Biemer & Lyberg, 2003; Fowler, 2002).

In complex national surveys, a week or more of initial and supplementary training may be necessary. The effects of five half-days of interviewer training have been found to be particularly significant for factual questions that required a great deal of activity on the part of the interviewer, such as giving instructions, probing, or providing feedback to the respondent (Billiet & Loosveldt, 1988). It may be particularly advantageous to use a longer training period (two to three weeks of training followed by periodic refresher classes) to train interviewers who have less training or experience to administer surveys to particularly at-risk populations (Beals, Manson, Mitchell, Spicer, & AI-SUPERPFP Team, 2003).

Standardized survey interviewing practices have been emphasized as the norm of the survey research trade for over forty years (Cannell, Miller, & Oksenberg, 1982; Fowler & Mangione, 1990; Hyman, 1955; Kahn & Cannell, 1957; University of Michigan Survey Research Center and National Center for Health Services Research, 1977). In standardized interviewing, interviewers use identical methods to the maximum extent possible in carrying out field procedures, asking questions, probing, and recording responses.

There has been criticism of the artificiality of the standardized interviewing process and the impact that it might have on the accuracy and completeness of answers that respondents provide. Standardized interviewing has been viewed as an essentially stimulus-response approach to data gathering. Conrad and Schober (2000, p. 1) have, for example, argued that "more standardized comprehension may require less standardized interviewer behavior." Proponents of conversational interviewing argue that interviews should be conducted and analyzed as narrative accounts (or stories) that respondents are asked to tell in their own natural language. Otherwise the real meaning of the questions and answers to respondents is lost to the investigator. Narrative analysis procedures originally developed in the field of sociolinguistics can then be used to analyze the resulting data. These procedures involve looking at the narrative accounts provided by respondents in response to a question as stories for which semantics, syntax, and pragmatics can be examined as a way of understanding what respondents meant, how they said it, and how the social context of the interview itself affected the stories (Conrad & Schober, 2000; Houtkoop-Steenstra, 2000; Mishler, 1986; Smith, 1987; Schober & Conrad, 1997; Suchman & Jordan, 1990).

The application of the principles of cognitive psychology in the early stages of developing a more standardized instrument is a constructive and useful approach to addressing these concerns. "Focused" or "conversational" interviewing, in which interviewers are given the opportunity to rephrase the questions to make sense to respondents, if needed, is also an alternative for gathering relatively straightforward factual data (Merton, Fiske, & Kendall, 1990). Interviewers must, however, be trained to distinguish "deviation" (a query that is equivalent in meaning to the original question) from "error":

Original: What is the highest grade or year of school you have completed?

Deviation: How many years of school have you finished?

Error: How many years were you in school?

In either case, investigators should be clear about the approach they want to use in carrying out the interviews in their study and make sure that the interviewing staff is trained accordingly.

Supervising Fieldwork

An important aspect of carrying out a survey is to have well-trained interviewer supervisors. Supervisors are generally involved in training the interviewing staff. They are also in charge of notifying local newspapers and relevant community leaders or agencies about the study, overseeing the scheduling and assignment of interviews to interviewers, implementing the quality control procedures, and writing the time, effort, and expense reports for the interviewing staff. In most firms, interviewer supervisors are former interviewers who came up through the ranks and have a great deal of experience in carrying out and overseeing different types of surveys.

There are four important quality control tasks that supervisors are generally in charge of monitoring: (1) field editing, (2) interview validation, (3) interviewer observation, and (4) retrieving missing data.

Field Editing Questionnaires

In performing this task, supervisors examine the questionnaire before it is sent to data processing to make sure that the interviewer has not made any major mistakes in carrying out the interview. The supervisor may also need to determine whether any of the information has been falsified using techniques such as "curbstoning"—that is, an interviewer's figuratively sitting on a curb to fill out the questionnaire (Biemer & Lyberg, 2003). Interviewers are encouraged to examine the questionnaire before turning it in so that they can get back to the respondent right away if needed. Supervisors sometimes edit a sample of interviewers' work as it is returned or coordinate the transmission of the questionnaires to a staff of editors and then provide feedback, as necessary, to the interviewers on their performance. Supervisors' field editing role is largely eliminated with computer-assisted personal and telephone interview systems.

Validating Completed Interviews

A quality control procedure that may be particularly important in personal interview surveys is the validation of completed interviews. Validation requires the supervisor or a senior interviewer to call back a sample of the cases assigned to an interviewer and directly ask the individuals if they participated in the original interview or to readminister sections of the questionnaire to them. If significant inconsistencies are discovered during this process, other interviews completed by that interviewer could then be checked. Verification that interviewers have falsified cases should result in their immediate dismissal. All of their cases should then be validated and, if necessary, assigned to another interviewer. Telling interviewers that their interviews will be validated in this way will probably eliminate any tendency toward curbstoning. A particular advantage of telephone interviews is that there can be constant monitoring throughout the field period of the placement and outcomes of calls made by interviewers, virtually eliminating curbstoning in telephone-based studies.

Observing Interviewers

Interviewers can be observed during the field period. For example, a supervisor can accompany an interviewer to the field to conduct a personal interview or can ask the interviewer to tape-record the interview. The supervisors can use "behavioral coding" of interviewing behaviors as a means of detecting variations in the quality of interviewing. In behavioral coding, differences in question delivery and feedback that is provided to the respondent's, pacing, or clarity are identified (Biemer & Lyberg, 2003). In telephone interviews, the supervisor can listen in as the interview is being conducted. Observing interviewers in at least one of these ways may be a useful retraining device for interviewers who are encountering problems in the field. It also communicates to the interviewing staff the importance of maintaining consistently high standards throughout the field period.

Following Up to Obtain Missing Data

A fourth major quality control procedure is a protocol for deciding when respondents should be contacted and for what kind or magnitude of information missing when the questionnaire is returned from the field. In general, a list of critical questions should be compiled and incorporated into the field and interviewer training materials. Interviewers should be encouraged to make sure that those questions have been answered before leaving the respondent's home. If they have not been answered, a procedure should be developed for deciding who should follow up to get this information, how, and within what period of time. Computer-assisted personal and telephone surveys offer a greater opportunity to build these types of checks into the design and conduct of the interview itself and to deal with any problems that arise while the interviewer is still on the telephone or with the respondent.

Managing the Survey

Overall management of a project includes responsibility for formulating the tasks, schedule, and budget, as well as monitoring expenditures over the course of the study.

If researchers are carrying out the survey themselves, the principal investigator will have overall responsibility for both the conceptual design of the study and administrative oversight of the project itself. For a large-scale study, specific operational tasks may have to be delegated to a study director, assistant study director, field manager, or other project staff. If the project's principal investigator (PI) contracts with a survey firm, he or she will not have direct responsibility for the actual execution of the study. The PI or the PI's delegate, however, should have the opportunity to provide input and monitor quality at each stage of the survey's development and receive regular progress and financial reports on the project.

Schedule

The sample survey time line in Table 13.1 reflects the steps in designing and conducting a survey outlined in Figure 1.2 and elaborated in the corresponding chapters of this book. The estimated time reported for each stage in Table 13.1 is based on person-weeks, that is, the equivalent of one person working full time (forty hours per week), and is meant to be illustrative but not necessarily applicable to every study. The precise amount of time that each step may require will vary depending on the mode of data collection chosen and type of sampling required. It is also important to keep in mind contingencies that may occur in the design and implementation of the survey, such as the time to obtain funding or institutional review board approval for the study or to draw the sample, as well as unanticipated problems that may occur during the data collection and data analysis stages of the survey.

Budget

Perhaps the most important aspect shaping the scale and scope of a survey is the amount of money available to do it from within one's home institution or through external sources of funding (grants, contracts, cooperative agreements, and so forth). Researchers should clearly specify each of the major tasks associated with carrying out the study (sampling, data collection, data entry, and analysis); the personnel, services, equipment, supplies, and other items required for each of these tasks; the unit costs of the required resources or services; and any general institutional overhead costs associated with the survey. If the researcher contracts with

TABLE 13.1. SAMPLE SURVEY TIME LINE.

Activity (Chapter)	Number of Weeks of Person Effort
Think about the topic for the survey (Chapter One)	One to two
Match the survey design to survey objectives (Chapter Two)	One to two
Define and clarify the survey variables (Chapter Three)	One to two
Think through the relationships between variables (Chapter Four)	One to two
Choose the methods of data collection (Chapter Five)	One to two
Draw the sample (Chapters Six to Seven)	Two to three
Formulate the questions (Chapters Eight to Eleven)	Two to three
Format the questionnaire (Chapter Twelve)	Two to three
Monitor and carry out the survey (Chapter Thirteen)	Four to twelve
Prepare the data for analysis (Chapter Fourteen)	Four to twelve
Plan and implement the analysis of the data (Chapter Fifteen)	Four to twelve
Write the research report (Chapter Sixteen)	Four to twelve

Note: This sample survey time line reflects the steps in designing and conducting a survey outlined in Figure 1.2 and elaborated in the corresponding chapters of this book. The estimated time reported for each activity is based on person-weeks, that is, the equivalent of one person working full time (forty hours per week). The estimated number of weeks in the table is meant to be illustrative and will vary across studies. Also, some of these activities are quite likely to be going on simultaneously.

a survey research firm, the potential contractor should provide a detailed budget for each of the tasks that the firm will be responsible for carrying out. Accounting systems using spreadsheet software should be set up to monitor carefully the expenditure of project funds, relative to the original budget, throughout the course of the study.

Sample budgets for personal, telephone, and mail surveys are shown in Table 13.2 based on Figures 4.1 to 4.3 of Salant and Dillman (1994). If one chooses to use the approach to constructing survey budgets in these tables, wages and other direct costs, such as postage and transportation, would have to be updated and revised in terms of prevailing rates in the locality at the time the study is conducted.

As has been emphasized throughout this book, survey designers need to think through what they want to do before they knock on doors or call to conduct an interview. They also need to realistically consider what they can afford to do—*before* they start. Running out of money before the study is finished means that something does not get done—either well or at all.

TABLE 13.2. SAMPLE BUDGETS FOR MAIL, TELEPHONE, AND PERSONAL INTERVIEW SURVEYS.

A. Mail Survey with a Net Sample Size of 520

	Clerical Hours @ $8.40 per hour[a]	Other Costs (dollars)	Total Costs (dollars)
Prepare for survey			
Purchase sample list in machine-readable form		375	375
Load database of names and addresses	2		17
Graphic design for questionnaire (hire out)		100	100
Print questionnaires: 4 sheets, legal size, folded, 1,350 @ $.15 each (includes paper) (hire out)		203	203
Telephone		100	100
Supplies			
Mail-out envelopes, 2,310 @ $.05 each, with return address		116	116
Return envelopes, 1,350 @ $.05 each, preaddressed but no return address		68	68
Letterhead for cover letters, 2,310 @ $.05 each		116	116
Miscellaneous		200	200
First mail-out (960)			
Print advance-notice letter	3		25
Address envelopes	3		25
Sign letters, stamp envelopes	6		50
Postage for mail-out, 960 @ $.29 each		278	278
Prepare mail-out packets	16		134
Second mail-out (960)			
Print cover letter	3		25
Address envelopes	3		25
Postage for mail-out, 960 @ $.52 each		500	500
Postage for return envelopes, 960 @ $.52 each		500	500
Sign letters, stamp envelopes	12		100
Prepare mail-out packets	14		118
Third mail-out (960)			
Prestamped postcards, 4 bunches of 250 @ $.19 each		190	190
Address postcards	3		25
Print message and sign postcards	6		50
Process, precode, edit 390 returned questionnaires, 10 minutes each	65		546
Fourth mail-out (475)			
Print cover letter	3		25
Address envelopes	3		25

TABLE 13.2. SAMPLE BUDGETS FOR MAIL, TELEPHONE, AND PERSONAL INTERVIEW SURVEYS, *continued.*

	Clerical Hours @ $8.40 per hour[a]	Other Costs (dollars)	Total Costs (dollars)
Sign letters, stamp envelopes	3		25
Prepare mail-out packets	20		168
Postage for mail-out, 475 @ $.52 each		247	247
Postage for return envelopes, 475 @ $.52 each		247	247
Process, precode, edit 185 returned questionnaires, 10 minutes each	31		260
Total, excluding professional time	196	3,240	4,883
Professional time (120 hours @ $35,000 annual salary plus 20% fringe benefits)		2,423	2,423
Total including professional time		5,663	7,306

B. Telephone Survey with a Net Sample of 520

	Clerical Hours @ $8.40 per hour[a]	Interview Hours @ $6.48 per hour[b]	Other Costs (dollars)	Total Costs (dollars)
Prepare for survey				
Use add-a-digit calling based on systematic, random sample from directory	10			84
Print interview manuals	2		20	37
Print questionnaires (940)	4		50	84
Train interviewers (twelve-hour training session)		108		700
Miscellaneous supplies			25	25
Conduct the survey				
Contact and interview respondents; edit questionnaires; fifty minutes per completed questionnaire		430		2,786
Telephone charges			3,203	3,203
Total, excluding professional time	16	538	3,298	6,919
Professional time (120 hours @ $35,000 annual salary plus 20% fringe benefits)			2,423	2,423
Total, including professional time			5,721	9,342

C. Face-to-Face Survey with a Net Sample of 520

	Clerical Hours @ $8.40 per hour[a]	Interview Hours @ $8.10 per hour[b]	Other Costs (dollars)	Total Costs (dollars)
Prepare for survey				
Prepare map for area frame			200	200
Print interview manuals	2		12	29
Print questionnaires (690)	4		345	379
Train interviewers (twenty-hour training session)		140		1,134
Miscellaneous supplies			25	25
Conduct the survey				
Locate residence; contact respondents; conduct interviews; field-edit questionnaires; 3.5 completed interviews per eight-hour day		1,192		9,655
Travel cost ($8.50 per completed interview, interviewers use own car)			4,420	4,420
Office edit and general clerical (six completed questionnaires per hour)	87			728
Total, excluding professional time	93	1,332	5,002	16,570
Professional time (160 hours @ $35,000 annual salary plus 20% fringe benefits)			3,231	3,231
Total, including professional time			8,233	19,801

[a]$7.00 per hour plus 20 percent fringe benefits.

[b]$6.00 per hour plus 8 percent FICA = $6.48; $7.50 per hour plus 8 percent FICA = $8.10.

Source: Adapted from Priscilla Salant & Don A. Dillman, *How to Conduct Your Own Survey* (Figures 4.1–4.3, pp. 46–49). Copyright © 1994 John Wiley & Sons, Inc. Reprinted by permission of John Wiley & Sons, Inc.

Computer-Assisted Data Collection Systems

A variety of computer-assisted data collection systems are available (many of which allow for Web-based data collection) that are also designed to handle the array of data collection and monitoring tasks reviewed here. Computer-assisted data collection (CADAC) methods are becoming the fundamental tools of the trade for governmental, academic, and commercial data collection organizations. Programs used by large-scale governmental and private survey research organizations include commercially available packages, such as AGGIES (Todaro & Perritt, 1999), Autoquest (NORSTAT, n.d.), Blaise (Westat, 2005), CASES (University of California at Berkeley. Computer-Assisted Survey Methods Program, n.d.), WinCATI, and Sensus Web (Sawtooth Technologies, 2003a, 2003b).

In addition, there are computer-based data entry or data management programs for developing customized electronic data collection forms, customized electronic data collection, and customized data documentation processes. These packages include commercially available packages such as the Handheld Assisted Personal Interview (Nova Research Company, 2004a), the Questionnaire Development System (Nova Research Company, 2004b), Snap Surveys (Mercator Research Group, 2005), the Sphinx Survey (Sphinx Development UK, n.d.), The Survey System (Creative Research Systems, 2004), Zoomerang (MarketTools, 1999), and SPSS data entry (SPSS, 2005), as well as free software that is available in the public domain, such as EpiData (EpiData Association, 2000) and EpiInfo (Centers for Disease Control and Prevention, Division of Public Health Surveillance and Informatics, 2004). Many of these systems, which were initially developed for computer-assisted telephone interviewing, are increasingly being adapted and applied to computer-assisted personal and self-interview as well as Internet modes of data gathering.

Substantial investments are required to purchase, maintain, and update these systems. One would need to weigh the alternatives between launching a computer-based system and using traditional methods of data collection and data entry. For example, Harris (1996) noted that costs for editing the NCHS population-based surveys (for example, the National Health Interview Survey), the NCHS provider surveys (for example, the National Hospital Discharge Survey), and the NCHS followback surveys (for example, the National Mortality Followback Surveys) tended to be high and pointed out the advantages of the increasing adoption of computer-assisted data collection and processing methods in these studies. In spite of the underlying costs of such systems, computer-based systems allow decreased time between data collection and data delivery and can result in the production of more accurate and up-to-date data for users as a result of the decreased time in data processing (Ball, 1996). Survey researchers must carefully evaluate whether and what type of such a system would best meet their needs in the most cost-effective manner.

Regardless of whether CADAC systems or paper-and-pencil questionnaires are used to gather the data, successful survey implementation compels the systematic planning and monitoring of the data collection and monitoring procedures reviewed here.

Special Considerations for Implementing Internet Surveys

Special considerations may come into play as well in implementing Internet (e-mail and Web) surveys (Jones, 1999). As in the case of mail surveys, Dillman (2000) suggests that a prenotice e-mail is an important part of a multistage strategy for improving responses to e-mail surveys or Web surveys for which e-mail addresses are available. In fact, he notes that a prenotice e-mail takes on greater importance for Internet surveys as respondents are more likely to quickly discard e-mails after reading them. Dillman also suggests a shorter time lapse between the sending of the prenotice e-mail and the questionnaire than what is recommended for mail surveys (two to three days instead of one week).

Like mail surveys, multiple contacts may be needed to ensure an adequate response rates for Internet surveys. At a minimum, a reminder should be sent, and in some cases, an additional one or two reminders would be appropriate. For e-mail surveys, an advance e-mail would be followed by an e-mail with a cover letter and survey, which would then be followed by the transmission of a replacement questionnaire, along with a reminder to complete the survey. For Web-based surveys, an e-mail with a link that takes them directly to the Web page containing the survey may help to improve the response rate (Dillman, 2000; Umbach, 2004).

Although the need for field editing is minimized with computer-assisted interviewing systems, this issue may still be problematic in fielding Internet surveys. Depending on how the instrument is designed, it may be possible for respondents to mis-key (or type in) their responses to questions. In fact, it may be difficult or impossible to know that study participants have entered correct and accurate data in Web-based surveys (Im & Chee, 2004).

A second problem inherent in implementing an Internet survey is the limited ability to monitor problems that may occur as the respondent attempts to complete the survey. For example, respondents might encounter problems in attempting to download the questionnaire on their computer or, if the survey is not appropriately programmed, skip questions without answering them (Im & Chee, 2004).

A final issue is the possibility of selection bias since "the demographic group that continues to use the Internet most heavily continues to be made up of highly educated, high-income, White males" (Im & Chee, 2004, p. 161). Researchers may need to develop a sampling strategy to counter this potential bias as well as monitor the potential implementation of the data collection to ensure that other populations are adequately covered in the survey implementation process.

Special Considerations for Special Populations

Considerations of the demographics of data collection personnel often come into play when hiring interviewers or deciding which types of interviewers should be dispatched to interview in certain areas or with certain types of respondents. A broader look at the diversity and fit of personnel and procedures at all levels of designing and implementing the data collection process is, however, required, particularly in developing surveys of groups that do not mirror the modal demographic categories (racial and ethnic minorities or gay men with HIV/AIDS, for example).

For example, Leal and Hess (1999) found a relationship between the characteristics of the interviewer and the potential for being biased toward the respondent during the interview process. Interviewers were more likely to evaluate respondents with lower socioeconomic status than themselves as being less informed and less intelligent.

Input from individuals like those who are to be the focus of the study (as senior study personnel, members of community or technical advisory panels, participants in the pretest and accompanying questionnaire and procedures development process, as well as field staff and interviewers) is likely to yield the most fitting and informed approach to gathering data on those populations (Beals et al., 2003; McGraw, McKinlay, Crawford, Costa, & Cohen, 1992; Rhodes, 1994).

One of the issues to consider in implementing survey procedures in countries and communities that are not familiar with the survey process is that it may be important to take the time to learn about the state of the knowledge and information regarding that topic in that community before launching a survey there. There are historical or cultural factors that may shape the nature of types of responses that are provided by the respondents. For example, in some cultures, it may be inappropriate for men to display emotions. Thus, interviewers may obtain inaccurate responses to questions that focus on the expression of worry, anger, anxiety, or stress among men from these cultures, since their response to a question may not reflect how they actually feel. In other cultures, it may be inappropriate for a woman to talk about the topic of sex with a stranger. It may also be inappropriate to have a child serve as a translator for an adult in a study that focuses on asking questions about sensitive subjects such as sexual practices, since these types of conversations do not typically take place between an adult and child (Bulmer, 1998; Kuechler, 1998).

One may also need to be aware of the possibility that the mere presence of an interviewer in the community (as with coming to a home to conduct an interview) may have an effect on the community itself. This is especially important in tightly knit communities, where news of an interviewer's arrival spreads quickly. The nuances of religion (for example, Islam) may dictate the way in which men and women are allowed to interact with each other. For example, it may be inappropriate for men to enter a household to conduct an interview with a married female when the male spouse is not present in the room. Cultural sensitivity is an important consideration in designing and implementing survey data collection procedures with diverse populations (Bulmer, 1998; Newby, Amin, Diamond, & Naved, 1998).

Selected Examples

Detailed general and study-specific training and field procedures manuals were developed by for each of the surveys highlighted in Resources A, B, and C. The manuals for the CHIS and UNICEF MICS are available through the project Web sites (UCLA Center for Health Policy Research, 2005; UNICEF, 2000, n.d.). The cover letters and postcard reminder used in the dentist survey are included in Resource C.

Guidelines for Minimizing Survey Errors and Maximizing Survey Quality

To wind one's way through the data collection process successfully compels envisioning the forest as well as spotting the trees. The array of components in implementing a survey can be viewed as steps along a well-marked path. Fortunately, prominent and productive general and health survey research methodologists have provided useful guideposts for signaling the proper course. These include Don Dillman (Washington State University), Seymour Sudman (University of Illinois) and Norman Bradburn (University of Chicago), Charles Cannell (University of Michigan), Robert Groves (University of Michigan and University of Maryland), and Paul P. Biemer (University of North Carolina) and their respective and numerous colleagues. The schools of thought represented in the corpus of the work of these major investigators and their associates provide particularly useful guidance in thinking systemically and theoretically about the interrelatedness of the steps in carrying out a survey and how best to maximize the quality of the data resulting.

Don Dillman's tailored design method is rooted in exchange theory and a consideration of the rewards and costs presented to respondents in answering a survey questionnaire. His recommendations also incorporate a consideration of the influence of survey design and administration on a variety of types of errors (coverage, sampling, and measurement error), in addition to nonresponse error, which was the central focus of his pioneering contributions in mail survey design (Dillman, 1978, 2000; Salant & Dillman, 1994).

Sudman and Bradburn, as mentioned in Chapter Eight, introduced the notion of response effects in surveys—departures from accuracy that may be influenced by characteristics of the instrument, the interviewer, the respondent, or their interaction. This concept has been elaborated and extended and its empirical origins more fully examined in the substantial body of methodological research conducted by these researchers and their colleagues. They also undertook a fruitful extension of their work in exploring the contributions of cognitive psychology to understanding the effects of question and questionnaire design on survey responses (Bradburn et al., 1979, 2004; Schwarz & Sudman, 1996; Sudman & Bradburn, 1974; Sudman, Bradburn, & Schwarz, 1996).

University of Michigan investigators Charles Cannell and Robert Groves and their associates argued convincingly for the formulation of a fuller theoretical understanding of the interplay of the array of factors that influence respondents' participation in the survey process and the role that interviewers play in encouraging participation (Cannell et al., 1982; Groves et al., 1988, 1992, 2002; Groves & Couper, 1998).

The formulation of the components and costs of survey errors in the context of a total survey error and total survey quality perspective, developed by Groves and Biemer and their colleagues, provides a particularly helpful anchor and benchmark against which the complex decisions involved in designing and implementing surveys can be evaluated (Biemer, Groves, Lyberg, Mathiowetz, & Sudman, 1991; Biemer & Lyberg, 2003; Groves, 1989).

The data collection process and related response rates will be affected by how well the principles of question and questionnaire design highlighted in Chapters Eight through Twelve are dealt with. As summarized in Table 13.3, the key challenge in implementing and monitoring a survey is developing and using systematic procedures for tracking the data collection efforts as well as deciding how to convert nonrespondents. A multitude of sources are available on developing the types of procedures that can contribute to effective and efficient survey implementation (see listing below).

TABLE 13.3. SURVEY ERRORS: SOURCES AND SOLUTIONS— MONITORING AND CARRYING OUT THE SURVEY.

	Systematic Errors		*Variable Errors*
	Questionnaire Effects: Item Nonresponse Bias	**Questionnaire Administration Effects: Unit Nonresponse Bias**	**Interviewer Effects: Interviewer Variability**
Solutions to Errors	Employ the general and specific principles of question and questionnaire design (Chapters Eight through Twelve).	Develop and employ comprehensive and systematic follow-up procedures with nonrespondents.	Develop and employ comprehensive and systematic interviewer training and monitoring procedures.

Supplementary Sources

For additional detail on designing personal or telephone surveys, see Frey and Oishi (1995), Lavrakas (1993), and Stouthamer-Loeber and van Kammen (1995). For mail and self-administered surveys, see Bourque and Fielder (2003) and Mangione (1995). Dillman (1978, 2000) and Salant and Dillman (1994) provide useful guidance in terms of the total design method for both interviewer- and self-administered surveys. The *Handbook of Interview Research: Context and Method* (Gubrium & Holstein, 2002) provides a review of the methods used in standardized, conversational, computerized, and a variety of other types of interviewing. Also, consult Web sites for the Federal Committee on Statistics and Methodology, the National Center for Health Statistics, the National Science Foundation, the Census Bureau, and other federal statistical agencies for methodological reports on the design and implementation of surveys (see Resources D and E).

CHAPTER FOURTEEN

PREPARING THE DATA FOR ANALYSIS

Chapter Highlights

1. Coding survey data involves translating answers into numerical codes that can then be used in computer-based data analyses.
2. Data may be entered and stored on computerized media, such as disk storage space in the body (hard drive) of the computer or portable disks, such as compact disks (CDs), digital video disks (DVDs), zip disks, jump drives, flash drives, or other machine-readable storage media.
3. Both range and consistency checks should be conducted to detect and clean (or correct) errors in the data once the data have been computerized.
4. Before analyzing the data, researchers must decide how to deal with questions for which responses are missing because the respondent neglected to provide the information or the interviewer failed to ask the question properly.
5. External data sources can be used to estimate information for analytical variables of interest in the survey.
6. Analysts should anticipate other data transformations that may be required before implementing the analysis plan.

The rapid development and growth of computer technologies and the Web have had a significant impact on the design, implementation, and analysis of surveys. In particular, the evolution of microcomputers, personal digital assistants (PDAs), and the Internet have made possible the development of high-speed, computer-based systems for collecting, processing, and analyzing survey data (Bourque & Clark, 1992; Couper et al., 1998; Jones, 1999). Computer-assisted and Internet-based personal, telephone, and self-administered data-gathering methods were described in Chapter Five. Many surveys still use paper-and-pencil data collection methodologies, but almost all survey designers now rely on computers in preparing and executing their analyses. Computers have their own technical languages for translating and interpreting information. Survey designers therefore need to know how to process (or transform) the information collected from survey respondents into the symbols, language, and logic of computers if they are to make effective use of this powerful and important technology.

This chapter presents approaches for (1) coding or translating survey responses into numerical data, (2) entering these data into a computer, (3) cleaning or editing the data to correct errors, (4) imputing the answers that either respondents or interviewers fail to provide, (5) using information from other sources to estimate values for certain analytical variables of interest, and (6) anticipating transformations of the data that may be required before executing the analysis plan.

Coding the Data

Coding the data involves translating the information that survey respondents provide into numerical or other symbols that can be processed by a computer. Different approaches are generally involved in coding closed-end and open-ended survey questions. With closed-end questions, for example, response categories are provided to respondents or interviewers to use in filling out the questionnaire. It is advisable that numerical codes be assigned to each of these categories, with instructions to circle or check the number that corresponds to the respondent's answer to that question:

(Circle the number that corresponds to your answer):

Yes   1

No   2

Failure to associate a code with an answer on the questionnaire (for example, simply placing a line to check by each response on a paper-and-pencil questionnaire) will make errors more likely when this response is translated into numbers that can be entered into a computerized data file. With computerized data collection systems, the codes assigned to particular response categories are programmed so that a response is automatically coded when it is entered (typed in on a keyboard by the interviewer or respondent). While nonnumeric characters (such as letters of the alphabet) can also be used as codes or symbols for respondents' answers, it is generally advisable not to do so because they may cause problems when used in certain analysis software packages.

As discussed in Chapter Eight, open-ended questions ask respondents to use their own words in answering. These questions thus yield verbatim or narrative information that has to be translated into numerical codes. Open-ended questions are sometimes asked in pilot studies to elicit responses that can be used to develop categories for coding the data from these questions or to derive closed-end answer formats for the questions in the final study.

To develop codes for open-ended questions, researchers draw a sample of cases in which the question was asked. The actual number of cases to review will vary (say, from twenty-five to one hundred), depending on the sample size for the study as a whole and the variability anticipated in responses to the questions across respondents. The answers to the questions should be reviewed in the light of the concepts or framework to be operationalized in the survey. It may be important to code the answers using a number of dimensions to capture complex study concepts.

Survey designers should consider whether answers reflect broad groupings as well as whether specific responses seem to cluster within general dimensions or even form separate subdimensions within them. For example, in an evaluation of the delivery of case management services to Baltimore Needle Exchange Program recipients, a conceptual model of case management services delivery—the strengths-based case management model (SBCM) developed by Charles Rapp (1998)—was used to guide the approach that case managers used for meeting the needs of these injection drug users. This model also served as the guiding framework for the classification and coding of the various types of case management services (Cornelius et al., 2006).

In the Baltimore Needle Exchange Program evaluation, the case managers used open-ended questions to record specific skills, talents, abilities, and "helping habits" of each client (for example, the client had a high school diploma or consistently participated in a program) according to the SBCM. At the same time, the interests, desires, and goals of the client for various life domains (daily living situations, financial and employment, jobs and education, social support, health, and spirituality) were recorded on charts to which both the case manager and the client contributed. Both past and present attempts of addressing these goals were discussed, including obstacles for overcoming the barriers to achieving these goals.

The information that was recorded on the charts was reviewed for consistency by three licensed senior social workers and a data manager who were trained in the use of the SBCM. The responses under each of these domains were then used to organize and classify and code respondents' specific answers. Responses that fit within each of these categories were identified, and numerical codes were assigned to each. The distributions of responses were tabulated in reporting the answers to this question.

Survey designers should thus be involved in developing codes for open-ended questions because they presumably can specify the most useful form and content of the data for subsequent analyses. Once an initial coding scheme has been developed and a sample of answers has been coded by means of this scheme, another coder should be asked to classify the same responses using the same codes independently. Discrepancies between the two coders should be discussed and the coding scheme then revised as necessary or appropriate training or validation procedures developed to ensure a standardized approach to the treatment of respondents' answers across coders.

Special coding staffs are often trained to deal with open-ended questions. For example, in the California Health Interview Survey, a detailed series of questions are asked about the jobs people hold, and their occupations are then coded according to a scheme developed by the Census Bureau (CHIS 2001, section K, questions AK5–6).

Closed-end questions that ask respondents or interviewers to write in or specify "other" responses not explicitly reflected in the response categories represent a special case of open-ended coding. Coders may be asked to record these responses in a separate file (in which the questionnaire ID number and response are recorded); in computerized data collection systems, space may be provided to input such responses, which are then stored in separate files for subsequent coding or processing. These responses can be periodically reviewed to see if some answers appear with sufficient frequency to warrant developing unique codes to distinguish them from the "other" responses.

Interviewers may also be asked to do field coding of survey responses. With field-coded questions, respondents are not provided a list of categories from which to choose but are asked the question and the interviewer codes their answers according to precoded categories available only to the interviewer. This is an alternative to entirely open-ended coding, which is often costly and time-consuming to do. It can, however, introduce response errors if the interviewers are not accurate or consistent in using the codes provided. With computer-assisted (especially telephone) interview methods, respondents' verbatim answers can be recorded and interviewers' coding independently validated by the interviewing or coding supervisor.

Like survey interviewers, survey coders should be well trained and their work checked periodically. They should also be provided with clear instructions (documentation) for coding each question in the survey and dealing with problems that arise during coding.

The key source document for coding survey data is the survey codebook. The codebook provides detailed instructions for translating the answers to each question into codes that will be read by the computer, and it notes any special instructions for handling the coding of particular questions. These codebooks should be developed for paper-and-pencil surveys. They are generated by commercial and proprietary software used to set up computer-assisted data collection (CADAC) or data entry (CADE) procedures.

The column or columns required to reflect the answers to a question are referred to as the *data field* or the *field size* for that question in the data file. The codebook for the survey usually contains general instructions for approaching the coding process as well as the following specific information for each data field: the questions from which the data were gathered, the codes or numbers to be used in coding answers to these questions, and any special instructions required for coding the item.

The names and descriptive labels for variables constructed from a question can be incorporated into the codebook to facilitate the preparation of documentation for these variables in designing programs to analyze the data (VARIABLE NAMES and VARIABLE LABELS statements in SPSS, for example). Directly incorporating the original question number into the names or labels developed for variables based on these items makes it easier to relate the variables used in the analyses to the source questions on which they are based. Another option to consider is developing variable names that relate directly to content of the question (for example, RATEHLTH for a rating of self-reported health status), which would also make it easier to keep track of the variable during data analysis.

The codes are the numbers that have been assigned to or developed for each of the response categories for closed-end or open-ended questions, respectively. Once again, attention can be given to developing mnemonics for the labels that can be used in documenting what each of the codes means later when the analysis program is designed (VALUE LABELS statements in SPSS).

Finally, special instructions or information may be needed in coding a particular item, such as which questions should be skipped if certain answers are given to that question, whether answers to this question should agree with other answers in the questionnaire, or whether this is a critical question about which respondents should be recontacted if they provide incomplete or unclear information.

In general, the first few columns of a record should contain study and respondent ID information. It is desirable to zero-fill multiple-column fields—for example, coding three days of the disability during the year as "003" in a three-column field for that question—because it is easier to keep track of columns in which data are being entered and some software packages handle blanks differently from zeros in processing the data. Verbatim responses to open-ended questions or "other" responses besides those listed for closed-end items can be coded by means of categories developed for this purpose or listed verbatim for the researcher to refer to later. Uniform conventions for coding different types of missing data should also be developed and documented in the codebook:

Type of Missing Data	Length of Field (Column)		
	1	2	3
Respondent refused to answer	7	97	997
Respondent did not know answer	8	98	998
Question skipped (error)	9	99	999

The codebook should be used as the source document for training coders. Coding supervisors should routinely check samples of the coders' work throughout the study and assist them in resolving any problems that arise in coding.

Entering the Data

Survey data must be entered onto a medium that can be read by a computer. These media include disk storage space in the body (hard drive) of the computer or portable disks, such as compact disks (CDs), digital video disks (DVDs), zip disks, jump drives, or flash drives.

There are two main types of data entry: *transcriptive* and *source* data. Transcriptive data entry involves coding the data onto a source document, which is then used as the basis for entering the information into a machine- or computer-readable medium. The main types of transcriptive data entry use transfer sheets, edge coding, and punching directly from a precolumned questionnaire. In source data entry, the data are coded and entered directly into a machine-readable medium. Source data entry methods include Web-based data entry, optical mark readers, computer-assisted interviewing, and CADE (Couper et al., 1998). Source data entry techniques have evolved in response to the computerization of surveys.

Transcriptive Data Entry

Transfer sheets are sheets that are generally ruled off into a series of columns that reflect the format for the data file. Working from the survey questionnaire and codebook, coders assign codes for each question, and these codes are then entered in the appropriate columns of the transfer sheets. The transfer sheets are used as the basis for entering data onto a computerized medium, such as a database software package.

Edge coding involves reserving space along the margin of each page of a questionnaire—space in which the codes for the answers to each question can be recorded. This space is generally headed with the statement, "Do not write in this space—for office use only." The column numbers for each question are indicated beside or underneath boxes or lines. The codes corresponding to the answers to each question are then recorded in the boxes or on the lines.

Entering data from a precolumned questionnaire is similar to edge coding in that the questionnaire itself serves as the basic source document for coding and entering the data. With precolumned questionnaires, however, the location for the answer to a particular question is clearly indicated, generally along the right margin and as close as possible to the response categories for the question on the questionnaire itself. (See Aday, 1996, Resource A, for an example, based on the National Center for Health Statistics-Health Interview Survey.) For closed-end items, the code for the response category that is circled or checked on the questionnaire is the code that should be entered in the computer for that question. For open-ended questions, coders can write in the codes that have been developed and documented in the codebook, which represent the answers to that question, beside the corresponding column number for the question on the questionnaire.

All three of these transcriptive data entry approaches assume that a codebook has been designed to identify the fields into which the data for a particular question should be recorded. The questionnaires should always be carefully edited before being sent to coding, and the codebook should be used as the basis for identifying the appropriate codes to assign to the answers that respondents have provided. The three transcriptive data entry methods differ principally in the extent to which coders have to transfer information reported in the questionnaire to another location or source for entering. Transfer sheets require transfer of the greatest amount of information and precolumned questionnaires the smallest amount. The more complex the information is to be transferred, the greater is the chance of error. Precolumned questionnaires should be carefully designed so that it is clear what information is to be entered in what fields and what conventions are to be used to provide additional instructions to the data entry personnel for entering this information (such as using red pencils to strike through the columns to be left blank because a question was legitimately skipped or editing responses to a question when the respondent mistakenly circles more than one response code).

Electronic spreadsheet packages such as EXCEL and database management systems such as ORACLE or ACCESS can be used to enter the data onto a computerized file. These software packages are readily available to most computer users and are relatively easy to use. They do not, however, have procedures for data checking and cleaning built in as standardized features, as do the proprietary data entry packages.

Transcriptive data entry methods, especially transfer sheets, have been supplanted by computer-assisted source data entry approaches.

Source Data Entry

Source data entry methods largely eliminate the intermediate step of coding or transferring information to another source or location before entering it onto a computerized medium (Bourque & Clark, 1992; Couper et al., 1998).

One type of source data entry makes use of optical mark readers that read a pattern of responses to boxes or circles that have been penciled in to reflect the respondent's answer to the question. This approach has been used widely in administering standardized tests to students in classroom settings. The type and complexity of questions that can be asked using this approach are limited. This approach also depends heavily on the willingness of respondents or interviewers to record carefully the answers in the spaces provided and on the availability of the equipment required for reading the "mark sense" answer format used in this approach.

Two other direct data entry methods offer much more promise for computerizing survey data and have gained greater prominence with the increasing computerization of the entire survey data collection and analysis process. These are computer-assisted data collection—computer-assisted telephone interviewing (CATI), computer-assisted personal interviewing (CAPI), and computer-assisted self-interviewing (CASI)—and CADE approaches. (The computerized telephone, personal, and self-administered data collection methods, along with the relative advantages and disadvantages of each in coding and computerizing survey data, were described in Chapter Five.)

Computerized data entry is a variation on these data-gathering approaches (Pierzchala, 1990). Paper-and-pencil questionnaires are used to gather the data, and programmed approaches are used to enter the data into a computerized medium for analysis. With this approach, a question (or prompt) displayed on a computer terminal video screen asks for the code that should be entered for the response to that question in a given case. Using the survey's codebook and the completed questionnaire, the coder determines the appropriate code and types it in at the terminal keyboard. The screen then prompts the coder to supply the next item of information and so on, until relevant codes for every item in the questionnaire have been entered. The format of the prompts may be in terms of a form that mirrors the survey questionnaire or a spreadsheet that takes on the appearance of the record for a given respondent, with each row being a respondent and the columns fields of data for each respondent. As with computer-assisted data collection methods, checks can be built into the program to signal discrepancies or errors that seem to exist when the data are entered for a given question and decision rules can be programmed in or applied to deal with these problems. Furthermore, computer-assisted data entry packages require that the appropriate questions and instructions be programmed and tested before the data are entered.

Most large-scale survey firms have designed their own proprietary data entry packages or purchased CADE software for this purpose. SPSS (Chicago), SAS (Cary, North Carolina), STATA (College Station, Texas), and EpiInfo (Stone Mountain, Georgia) have data entry and management components that are fully integrated with their statistical analysis packages. (Also, review the variety of proprietary and public domain survey design and collection packages in Chapter Thirteen.) An advantage of many of these packages is that they have statistical analysis procedures within their family of programs that can be executed on the data by means of the associated data entry software package.

Cleaning the Data

Data cleaning refers to the process for detecting and correcting errors during the computerization of survey data. There are two major types of computerized error checking: range checking and contingency checking.

Range Checking

Range checking refers to procedures for verifying that only valid ranges of numbers are used in coding the answers to the questions asked in a survey by computing and reviewing frequency distributions of responses to the survey questions. For example, if the codebook shows that answers to a question are either yes or no (coded as 1 and 2, respectively), then a code of 3 for this question would be in error. Decision rules have to be developed for dealing with these errors: for example, by consulting the original questionnaire to determine the correct answer, assigning a code based on the responses to other questions, or assigning a missing value code (such as 9) to indicate an indeterminate response to the item.

As indicated earlier, when using a computerized data entry system, such as CATI, CAPI, or Internet survey, inconsistencies in data collection due to the recording of out-of-range responses are dealt with beforehand in the design of constraints built into the system initially. However, it is still prudent to perform some quality control checks after the data have been entered to verify their integrity. For example, in the California Health Interview Survey (CHIS), while the data were being collected in the field, a small cluster of staff identified and corrected interviewer, respondent, and CATI errors and updated the files accordingly. Along the lines of what was done in CHIS, it may be useful to develop decision logic tables to guide data editing and cleaning. These tables can help sort out the types of problems and develop a consistent strategy for resolving them. These decision logic tables then become part of the permanent data-processing record for the data set.

Contingency Checking

In data cleaning by contingency checking, responses are compared between related questions by computing a cross-tabulation or other internal checks between two or more variables. For example, if a question or series of questions should be skipped because of the answer provided to a prior (filter) question (about the person's age, for example), a series of steps can be programmed to check whether these questions have been answered. More substantive contingency checks between questions can also be built into cleaning the data. Individuals who said they saw a doctor five times during the year for treatment associated with a particular chronic condition would be expected to report at least this many doctor visits in total when asked about all the times they had been to a doctor in the past year. As with the range-check cleaning procedures, decision rules should be developed for resolving errors that are detected when these contingency checking procedures are used.

The advantage of the computer-assisted data collection and data entry procedures described earlier is that both range and contingency checks can be built in and major problems can be identified and corrected at the time the data are actually being entered (assuming all the software, programming, and hardware details have been worked out in setting up the computer-assisted data entry system). In the past, when transcriptive data entry procedures were used, most data cleaning was carried out after the data were collected and entered, which often meant that a large number of problems had to be resolved long after the study was out of the field. Even when computer-assisted data collection is used, the researcher may still want to develop and execute supplementary data cleaning procedures after they are entered if the data are particularly complex or more extensive checking is desired. To do this, he or she would use the basic computer-assisted data entry checking procedures, although extensive checking of this kind is quite likely to increase the cost of the study and delay the final analyses of the data.

Another approach to checking the accuracy of data entry that is particularly appropriate for transcriptive data entry procedures is to verify all or a sample of the data entry for the questionnaires. This means asking another data entry clerk to punch in the information for the questionnaires on the computerized medium a second time. If any discrepancies occur in repunching the data, they should be flagged and any problems resolved. If certain data entry clerks have high error rates when their work is verified in this way, they may have to be retrained or even removed from the study if their performance does not improve.

Imputing Missing Survey Data

Survey respondents often may not know or may refuse to provide answers to certain questions (such as their total income from all sources during the past year), or interviewers may inadvertently skip questions during an interview. When there are a large number of cases with missing information on a particular question, the result can be biased (or inaccurate) estimates for the variables based on that question or the elimination of cases with missing data from analyses that examine the relationships of this variable to other variables in the study.

Techniques have been developed to impute values on variables for which data are missing, using information from other cases in the survey. These include deductive, cold-deck, hot-deck, statistical imputation, and multiple imputation procedures (Brand, van Buuren, Groothuis-Oudshoorn, & Gelsema, 2003; Groves, Dillman, Eltinge, & Little, 2002; Kalton & Kasprzyk, 1986; Little & Rubin, 1989, 2002; Marker, Judkins, & Winglee, 2002; National Research Council, Committee on National Statistics, Panel on Incomplete Data, 1983; Rubin, 1996, 2004; Schafer & Graham, 2002). Although these techniques vary in complexity, they all attempt to take typical values for the sample as a whole or subgroups within it or for comparable cases for which data are not missing. They then use the values derived from these sources to arrive at estimates for the cases for which the data are missing.

Decisions about whether to impute missing data should be dictated by the importance of the variable in the analyses, the magnitude of the missing information, the time and costs involved in the imputation process, and the study resources available for this process. In general, priority should be assigned to imputing data for the major variables in the analysis. Major variables for which information is missing on 10 percent or more of the cases could be the principal candidates for imputation. Researchers would then have to determine which types of imputation procedures would be most appropriate, how long the process would take, and how much it would cost. Final decisions about imputation would depend on the availability of trained project staff and funds. Also, if the proportion of missing values for a given item is substantial (25 to 50 percent or higher), the investigator should consider excluding the variable from the analysis altogether. It is not necessary to impute values for all the variables that may have missing values but only for those that are of key analytical importance and have a large number of missing values (10 percent or more).

The basic premise of imputation is that fewer biases are introduced by estimating reasonable values for cases for which data are missing than by excluding them from the analyses altogether. To test whether this assumption is correct, researchers can compare two estimates to a criterion source: (1) the estimate for analyses in which cases with missing values are included and (2) the estimate for analyses in which values are imputed (or assigned). This comparison should indicate which estimate is closer to the "real" value. In the absence of such a validating source, researchers can also compare the results for the variables, excluding cases that had missing values with the results obtained by including those cases for which values have been imputed. This comparison could at least provide some indication of whether the substantive results of the study would vary if different approaches to handling these cases were used.

Deductive Imputation

Deductive imputation is similar to editing a questionnaire and filling in those questions for which information is missing (such as the sex of the respondent) by using other information in the questionnaire (his or her name).

Cold-Deck Imputation

Cold-deck imputation procedures use group estimates, such as means, for the sample as a whole or for subgroups within it as the source of information for the values to assign to those cases for which data are missing.

In overall mean imputation, the overall mean for the study sample as a whole on the variable of interest is estimated for everyone for whom information is available. This mean is then assigned to each case for which information is missing.

Class mean imputation is a refinement of the overall mean imputation procedure. With this procedure, the entire sample is divided into a series of classes or groups based on a cross-classification of relevant variables (family size and occupation, for example). The mean on the variable of interest (family income) is then computed for each subgroup resulting from this cross-classification using the data for those for whom the information is available. This value is assigned to all the people in that group for whom it is not available.

Hot-Deck Imputation

Hot-deck procedures use the actual responses provided by particular individuals in a study as a basis for assigning answers to those persons for whom information is missing.

One of the simplest hot-deck procedures is that of random overall imputation. With this procedure, a respondent is selected at random from the total sample for the study, and the value for that person (his or her income, for example) is assigned to all the cases for which this information is missing.

Random imputation within classes is similar to random overall imputation except that the former procedure takes the selected respondent's value from a randomly chosen respondent within certain classes or groups of respondents (by age, sex, and race, for example). This means that the value chosen is taken from someone in the study for whom the variable of interest (such as income) is not missing and who matches the characteristics of the person for whom a value is being estimated (an African American female twenty-five to forty years of age, for example).

A sequential hot-deck imputation procedure is basically a variation of the random imputation within classes procedure. It begins with a set of groups and then assigns a value to each group by means of one of the cold-deck procedures described earlier. The cases in the file are ordered sequentially so that, as far as possible, cases that are related in some way (clustered in the same U.S. census tract or telephone exchange, for example) appear together. The first record within the group for which values are to be imputed (for example, African American females twenty-five to forty years of age) is examined. If it is missing, then the preassigned (cold-deck) value replaces the missing value. If a real value exists for this first case, it replaces the cold-deck value for this imputation class. The next record is examined. If it is missing, the new hot-deck value is used to assign a value to the case; if it is real, the hot-deck value is replaced. The process continues sequentially until all missing values are replaced by real values donated by the case preceding it within the same class or group.

Hierarchical hot-deck imputation procedures attempt to deal with problems that can arise with the sequential hot-deck procedure when, within an imputation class, a record with a missing value is followed by one or more records with missing values. In such instances, there will not be enough donor cases to match with real values within a class or a number of cases might be assigned the same value from the same donor case. In the hierarchical procedure, respondents and nonrespondents are grouped into a number of subclasses (age by sex by race) based on cross-classifications of broader groupings (age, sex, race). If a match cannot be found in one of the more detailed subclasses (age by sex by race), the subclasses are then collapsed into one of the broad groupings (age only) and a match is attempted at that level.

Statistical Imputation

Other data imputation procedures that rely on statistically generated values are regression or maximum likelihood imputation and distance function matching (Chen & Shao, 2000; Schafer & Graham, 2002). With the regression and maximum likelihood procedures, equations are used to predict values or the likelihood of values on the variable for which information is missing; in the distance function matching procedure, a nonrespondent is assigned the value of its nearest neighbor, where "nearest" is defined in terms of a statistically derived distance function.

Multiple Imputation

An important limitation of many of these approaches to imputation is that they may introduce other errors through, for example, reducing the variance as well as increasing the bias of the resulting estimates by providing only one imputed value to replace the missing value, derived from information from the subset of cases for which information is available (which may differ from those for whom it is missing). Multiple imputation generates more than one acceptable value for the items that are missing, creates different complete data sets using these different imputed values, and then combines the estimates resulting from these multiple iterations (Rubin, 1996, 2004).

The hot-deck, regression, and multiple imputation approaches have been used most often in large-scale national health surveys. The hot-deck and regression methods tend to generate similar distributions and results. An advantage of the hot-deck method is that it deals more effectively with estimating categorical (or nominal) data since they borrow real (rather than estimated) values from donor cases. Research has demonstrated that multiple imputation does address the variance and bias problems associated with these single-imputation methods, but these and related statistical imputation methods are continuing to be developed and refined (Chambers & Skinner, 2003; Little & Rubin, 2002; Rubin, 1996, 2004; Schafer & Graham, 2002).

Computer software for implementing these various procedures is increasingly available. Experienced programmers can also design or adapt programs to implement these various procedures. If the programming expertise or resources needed to implement these procedures successfully are not available, however, researchers may need to rely on the simpler deductive or cold-deck imputation procedures to estimate missing data on key study variables. It is advisable that flags (or special codes) be developed and entered into the data file to identify the imputed variables for each case in the file. Analyses could be replicated, including and excluding the "made-up" data, to see what effect imputing versus leaving out cases with missing information has on the substantive interpretation of the findings.

Estimating Survey Data

Imputation makes use of data internal to (from) the survey to construct a complete set of information on the analysis variables in the survey. Estimation implies the use of data external to the survey to construct analysis variables not directly available in the survey.

For example, an investigator may want to estimate the total charges for physician and hospital services that respondents reported receiving. The respondents themselves, however, may have little or no information on the charges for these services, especially if the providers were reimbursed directly by a third-party public or private insurer through which the respondent had coverage. The researcher could ask the respondent for permission to contact the providers directly to obtain this billing information or use data available from the American Medical Association, the American Hospital Association, or other sources on the average charges for these services in the community, state, or region in which the study is being conducted. The data obtained from these external sources could then be used to estimate the total charges for the services that study respondents reported receiving.

Anticipating the Analysis of the Data

A first step, before analyzing survey data, is to generate basic descriptive statistics to profile the characteristics of the sample as a whole or selected subgroups within it as part of the data cleaning and editing process. In addition to providing a profile of the members of the sample, the frequencies alert the researcher to (1) whether there is a large proportion of missing values for a particular variable, which could preclude the analysis of that variable or suggest the need for procedures to impute values for the cases for which values are missing; (2) whether there are too few cases of a certain kind to conduct meaningful analyses for that group or whether it would make sense in some cases to combine certain groups for the analyses; and (3) whether there are outliers, that is, cases with extremely large or extremely small values on a variable compared with the rest of the cases. The researcher may want to consider excluding these outliers or assigning them a maximum value for certain analyses.

If there is a concern with possible nonresponse bias in the survey sample, this is the stage at which analyses could be run comparing the composition of the survey sample with the original target population on selected characteristics for which corresponding data on the study universe are available. Response rate or post-stratification weighting adjustments, as well as any other weights required to adjust for disproportionate sampling, could be computed and added to the data file (see Chapter Seven).

If the intent is to develop summary indexes or scales to operationalize the major study concepts, then reliability and validity testing of these scales may also be undertaken before using them in analyses to address the principal study objectives or hypotheses. It may be particularly useful to conduct internal consistency reliability analysis or factor analysis of multi-item scales to confirm their coherence or to drop items from the final summary scale if warranted (see Chapter Three).

It may be necessary to transform the data in other ways as well to make sure the data better fit the assumptions required for a particular analytical procedure. A highly skewed distribution of a key study variable may, for example, require a logarithmic or other arithmetic transformation to ensure it better matches the (normal) sampling distribution required for certain procedures (such as multiple regression).

There are also conventions for converting nominal or ordinal variables into dummy (interval) variables for the purposes of using them in regression procedures that assume an interval or interval-like level of measurement. For example, if one wanted to use a four-category race and ethnicity variable as a predictor in a regression equation, four different dichotomous (interval-like) variables would need to be created to reflect whether the respondent was a member of one of the racial categories:

original race variable (nominal)

RACE: 1 = White; 2 = African American; 3 = Hispanic; 4 = Other

dummy variables (interval-like)

RACE1: 1 = White; 0 = African American, Hispanic, or Other
RACE2: 1 = African American; 0 = White, Hispanic, or Other
RACE3: 1 = Hispanic; 0 = White, African American, or Other
RACE4: 1 = Other; 0 = White, African American, or Hispanic

One of the dummy variables can then be chosen as the reference category (the group to which the other groups are compared). Procedures for recoding the categories from one variable into a series of dummy variables are available in most conventional statistical packages. To effect this using regression analysis, that variable (RACE1, which designates whites, for example) would not be included as a predictor variable, but all of the other dummy variables representing different categories of race and ethnicity (RACE2, RACE3, RACE4) would be. The regression coefficients for these variables would then effectively examine the effect of being a member of the respective minority groups (African American, Hispanic, or other), compared with being a member of the white majority, on predicting the outcome of interest (seeing a physician in the year).

The study design and objectives may also require systematically linking data from other sources (medical records or insurance claims, for example). This step should be anticipated early on, required permissions obtained, and adequate information gathered to match data from survey respondents accurately with information from these other sources.

Once the data are coded, computerized, and cleaned and missing data are imputed or estimated, the resulting data set should then be ready for analysis (Chapter Fifteen).

Special Considerations for Special Populations

Special populations may present special challenges during the coding, cleaning, editing, and imputation processes. In surveys of diverse populations, open-ended questions are likely to yield a comparably diverse array of responses that must be accommodated in the coding schemes for these questions. Questions that respondents had trouble interpreting or answering will surface as having high rates of missing values. Differential item (question) nonresponse rates compound the concerns with the effects of imputing (or not imputing) data on the bias (systematic error) in the survey estimates.

If there is a concern with the quality and completeness of the data that are likely to be obtained for certain subgroups, then the pretest and pilot study phases of the study should be expanded to allow adequate testing of the questionnaire as a basis for revising or deleting those questions that are particularly problematic prior to the final study. This may be especially important as it relates to the willingness or lack of willingness of some respondents to answer questions under any circumstances; for example, forcing respondents in a substance abuse treatment program to answer questions about their substance abuse history may pose some problems if doing so creates a risk of remission or recidivism for the client.

Selected Examples

In the UNICEF Multiple Indicator Cluster Survey study, several activities were recommended to the researchers implementing the study in their country to facilitate the data-processing activities. Researchers were first advised to archive a copy of the original data that come from the field before performing any edit checks. They were then asked to check the raw data against the questionnaires for consistency. This was to be followed by a series of checks of the ranges of responses provided for each question, a check to ensure that the correct number of questionnaires was entered into the database, and a check to ensure that the data were recorded in the correct fields in the database. Once this was done, the researchers were asked to complete a series of logical edits of the data, following the guidelines specified in the manual (UNICEF, 2000).

In the CHIS study, the CATI system was programmed upfront to handle potential data entry errors, incorrect data entry (that is, data outside of the range for that questions), or data that were not internally consistent with other data entered previously. This still left some situations where it was necessary to seek out a supervisor to obtain advice regarding how to resolve a data entry problem (for example "respondent wanted to change several answers, I was unable to backup properly") (UCLA Center for Health Policy Research, 2002c, p. 2-2). The interviewer used either a problem sheet (hard copy) or a comments field in the database to communicate these types of problems to the central data management office, which resolved the case.

In addition to these series of data entry activities, three types of imputation were performed by the CHIS staff. First, geographical data were used to code missing responses for the question regarding the respondent's county of residence. Next, in a small percentage of cases, data randomly selected from nonmissing cases were imputed for missing responses. For example, when the value for self-reported age was missing, a randomly selected value for the respondent's age was selected from the distribution of an adult, child, or adolescent respondent. Finally, a hot-deck imputation was performed to impute race, ethnicity, and household income. In this case, the data were split according to respondents who had the complete data (donors) and the respondents who were missing the data (recipients). A recipient was then matched to a subset pool of donors with the same type of household structure. "The recipient is then randomly imputed the same income, race/ethnicity (depending on the items that need to be imputed) from one of the donors in the pool" (UCLA Center for Health Policy Research, 2002c, p. 1–8). Beginning with CHIS 2003, missing values for all source variables in the data file were imputed.

Guidelines for Minimizing Survey Errors and Maximizing Survey Quality

Systematic errors (or bias), especially item nonresponse, are of principal concern at this stage of survey implementation. Systematic errors may occur as a result of not using a framework that would allow one to systematically identify and resolve problems that may occur during the data collection or data-processing phases. Random errors can occur during the coding and data entry process (Table 14.1). These random errors, however, can be minimized through adequate training and supervision of the data collection and processing staff; development and implementation of quality control monitoring systems; developing a decision logic model for reducing inconsistencies in the coding of the data; and reverification of data that have been input by reentering them, in the instance of paper-and-pencil questionnaires.

More troublesome are variables for which information is missing (either the interviewer or respondent did not record an answer or the respondent did not know how or refused to answer). One can choose to exclude cases with missing data from analyses using the affected variables or impute values for those cases using the cases for which data are available. Nonetheless, the cases that have complete information may differ from those that do not. To attempt to minimize the possible biases in the estimates generated from the data, the investigator can use several different approaches to imputation, compare findings based on imputed and nonimputed data, and document whether the substantive results emanating from the various methods are confirmed.

TABLE 14.1. SURVEY ERRORS: SOURCES AND SOLUTIONS— PREPARING THE DATA FOR ANALYSIS.

	Systematic Errors: Imputation/ Estimation Errors	Variable Errors: Data Coding, Editing, or Data Entry Errors
Solutions to Errors	Compare the estimates based on alternative imputation procedures.	Develop and implement quality control monitoring systems.
	Compare the estimates based on imputed and nonimputed data.	Develop a decision logic model for reducing potential inconsistencies in the coding of the data.
		Reenter the data to identify variable errors in data entry.

Supplementary Sources

For an overview of data processing in general, see Biemer and Lyberg (2003). For computer-assisted interviews in particular, see Couper et al. (1998), and for Internet surveys, see Jones (1999). For a discussion of the issues underlying imputation, see Rubin (1996) and Schafer and Graham (2002).

CHAPTER FIFTEEN

PLANNING AND IMPLEMENTING THE ANALYSIS OF THE DATA

Chapter Highlights

1. A measurement matrix shows how the items asked in a survey questionnaire will be used to create variables to address the study's specific objectives and hypotheses.
2. Univariate statistics, such as measures of central tendency (mode, median, and mean) and dispersion (percentiles, range, and standard deviation), are used to describe the distribution of a single variable in a study.
3. Bivariate statistics enable the researcher to test hypotheses about the existence or strength of the relationship between *two* variables.
4. Multivariate statistics permit tests of hypotheses about the relationships between two or more variables while controlling for other variables.
5. The criteria for selecting the appropriate statistical procedures are based on the variables and the relationships between them implied in the study's research objectives and hypotheses.
6. Constructing mock tables designed to show how the data will be reported forces researchers to specify the types of information they need to collect and what they will do with it before they begin the study.

This chapter provides an overview of the process for developing an analysis plan for a study. A well-articulated analysis plan that describes what the researcher plans to do with his or her data is a way of making sure that all the data needed to answer the principal research questions will be gathered and that those items for which there is no clear analytical purpose will not be asked.

Failure to develop an analysis plan is the weakest point in the design of most surveys. Often both experienced and inexperienced survey designers do not have a clear idea of how they will use all the information they gather or they find that they wish they had included other items once they start to analyze the information they did gather. A clear picture of the variables that will be constructed from the questions asked in the survey and the procedures that will be used in analyzing them provides an invaluable anchor and point of reference for the researcher in deciding what to include in the survey questionnaire. This chapter places particular emphasis on determining which procedures are most appropriate for which types of study designs and variables.

Constructing a Measurement Matrix

In the process of developing and finalizing the survey questionnaire, the analyst should construct a matrix that displays how each item in the survey will be used to address the major study concepts. An example of this measurement matrix for the National Dental Malpractice Survey (which is shown in Resource C) is provided in Table 15.1.

This kind of matrix, at a minimum, lists each question and identifies the major study concept the item is intended to operationalize, the level of measurement it represents, and the specific objective or hypothesis it most directly addresses. Other information can be added to the matrix as well, such as an indication of the transformation of survey items or the construction of indexes or scales to measure key study constructs; other studies or scales from which the questions were drawn; and what is known (if anything) about their reliability and validity.

This matrix is intended to discipline the investigator to consider how each survey item is useful as well as whether other items may need to be added to address the study objectives adequately. It can be a helpful guide for deciding which survey questions might be eliminated to reduce the length or complexity of the questionnaire if a clear application of the questions in terms of the study objectives cannot be identified. Analysts should give thought to alternative ways of measuring the concepts they incorporate in their studies as well as the types of simple or complex variables they would like to construct for an empirical examination of the relationships between these concepts. The level of measurement that study

TABLE 15.1. MEASUREMENT MATRIX BASED ON
THE NATIONAL DENTAL MALPRACTICE SURVEY.

Question	Concept	Level of Measurement	Objective
1	Doctor-patient communication: satisfaction with practice	Ordinal	3
2	Doctor-patient communication: percentage of visits that are frustrating	Ordinal	3
3	Doctor-patient communication: characteristics of unsatisfactory patient encounters (Likert scale)	Ordinal (interval)	3
4	Practice characteristics: how clinical problems are handled	Ordinal	3
5	Practice characteristics: occurrence of problem situations	Ordinal	3
6	Practice characteristics: number of dental operatories	Interval	3
7	Practice characteristics: average length of appointment for adult prophylaxis	Ordinal	3
8	Practice characteristics: average length of appointment for new patient examination	Ordinal	3
9	Practice characteristics: average time in advance to schedule appointment for new patient examination	Ordinal	3
10	Practice characteristics: average office waiting time for patient	Ordinal	3
11	Practice characteristics: dentist employment status	Nominal	3
12	Practice characteristics: bases for dentist remuneration	Nominal	3
13	Practice characteristics: average hours at chairside per week	Interval	3
14	Practice characteristics: number of other full-time dentists	Interval	3
15	Practice characteristics: number of other part-time dentists	Interval	3
16	Practice characteristics: number of other full-time or part-time employees	Interval	3
17	Practice characteristics: number of patient visits in typical week	Interval	3
18	Practice characteristics: hourly rate for primary dental asst.	Interval	3

Question	Concept	Level of Measurement	Objective
19	Practice characteristics: percentage of time devoted to selected procedures in typical week	Interval	3
20	Practice characteristics: referral rates for selected procedures	Ordinal	3
21	Practice characteristics: percentage of dental hygienist visits checked	Ordinal	3
22	Practice characteristics: busyness of practice	Nominal	3
23	Practice characteristics: ADA dental procedures performed	Nominal	3
24	Practice characteristics: frequency of selected office practices	Ordinal	3
25	Practice characteristics: office policies and equipment	Nominal	3
26	Practice characteristics: new patient procedures	Interval	3
27	Practice finances: patient awareness of costs	Ordinal	3
28	Practice finances: percentage of patients with insurance coverage	Interval	3
29	Practice finances: fees for selected procedures	Interval	3
30	Malpractice insurance: type	Nominal	1, 2, 3
31	Malpractice insurance: company	Nominal	1, 2, 3
32	Malpractice insurance: policy limits	Ordinal	1, 2, 3
33	Malpractice insurance: premium adjustments	Nominal	1, 2, 3
34	Malpractice insurance: premium	Ordinal	1, 2, 3
35	Malpractice insurance: number of complaints	Ordinal	1, 2, 3
36	Malpractice insurance: most recent incident—date	Ordinal	1, 2, 3
37	Malpractice insurance: most recent incident—result in claim or not	Nominal	1, 2, 3
38	Malpractice insurance: most recent incident—area of dentistry	Nominal	1, 2, 3
39	Malpractice insurance: most recent incident—allegations involved	Nominal	1, 2, 3
40	Malpractice insurance: most recent incident—resolved or not	Nominal	1, 2, 3

TABLE 15.1. MEASUREMENT MATRIX BASED ON
THE NATIONAL DENTAL MALPRACTICE SURVEY, *continued.*

Question	Concept	Level of Measurement	Objective
41	Malpractice insurance: most recent incident—dollar amount paid	Interval	1, 2, 3
42	Malpractice insurance: most recent incident—signed agreement to settle	Nominal	1, 2, 3
43	Malpractice insurance: most recent incident—company	Nominal	1, 2, 3
44	Malpractice insurance: second most recent incident—yes or no	Nominal	1, 2, 3
45	Malpractice insurance: second most recent incident—date	Ordinal	1, 2, 3
46	Malpractice insurance: second most recent incident—result in claim or not	Nominal	1, 2, 3
47	Malpractice insurance: second most recent incident—area of dentistry	Nominal	1, 2, 3
48	Malpractice insurance: second most recent incident—allegations involved	Nominal	1, 2, 3
49	Malpractice insurance: second most recent incident—resolved or not	Nominal	1, 2, 3
50	Malpractice insurance: second most recent incident—dollar amount paid	Interval	1, 2, 3
51	Malpractice insurance: second most recent incident—signed agreement to settle	Nominal	1, 2, 3
52	Malpractice insurance: second most recent incident—company	Nominal	1, 2, 3
53	Demographics: age	Interval	2, 3
54	Demographics: gender	Nominal	2, 3
55	Demographics: race/ethnicity	Nominal	2, 3
56	Demographics: number of dental office locations	Interval	2, 3
57	Demographics: number of years in practice at primary location	Interval	2, 3
58	Demographics: zip code and county of primary practice	Nominal	2, 3
59	Demographics: dental school attended	Nominal	2, 3
60	Demographics: continuing education in past twelve months	Nominal	2, 3
61	Demographics: hours of continuing education in past twelve months	Interval	2, 3

variables represent has important implications for the choice of analytical procedures and transformations in the form of the variables that may be required to use certain procedures.

The primary research objectives for the dental preferences study are summarized in Table 2.3 (see Chapter Two). The measurement matrix for this study (Table 15.1) displays how each item in the survey questionnaire would be used to operationalize the major study concepts reflected in these objectives (doctor-patient communication, practice characteristics, practice finances, malpractice insurance, and demographics).

Objective 1 for the survey was concerned with estimating dental malpractice insurance experience in a representative sample of U.S. dentists. Objective 2 compared dental malpractice experience by the dentist's demographic characteristics, and objective 3 analyzed the relative importance of an array of predictors in understanding dental malpractice experience.

The questions asked in the dentists' survey are a mix of nominal, ordinal, interval, and ratio measures. Ratio measures are principally distinguished from interval measures based on whether a zero value is a theoretically possible response to the question (number of times a specific procedure was performed each week). As indicated in the matrix, a Likert summary scale could be created to summarize a series of measures intended to capture the characteristics of unsatisfactory patients (question 3). The individual items are clearly ordinal-level measures, based on a scale ranging from 1 to 5 indicating whether respondents thought the statement was very typical (1) or not at all typical (5) of unsatisfactory patient encounters (Mellor & Milgrom, 1995). However, methodological research in the social and behavioral sciences suggests that it is acceptable to treat these types of ordinal items, and the summary scales produced from them in particular, as interval-level data to permit their use with more powerful statistical procedures (DeVellis, 2003; Nunnally & Bernstein, 1994).

Reviewing Potential Analytical Procedures

Alternative analysis techniques are presented here to acquaint the researcher with (1) the basic types of procedures available to answer a given research question, (2) how they can be used to answer that question, and (3) which procedures are most appropriate to use with what types of data. This chapter also outlines the criteria to apply in deciding what type of statistical procedure best addresses the questions that the study was designed to answer.

The major dimensions to take into account in weighing the relevance of different types of procedures for one's study purposes, reflected in the tables and figures summarizing these procedures (Tables 15.2 and 15.3 and Figures 15.1 to 15.3), include the applicability of descriptive versus inferential statistics; univariate, bivariate, and multivariate analyses; parametric versus nonparametric procedures; tests of the existence of an association as well as measures of the strength of an association; and whether the design is based on independent or related samples. The researcher should have the target audience for the study (such as public health practitioners, academicians, or policymakers) clearly in mind in formulating the study objectives and related analysis plan. For some, simple descriptive statistics to document or define a problem (such as the magnitude of the problem of the uninsured) may be sufficient, but for others, more analytical model development or hypothesis testing to advance a field of study or practice might be appropriate.

Descriptive Versus Inferential Statistics

Descriptive statistics summarize the characteristics of a particular sample. Inferential statistics enable the researcher to decide, on the basis of the probability theory (sampling distribution) underlying a given test statistic, the level of confidence that he or she can have in inferring the characteristics of the population as a whole on the basis of the information obtained from a particular sample. Analytical study designs are essentially distinguished from descriptive designs through the use of tests of significance and related inferential test statistics (such as a chi-square, t-test, or F-test, for example) to reject or confirm specific statistical hypotheses (see Chapter Two). These tests are fundamentally grounded in theories of probability regarding the likelihood of a given value on the test statistic if the hypothesized assumptions are true in the population from which the sample was drawn.

Test statistics are inferential rather than descriptive. They are used to test statistically how often the differences or associations observed between two (or more) groups are likely to occur by chance if a hypothesis about this relationship is true for the populations from which the groups were drawn. Different test statistics are used with different statistical procedures. Test statistics (such as the chi-square, t-test, and F-test statistics) are assumed to have specific types of "sampling distributions," which are based on the size and randomness of the sample for the study, the level of measurement of the study variables being tested, and the characteristics of the population from which the sample was drawn.

Application of the normal sampling distribution for testing hypotheses about the characteristics of the population is discussed in Chapter Seven. An analogous process is involved in testing hypotheses by means of test statistics that have other types of sampling distributions. Appropriate adjustments should be made to the test statistics when complex sample designs are used (American Statistical Association, Section on Survey Research Methods, n.d.-b; Lee, Forthofer, & Lorimor, 1989).

Since the "truth" of a theoretical hypothesis can never be known with certainty when researchers use methods based on the probability of occurrence of the hypothesized result, statistical hypotheses are generally stated in terms of a "null" hypothesis; that is, there is said to be "no" difference or association between the variables. This is in contrast to the substantive research (or alternative) hypothesis, which states the relationship that one would expect to find given the theories or previous research in the area. If an association *is* found in a particular sample, the researcher would conclude that the null hypothesis of *no* difference or association hypothesized between groups is probably *not* true for the populations from which these groups were drawn.

Univariate, Bivariate, and Multivariate Analyses

Univariate statistics (such as frequencies, percentages, the mode, median, and mean) are useful descriptive statistics for profiling the characteristics of survey respondents and identifying potential problems with missing data, outliers, or small numbers of cases for selected categories of a survey variable. Bivariate statistics focus on examining the relationship between two variables and multivariate statistics on the relationship among an array of variables. These procedures are used directly in testing and elaborating study hypotheses, respectively (for which mock tables were displayed in Exhibit 4.1, Chapter Four).

Parametric Versus Nonparametric Procedures

Parametric statistics make certain assumptions about the distribution of the variables in the population from which the sample was drawn. Many of the parametric test procedures assume a normal distribution in the parent population and a simple random sample of a minimum size (generally at least thirty cases). (See Figure 7.1 and the related discussion of the normal sampling distribution in Chapter Seven.) Nonparametric procedures do not. Furthermore, more nonparametric procedures deal principally with analyses of nominal- or ordinal-level variables, whereas parametric procedures generally assume at least interval or ratio data (Conover, 1999).

Existence Versus Strength of Association

Researchers should decide whether they are principally interested in testing for the simple *existence of a relationship* (or association) between two variables or groups of interest, as displayed in mock tables (see again Exhibit 4.1 in Chapter Four), or the *strength of the relationship* (or association) between the two variables, or both. An array of statistical procedures and associated tests of significance (such as chi-square, *t*-tests, and analysis of variance) are used to test for the existence of a relationship between variables. Correlation coefficients appropriate to the level of measurement of the respective variables—most of which range between 0 and 1.0 or −1.0 to +1.0—can be used to measure the strength and direction of the relationship between variables (or groups).

Independent Versus Related Samples

Another factor to consider in reviewing potential analysis procedures is the basic study design for the survey—in particular, whether the groups (or samples) being compared are independent of one another. With longitudinal panel designs, the groups being compared at different points in time are not independent. In fact, they include the same people. Similarly, retrospective designs may contain some case-control features, such as looking at people before and after they became ill or matching those with and without the illness on other relevant characteristics. In those instances as well, the samples are correlated (or dependent), and tests appropriate to the related samples should be used. In cross-sectional surveys or other studies in which there is no effort to reinterview the same people or match and compare individuals, tests for independent samples are appropriate. Researchers must take into account whether the samples (or groups) being compared are correlated when choosing a particular procedure; some correlations between groups may already be built in because of the way in which the sample was drawn. The procedures used with related samples take any preexisting overlap between them into account in computing the statistics to test the relationships between such groups. This would be of particular importance when groups are matched in the instance of case-control designs or the same groups followed over time in longitudinal or experimental designs.

The reader should consult standard statistics and biometry texts for more information on a particular statistical technique of interest. (See the sources listed at the end of this chapter.) Some of the statistical software packages that are available include SPSS, SAS, STATA, and EPI-INFO. SPSS, SAS, and STATA are powerful and versatile packages that contain a variety of analysis procedures. EPI-INFO is readily available in the public domain and offers a wide range of applications for epidemiological research. The decision about which package to use should be based on the user's familiarity with a particular package, what is available at the institution in which the research is being conducted, and whether unique features of a particular package better satisfy the requirements for a given type of analysis. If a complex sample design was used in the study, then the analyses will need to be run using the software and procedures for handling associated design effects described in Chapter Seven.

Using Univariate Statistics to Describe the Sample

The first step in carrying out the analysis of any data set—regardless of the type of study design—is to analyze the sample by each of the major study variables of interest. Investigators may or may not report the basic distributions of and summary statistics on the study variables in their final report of the study. This documentation does, however, provide the starting point for determining what the data look like preparatory to constructing any other analytical variables or pursuing subsequent subgroup analyses. There have to be enough cases, for example, to carry out certain analytical procedures in a meaningful way.

Univariate statistics are summary measures used to describe the composition of one variable at a time, such as how many people with certain ranges of income, levels of perceived health, or numbers of physician visits constitute the sample. The particular types of univariate statistics to use depend on the level of measurement of the respective variables. The basic types of univariate statistics are summarized in Table 15.2.

Frequencies

Frequencies refer to the number and percentage of people with certain characteristics. We saw in Chapter Three that regardless of the level of measurement of any particular variable, numerical codes can be assigned to each category or value that is relevant for describing someone in the sample. For nominal variables, such as marital status, the codes simply identify categories of individuals—people who are currently married, widowed, divorced or separated, or never married, for example. For ordinal variables, the codes represent rankings on the level of the variable, such as the extent to which selected clinical problems are encountered in everyday dental practice—nearly always, often, sometimes, not often, almost never, and never (as in question 4 in the dentist survey shown in Resource C).

With interval scales, the codes refer to equal points along some underlying continuum, such as units of temperature. With ratio scales, some absolute zero reference point (the total absence of the characteristic, such as having no or "zero" visits to a physician in the year) can be a valid value for the variable. (In the example in Table 15.2, the analysis is limited to those who had at least one physician visit in the year.)

TABLE 15.2. USING UNIVARIATE STATISTICS TO DESCRIBE THE SAMPLE.

	Levels of Measurement		
Type of Univariate Statistic	Nominal	Ordinal	Interval or Ratio
Examples	*Marital status*	*Perceived risk of AIDS*	*Number of M.D. visits (those with 1+)*
Frequencies (number and percent of people in sample with the characteristics)	*Values* % (n) 1–Married 30% (30) 2–Divorced 20 (20) 3–Separated 10 (10) 4–Widowed 0 (0) 5–Never married 40 (40) Total 100% (100)	*Values* % (n) 1–Not at all 30% (30) 2 20 (20) 3 10 (10) 4 0 (0) 5–Extremely 40 (40) Total 100% (100)	*Values* % (n) 1 30% (30) 2 20 (20) 3 10 (10) 4 0 (0) 5 40 (40) Total 100% (100)
Measures of Central Tendency			
Mode (most frequent value)	5	5	5
Median (value with half of cases above and half below it)	Not applicable	2.5	2.5
Mean (Average) (sum of values/total *n*)	Not applicable	Not applicable	$[(1 \times 30) + (2 \times 20) + (3 \times 10) + (4 \times 0) + (5 \times 40)] \div 100 = 3$
Measures of Dispersion			
Range (maximum – minimum value)	Not applicable	Not applicable	$5 - 1 = 4$
Variance (average difference between each value and mean, as follows...) $\dfrac{\text{Sum (value} - \text{mean})^2}{n-1}$	Not applicable	Not applicable	$[30 \times (1 - 3)^2 + 20 \times (2 - 3)^2 + 10 \times (3 - 3)^2 + 40 \times (5 - 3)^2] \div 99 = 3.03$
Standard Deviation (square root of variance)	Not applicable	Not applicable	$\mathrm{SQRT}\ 3.03 = 1.74$

Frequencies refer to how often individuals with the given attribute appear in the sample and what percentage (or proportion) they represent of all the individuals in the study. As discussed in Chapter Fourteen, codes can also be assigned to represent data that for some reason are missing for an individual respondent.

In addition to providing a basic profile of the members of the sample, the frequencies alert the researcher to (1) whether there is a large proportion of missing values for a particular variable, which could preclude the analysis of that variable or suggest the need for procedures to impute values for the cases for which values are missing; (2) whether there are too few cases of a certain kind to conduct meaningful analyses for that group or whether it would make sense, in some cases, to combine certain groups for the analyses; or (3) whether there are outliers, that is, cases with extremely large or extremely small values on a variable compared with the rest of the cases. The researcher may want to consider excluding these outliers or assigning them a maximum value for certain analyses.

Running frequencies on variables for which different values are possible (number of disability days in the year) can produce a long list of values. However, univariate statistics are available to summarize these frequency distributions in a more parsimonious fashion.

Measures of Central Tendency

Measures of central tendency help the researcher identify one number to represent the most typical response found on the frequencies for a variable. There are three principal measures of central tendency: *mode, median,* and *mean.* Which measure to use to summarize the frequencies on a survey variable depends on the variable's level of measurement.

Mode. The mode or modal response is the response that occurs most often in the data, that is, the one that has the highest frequency or percentage of people responding. The modal response for each of the variables for which frequencies are displayed in Table 15.2 is five (40 percent of the one hundred respondents).

Median. A second type of univariate summary measure is the value that would split the sample in half if one were to order people in the sample from the highest to the lowest values on some variable of interest, such as lining up students in a class on the basis of their height. This measure—the median—assumes at least an ordinal level of measurement so that study participants can be ranked (or put in order) on the attribute. It would, for example, not make sense to put individuals identified through categories of a *nominal* variable into some order representing more or less of a characteristic such as race, sex, marital status, or region of the country. Sometimes the median value will have to be interpolated (or interpreted) as the midpoint between two values—in Table 15.2, for example, 2.5, which lies between the values of 2 and 3, is the median value—to specify most precisely the point both below and above which exactly half (50 percent) of the cases fall.

Mean. The most commonly used expression of the mean is the arithmetic mean. As indicated in the example in Table 15.2, the arithmetic mean is computed by adding up all the values on the variable for everyone in the sample and dividing this figure by the total number of people in the sample to get an "average" score. The median is sometimes preferred to the mean in expressing the typical value for interval- or ratio-level variables since the mean could be considerably skewed by cases with extreme values (outliers).

Mean estimates are not meaningful for nominal- and ordinal-level variables. It does not make sense, for example, to add up the ethnic statuses of people in the sample and divide the result by the number of people in the sample to get an average ethnicity. In contrast, one could speak of the modal category of ethnic status in the sample, that is, the largest ethnic group in the study. Ordinal-level measures do not make assumptions about the exact distance between points on a scale that simply ranks individuals on some characteristic of interest. Computing averages using ordinal-level variables would be much like calculating the heights of a group of students in inches by means of a ruler on which the distances between each of the "inch" markers were all a little different.

Measures of Dispersion

A second major category of univariate statistics useful for describing the basic sample is measures of dispersion, which summarize how much variation there is across people in the sample in the answers they provide to a given survey question. The main types of measures of dispersion are the *range, variance,* and *standard deviation.*

Range. The range is the difference between the highest (maximum) and lowest (minimum) values that appear on the frequency table. For example, in Table 15.2, in which the values extend from one to five, the range is four (that is, five minus one). The range may be expressed by either the actual difference (four) or the two extreme scores (one to five). The computation of the range assumes at least an interval level of measurement. For nominal-level measures, a variation ratio can be computed, which is the percentage of people who are not in the modal category (60 percent in the example in Table 15.2). For ordinal-level variables, decile or interquartile ranges are used. These are based on dividing the distribution of cases into ten equal parts (deciles), each containing 10 percent of the cases, or into four equal parts (quartiles), each containing 25 percent of the cases. The decile or interquartile range is expressed as the values for the cases that define the cutoff for the highest and lowest deciles (10 percent) or quartiles (25 percent) of the distribution of cases (not shown in Table 15.2).

Variance and Standard Deviation. The measures used most often in reflecting the degree of variation for interval or ratio data are variance and standard deviation measures. These are ways of looking at how much the values for the respondents in the sample differ from the typical value (generally the mean) for the sample. The variance is computed by calculating the difference between the value for each case in the sample and the mean on the characteristic for the sample, squaring these differences (so that positive and negative values do not cancel one another), adding these squared values for all the cases in the sample, and then dividing this sum by the total number of cases in the sample less one $(n-1)$ or by the sample size itself (n) for larger samples (more than thirty cases). The standard deviation is the square root of the variance.

Using Bivariate Statistics to Test for Relationships Between Variables

After the basic composition of the sample has been described, the next step in analyzing most survey data is to look at the relationship between two or more variables. In simple cross-sectional descriptive studies, investigators may want to look at differences between subgroups on variables related to the principal study objectives. For example, in the case of the alternative designs for addressing different research questions related to high school seniors' smoking behavior (see Table 2.2 in Chapter Two), researchers might be interested in looking at the prevalence of smoking among seniors in different age, sex, and race groups as well as among seniors as a whole.

Group-comparison studies explicitly build in primary comparisons between certain groups in the design of the samples and selection of the samples of individuals to be included in the survey. These types of comparisons and related bivariate analyses underlie the approach to testing a simple hypothesis regarding the relationship between two variables displayed in Figure 4.1 in Chapter Four. Longitudinal studies focus on comparisons of data gathered at more than one point in time. In panel-type longitudinal designs, these comparisons involve data gathered from the same people at different times. Finally, analytical surveys are explicitly concerned with testing hypotheses about the relationship between at least one independent and one dependent variable by means of cross-sectional, prospective, or retrospective survey designs. Figures 15.1 and 15.2 provide a summary of different bivariate statistical procedures for looking at the relationship between two survey variables. (Figure 15.2 appears in the following section.)

Nonparametric Procedures

Nonparametric procedures are principally used to analyze nominal and ordinal data.

Nominal. As displayed in the first example in Figure 15.1, the simplest procedure for examining the relationship between two variables based on a nominal level of measurement is a cross-tabulation of the variables. A relationship between the variables is suggested by the fact that people in the sample cluster in systematic ways in certain cells of the table, as with the examples cited earlier in Chapter Four.

The Pearson chi-square is one test statistic used to examine the statistical significance of such a relationship for independent samples. It basically looks at the goodness of fit between the distribution that is *observed* in each of the cells compared with the distribution that would be *expected*, given the number of people in the sample with the respective characteristics (X and Y), and assuming the variables are not related. The less that the pattern observed in the table matches the expected distribution, as measured by the Pearson chi-square test statistic, the less support there is for the null hypothesis that there is no relationship between the variables in this particular sample. Fisher's exact test can be used for tables that have only two rows and two columns and in which the expected number of cases in some cells of the cross-classification table is less than five.

The McNemar test is designed for use with related samples or before and after experimental designs to detect any significant changes in the status of subjects over time, such as whether employees who formerly smoked quit smoking after a work site health promotion campaign. One would expect to find a higher proportion of nonsmokers after the campaign than before it.

The Cochran Q-test is used when three or more related groups are compared on some dichotomous variable, such as the proportion of enrollees in a new prepaid dental plan who had been to the dentist at least twice during the year for a preventive visit, in a longitudinal panel study of people interviewed annually over a three-year period. The underlying objective might be to see if there is an increased tendency to seek preventive dental services over time as a function of enhanced plan coverage and patient education efforts.

A variety of measures of the strength of the association between variables, based on cross-tabulations between nominal variables, are available. Some are based on modifications of the chi-square test statistic so that they range from 0 to 1, with

FIGURE 15.1. USING NONPARAMETRIC BIVARIATE STATISTICS TO TEST FOR RELATIONSHIPS BETWEEN VARIABLES.

		Bivariate Statistics		
		Tests of Association Between Variables		Measures of Strength of Association Between Variables
Type of Measurement	Example	Independent Samples	Related Samples	
Nominal (cross-tabulation of dependent variable by independent variable)	Independent Variable (X) X = 1 X = 2 Dependent Variable (Y) Y = 1 Y = 2	Fisher's exact test (2 × 2 table) Chi-square contingency table analysis	McNemar test for significance of changes (2 × 2 table) Cochran Q-test	Phi coefficient Yule's Q (2 × K table) Coefficient of contingency Cramér's V Lambda Odds ratio
Ordinal (association of ranks between two variables)	Ranks Case ID Variable X Variable Y 001 5 1 002 5 1 003 5 1 004 5 1 005 5 1	Chi-square contingency table analysis		Goodman and Kruskal's gamma Kendall's tau-a, tau-b, tau-c Somer's d Spearman rank order coefficient
Mixed (differences in ranks between groups)	Groups Group X = 1 Group X = 2 Variable Y 5 1 5 1 5 1 5 1 5 1	Median test Mann-Whitney U test Kolmogorov-Smirnov Wald-Wolfowitz runs test Kruskal-Wallis (3+ groups)	Sign test Wilcoxon matched-pairs signed ranks test Friedman two-way analysis of variance (3+ groups)	Lambda Uncertainty coefficient Goodman and Kruskal's gamma Somer's d Eta coefficient

0 corresponding to no association and 1 to perfect association between the variables. The phi coefficient, Yule's Q, the coefficient of contingency, and Cramér's V are examples of chi-square–based measures of association.

Other measures of association based on cross-tabulations of nominal variables are termed *proportional reduction in error* (PRE) statistics. PRE measures are based on formulas for computing how well the value of a dependent variable (Y) can be predicted from knowing the value of an independent variable (X). These statistics basically compare (1) a situation where the value of the dependent variable (such as being insured versus being uninsured) for any given case in the sample is estimated simply by determining how many people there are in the sample in each group of the dependent variable with (2) a situation in which the information on the value of the independent variable (such as whether the person works or not) is also used in estimating the value of the dependent variable for that case.

Odds ratios for case-control studies (discussed in Chapter Four) and relative risk estimates for cohort designs are used in epidemiological studies in particular for summarizing the strength of a given risk factor (or exposure) as predictive of a particular disease outcome (Kahn & Sempos, 1989; Kleinbaum, 2003).

Ordinal. The second major type of analysis procedure for examining the bivariate relationship between (two) variables or groups is one that assumes an ordinal level of measurement of the study variables. As shown in Figure 15.1 for the example relating to the bivariate analyses of ordinal variables, the variables X and Y take on values of one to five. A respondent (case ID 005) might, for example, say in response to a survey question that he thought he was *extremely likely* to get HIV/AIDS—for a rank of five on that variable (X)—but indicate in response to another question that he would *not be at all ashamed* to get it—for a rank of one on that indicator (Y). To calculate the overall correspondence between these two ordinal variables (fear and shame of the disease), the researcher would compare the differences and similarities in the rankings of the two variables for all the cases in the sample (cases 001, 002, 003, 004, and 005 in the example in Figure 15.1). The more the rankings of these variables correspond (either in a perfectly positive or perfectly negative direction), the more likely these ordinal test statistics are to indicate that a direct or inverse relationship exists between the variables.

The investigator might also be interested in comparing two groups (homosexuals and heterosexuals) to see if they differ on an ordinal variable (level of fear of HIV/AIDS). In that case, mixed procedures, based on nominal-level classification of individuals into the groups being compared, would be appropriate. Chi-square procedures are also used with ordinal data, particularly if the variables being considered have a limited number of categories and if there is no particular concern with an ordinal interpretation of the values for each variable.

The use of related sample tests would be relevant if the study design called for certain observations to be paired, as in a study of a sample of patients before and after they were told they had HIV/AIDS to see how they would rate their fear of the illness. The paired comparisons of the rankings of the patient and control cases on this fear scale would help test a hypothesis about the fear-arousal consequences of being diagnosed as having HIV/AIDS.

Parametric Procedures

Parametric procedures are based on the assumption that the distribution of the dependent variable of interest (Y) in the population from which the sample was drawn follows a particular pattern, such as the normal distribution (see Figure 15.2).

Interval or Ratio. One of the most popular parametric procedures for independent and dependent variables that assume an interval level of measurement is regression analysis. This form of analysis looks at the extent to which an interval-level variable Y (such as blood cholesterol level) is predicted by another interval-level variable X (the average daily intake of grams of fat).

Regression coefficients are generated that estimate the change in the dependent variable Y (cholesterol level) that results from a change in the independent variable X (grams of fat). Underlying the computation of the regression coefficient is the assumption that the X and Y values for each case can be plotted on a graph and a line drawn through these points that minimizes the squared difference between each of the points and this line—referred to as the "least squares" line (see the example in Figure 15.2). The hypothesis being tested is whether a linear relationship between the variables exists, based on how well this line fits the data. The t-test and F-test statistics are used to test the statistical significance of the hypothesized relationship.

The dependent variable used in regression analysis when the variables are based on samples that are not independent is a difference computed between measures at different points in time for the same people or between matched cases. Examples would be comparisons before and after an intervention for the same people or comparisons between matched cases and controls in matched case-control designs.

The Pearson correlation coefficient, which is a measure of the strength of association between the two variables, ranges between -1.0 and $+1.0$. These procedures are powerful and useful and can serve as the basis for more sophisticated multivariate procedures (see Table 15.3 in the following section) that enable the impact of a number of other control variables also to be considered in the analyses.

FIGURE 15.2. USING PARAMETRIC BIVARIATE STATISTICS TO TEST FOR RELATIONSHIPS BETWEEN VARIABLES.

| | | Bivariate Statistics | | |
| | | Tests of Association Between Variables | | Measures of Strength of Association Between Variables |
Type of Measurement	Example	Independent Samples	Related Samples	
Interval or Ratio (extent to which Y has a linear relationship to X)	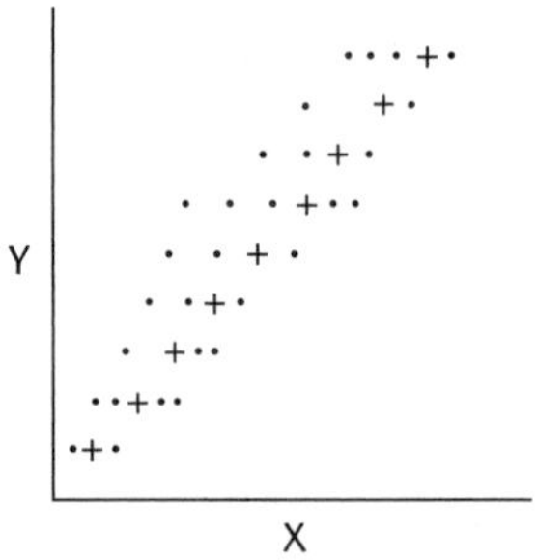 Y $\vert$ [scatterplot of X vs Y] X	Bivariate regression	Bivariate regression	Pearson correlation coefficient
Mixed (differences in means between groups)	*Variable X* *Mean of Y*	T-test of difference of means (2 groups)	Paired t-test of difference (2 groups)	Biserial correlation
Y = Interval or ratio X = Nominal	Group X = 1 $\bar{y}1$	One-way analysis of variance	One-way analysis of variance with repeated measures	Point biserial correlation
	Group X = 2 $\bar{y}2$			Eta coefficient
	Group X = 3 $\bar{y}3$			

Mixed. The final procedure reviewed in Figure 15.2 is a mixed one, where the dependent variable is an interval-level variable and the predictor variable is nominal. For example, one might be interested in looking at the level of blood cholesterol (Y) for African American and white children (X) and determining whether there are statistically significant differences between the two groups. This type of analysis can be conducted by using a t-test statistic of the difference between two means. Biserial or point biserial correlation coefficients can be computed to measure the association between the interval-level dependent variable and the dichotomous independent variable.

If there is interest in comparing means among more than two groups (African American, white, and Hispanic children, for example), then the one-way analysis of variance procedure, which uses the F-test statistic, is more appropriate. Analysis of variance is discussed in more detail later in this chapter.

Using Multivariate Statistics to Explain Relationships Between Variables

The procedures summarized in Figure 15.3 and Table 15.3 are used when researchers want to add one or more additional variables to the analysis in an effort to further understand the relationship between two variables examined in the bivariate analyses. These procedures can be viewed as the statistical devices for carrying out the elaboration of the study hypotheses, which were discussed in Chapter Four and displayed in Figures 4.2 through 4.5.

Nonparametric Procedures

Nonparametric multivariate procedures are designed to analyze data for which the dependent variable and related predictors are all either nominal, ordinal, or a combination of nominal and ordinal.

Nominal. The Pearson chi-square procedure could be expanded to include the analysis of a third nominal variable to see if the original relationship between X and Y holds when this control variable, expressed by an elaboration of the study hypotheses, is added. It may not be meaningful to expand the analysis in this way because the number of cases in some cells of the tables resulting from this cross-classification process may become very small. If more than 20 percent of the resulting cells have expected values of fewer than five cases, it is not meaningful to use the chi-square test statistic.

Log-linear analysis and weighted least squares (WLS) procedures are more appropriate procedures to use when all the predictors for a categoric dependent variable are also nominal-level variables. The Mantel-Haenszel procedure is used quite frequently in epidemiological analyses of dichotomous independent and dependent variables. It combines data from several 2×2 tables (resulting from cross-classifications of dichotomous variables) into a single estimate (expressed as an odds ratio) of the probability of having a disease (yes/no), based on the status of the respondents' exposure (yes/no) to a number of risk conditions (Rosner, 2000).

Ordinal. The Kendall coefficient of concordance expresses the strength of association among three or more ordinal-level variables. Several procedures (previously

FIGURE 15.3. USING NONPARAMETRIC MULTIVARIATE STATISTICS TO EXPLAIN RELATIONSHIPS BETWEEN VARIABLES.

| | | Multivariate Statistics | | |
| | | Tests of Association Between Variables | | Measures of Strength of Association Between Variables |
Type of Measurement	Example	Independent Samples	Related Samples	
Nominal (cross-tabulation of dependent variable by independent variable by control variables)	*(see contingency table example below)*	Chi-square multidimensional contingency table analysis Loglinear analysis Weighted least squares Mantel-Haenszel chi-square	Cochran Q-test	Coefficient of contingency Cramér's V Lambda Symmetric lambda Odds ratio
Ordinal (association of ranks between three or more variables)	*(see ranks example below)*	Chi-square multidimensional contingency table analysis		Kendall coefficient of concordance

Example (Nominal):

Z = 1

	X = 1	X = 2	X = 3
Y = 1			
Y = 2			

Z = 2

	X = 1	X = 2	X = 3
Y = 1			
Y = 2			

Example (Ordinal), Ranks:

Case ID	Variable X	Variable Y	Variable Z
001	1	5	3
002	2	4	2
003	3	3	1
004	4	2	5
005	5	1	4

TABLE 15.3. USING PARAMETRIC MULTIVARIATE STATISTICS TO EXPLAIN RELATIONSHIPS BETWEEN VARIABLES.

Type of Measurement	Example	Multivariate Statistics		Measures of Strength of Association Between Variables
		Tests of Association Between Variables		
		Independent Samples	Related Samples	
Interval or Ratio (extent to which Y has a linear relationship to X, Z, and so on)	$Y = a + b_1X + b_1Z_1 + b_2Z_2 + b_nZ_n + e$	Multiple regression	Multiple regression of difference scores	Multiple correlation coefficient
Mixed (differences in means between groups, controlling for other characteristics)	*Mean of Y* *Variable X and Variable Z*			
Y = Interval or Ratio X = Nominal Z = Nominal	X = 1 by Z = 1 $\overline{y}11$ X = 1 by Z = 2 $\overline{y}12$ X = 2 by Z = 1 $\overline{y}21$ X = 2 by Z = 2 $\overline{y}22$	Analysis of variance	Analysis of variance with repeated measures	Multiple correlation coefficient
Y = Interval or Ratio X = Nominal Z = Interval	X = 1 with Z $\overline{y}1adjZ$ X = 2 with Z $\overline{y}2adjZ$	Analysis of covariance	Analysis of covariance with repeated measures	Multiple correlation coefficient
(differences in percent between groups, controlling for other characteristics) Y = Dichotomy	*% of Y* *Variable X and Variable Z*	Logistic regression	Logistic regression of change in status	Odds ratio
X = Nominal Z = Mixed	X = 1 by Z = 1 y11% X = 1 by Z = 2 y12% X = 2 by Z = 1 y21% X = 2 by Z = 2 y22%			

listed as mixed procedures in Figure 15.1) are useful in comparing groups when the dependent variable does not meet the assumptions of interval- or ratio-level measurement. The Median and Kruskal-Wallis tests (for three or more groups) permit different groups, created by a cross-classification of the independent (X) and control (Z) variables, to be compared on an ordinal dependent variable (Y). The Friedman two-way analysis of variance procedure is used when the groups being compared are related.

Parametric Procedures

Parametric procedures assume interval- or ratio-level dependent variables.

Interval or Ratio. Multiple regression procedures may be used when two or more interval-level measures serve as predictors of some normally distributed interval-level dependent variable (see Table 15.3). In this procedure, the regression coefficient for any particular independent variable (X) represents the change in the dependent variable (Y) associated with a one-unit change in X, while the levels of the control variables ($Z1$, $Z2$, and so on) are held constant.

Mixed. Analysis of variance (ANOVA) procedures are based on the same underlying statistical model used in regression. In fact, ANOVA is similar to dummy variable regression, in which a series of dichotomous variables are used to represent the categories of a nominal variable. In contrast to regular regression procedures, analysis of variance focuses on comparing the means for cross-classifications of two or more groups of people, not on estimating coefficients that reflect the magnitude of change in the dependent variable associated with a unit change in the independent variables.

For example, one may want to look at the differences in the average cholesterol level for African American and white children (X), while controlling for whether the children are poor or not (Z) (referred to as two-way analysis of variance since the effects of two predictor variables are being examined). An F-test statistic can be used to summarize the difference in the variances between and within the resulting groups on the dependent variable (Y) of interest. The greater the variances *between* groups compared with the variance *within* groups, the more likely it is that the differences between the groups are significant. Analysis of variance can be used to test these relationships for independent and related samples as well as to compute a multiple correlation coefficient to measure the strength of the association between the dependent variable and a linear combination of the independent variables.

For analysis of covariance procedures, means on the dependent variable Y (cholesterol level) are compared for groups of individuals identified by a nominal variable X (African American versus white children), using some interval-level control variable Z. In the example just cited, an interval-level control variable Z (family income), rather than the nominal-level variable Z (poverty status), could be used. In that case, an analysis of covariance procedure would be more appropriate than an analysis of variance procedure. The analysis of covariance procedure then statistically controls or adjusts for the fact that the relation between the continuous dependent variable and race is also affected by this continuous control variable.

When the dependent variable of interest is *dichotomous* (whether the cholesterol reading is high or not, as determined by a normative cutoff point) rather than interval level (the cholesterol reading itself), and a variety of nominal, interval, or ratio measures are used as independent or control variables, it is appropriate to use probit or logistic regression procedures (Hosmer & Lemeshow, 2000; Kleinbaum, Klein, & Pryor, 2002). The test statistics for these procedures do not assume the same underlying sampling distributions found in the multiple regression approach for analyzing continuous dependent variables. The regression coefficients become estimates of odds ratios, which can be converted to estimates of the probability that a certain outcome (Y) will occur, based on its relationship to other variables (X, Z). A chi-square statistic can be used to test the statistical significance of these coefficients. Hanley (1983, p. 172) accurately observed that logistic regression "now stands in the same relation to binary (dichotomous) response data as classical regression does to continuous (interval) response data" in the analysis of epidemiological data.

Many other procedures are also available to researchers. Path analysis and LISREL *(LInear Structural RELations)* are powerful procedures for modeling the causal linkages between variables implied in complex conceptual frameworks and, in the instance of LISREL, for quantifying the validity and reliability of the variables used to measure the multidimensional constructs in these models (Jöreskog, 2000; Jöreskog & Sörbom, 1996). Multivariate analysis of variance examines the relationship between multiple independent and dependent variables, such as several different measures of the health-related quality-of-life construct (Kutner, Nachtsheim, Neter, & Li, 2005).

Mapping Out the Analysis Plan

Constructing a measurement matrix and considering the relevance of alternative statistical procedures for measuring and modeling the study objectives sets the stage for the formulation of the analysis plan for the study (Fink, 2003). A sample guide for this process, based on the dentist survey, appears in Table 15.4.

TABLE 15.4. MAPPING OUT THE ANALYSIS PLAN.

Study Objective	Number and Type of Variables		Analytical Procedures
	Independent Variable	Dependent Variable	
	One variable (neither independent or dependent)		
1. To estimate dental malpractice insurance experience in a representative sample of U.S. dentists in 1991.	Ordinal: Number of complaints reported (never, once, twice, three or more times)		Frequency, percentage, mode, median
	One independent and one dependent variable		
2. To compare dental malpractice insurance experience by the dentist's demographic characteristics.	Nominal (2 categories): male versus female	Nominal: Number of complaints reported (never versus one or more)	Chi-square, Fisher's exact test
		Ordinal: Number of complaints reported (never, once, twice, three or more times)	Chi-square, median test, Mann-Whitney U-test, Kolmogorov-Smirnov, Wald-Wolfowitz runs test
		Interval (or interval-like): Number of complaints reported (0, 1, 2, 3)	t-test, one-way analysis of variance
	Nominal (3 or more categories): race/ethnicity	Nominal: Number of complaints reported (never versus one or more)	Chi-square
		Ordinal: Number of complaints reported (never, once, twice, three or more times)	Chi-square, Kruskal-Wallis
		Interval (or interval-like): Number of complaints reported (0, 1, 2, 3)	One-way analysis of variance
	Two or more independent variables		
3. To analyze the relative importance of doctor-patient communication, practice characteristics, practice finances, and dentist's demographic characteristics on dental malpractice insurance experience.	Nominal (all)	Nominal	Chi-square, log-linear analysis, weighted least squares, Mantel-Haenszel chi-square
	Nominal (all) Nominal and interval Interval (or Interval-like) Interval (or interval-like)	Interval (or interval-like) Interval (or interval-like) Interval (or interval-like) Nominal (dichotomy)	Analysis of variance Analysis of (co)variance Multiple linear regression Logistic regression, probit

The first and primary reference point for developing the analysis plan is the study's specific objectives (and hypotheses, if applicable). The objectives should clearly convey who and what represent the central focus of the study as well as the underlying study design with respect to the number of groups of interest and when (or how often) the data will be gathered. The study objectives for the dentist survey, as well as the others used as primary examples throughout the text, were displayed in Table 2.3 in Chapter Two.

Second, the number and types of variables used in addressing the study objectives must be considered. The measurement matrix (Table 15.1) serves as a useful reference for this step in the process. For descriptive purposes, discrete variables may be analyzed separately using simple univariate statistics. When two or more variables are used, independent and dependent variables should be distinguished in the analysis. In analytical and experimental studies, these should be clearly identified in the study hypothesis: the independent variable is hypothesized to cause or influence the occurrence of the dependent variable. With respect to descriptive studies, the designation of independent and dependent variables is relevant when there is a group comparison or longitudinal aspect to the design. In those instances, the groups being compared or the passage of time can be viewed as independent variables that are assumed to be associated with or predictive of some other attribute or outcome (dependent variable). Sample size estimation procedures (described in Chapter Seven) are also essential in ensuring there are sufficient cases available to conduct the required analyses.

The third and final step, based on the criteria reviewed earlier, is to choose the relevant analytical procedures that most appropriately mirror and model statistically what the study objectives are intended to convey substantively. The basic logic for formulating an analysis plan is illustrated in Table 15.4, drawing on the dentist survey as an example.

As indicated earlier in this chapter (and summarized in Table 2.3), the first principal objective of the dentist survey was to estimate dental malpractice insurance experience in a representative sample of U.S. dentists. The questions related to dental malpractice experience are arrayed in questions 30 through 52 of the survey questionnaire (Resource C). These questions represent an array of levels of measurement (nominal, ordinal, and interval). The example used in Table 15.4 is based on the response to question 35 in the dentist survey, "How many times over the past five years have you reported to your agent, your broker, or your insurance carrier a potential or actual complaint against you, *even if no formal claim was ever filed, or no attorney was involved?*" The ordinal response categories provided in the questionnaire were never, once, twice, or three or more times. As indicated in Table 15.4, frequency, percentages, mode, or median could be used to summarize responses to this question. If interval- or ratio-level responses were used, such as the actual number of complaints reported, means could be used to summarize the survey responses.

The second objective concerned comparing dental malpractice experience for dentists with demographic characteristics. The choice of a bivariate statistical procedure to address this objective would be influenced by the number of categories of demographic characteristics being compared (two versus three or more), as well as the form of the variable used for characterizing the malpractice experience. The analysis could, for example, focus on simply whether a complaint was reported. The bivariate cross-tabulation would then display the distribution of responses for dentists in different sociodemographic groupings (such as by gender or race/ethnicity), and a chi-square or Fisher's exact test could be used to test for the significance of the difference between groups. (The Fisher's exact test would assume that only two groups were being compared and that the four categories of responses in question 35 were collapsed into two—"never" versus "one or more complaint," for example.)

Another measurement alternative is to analyze the original ordinal-level response categories ("never, once, twice, three or more times"). These responses could then be examined across dentists in different sociodemographic groups using bivariate analytic procedures that assume an ordinal-level dependent variable.

A third approach is to construct an interval (or interval-like) mean of the number of complaints reported, based on the recoding of the original response categories to an interval-like level of measurement (0, 1, 2, 3), for dentists in different sociodemographic subgroups, using either a *t*-test (two groups) or one-way analysis of variance (three or more groups). It would be reasonable to recode the data in this fashion if there were no or very few cases that have more than three complaints, based on the survey data, available external evidence (such as insurers' records of complaints), and/or expert judgment (insurer advisory group). Other approaches may also be relevant depending on the underlying research question and associated variables of interest.

An implicit analytical objective, particularly before proceeding with multivariate analysis procedures, may be to examine the bivariate correlations between potential predictor variables and the dependent variable to be considered in those analyses. This can serve as a basis for identifying and screening in (using) only those variables that are significantly correlated with the dependent variable into the multivariate stage of the analysis. An array of nominal- and ordinal-level correlational statistics is available (see Figures 15.1 and 15.2). The Pearson correlation coefficient is used with interval-level data.

The third major analytical objective of the dentist survey concerned the relative importance of doctor-patient communication, practice characteristics, practice finances, and dentists' demographic characteristics as predictive of dental malpractice experience. As displayed in Table 15.4, different forms of the candidate independent and dependent variables would dictate the choice of analytical procedures. The investigators in the National Dental Malpractice Survey used multiple regression to examine the extent to which an array of characteristics influenced a series of interval-level measures constructed from the survey reflecting the quality and volume of dental practice (Conrad, Milgrom, Whitney, O'Hara, & Fiset, 1998). Not all of the procedures displayed as examples in Table 15.4 would be executed in a single study.

Setting Up Mock Tables

Before considering any particular statistical approach to analyzing data, the researcher should give thought to the kinds of tables appropriate to displaying the data for purposes of addressing the study objectives or hypotheses. Constructing mock tables—tables formatted in the way that the data will eventually be reported but not filled in until the data are analyzed—forces the investigator to think concretely about how the information that is gathered in the study will actually be used. Running computer programs to conduct fancy statistical analyses without a clear idea of the specific relationships that need to be examined will waste the researcher's time and resources and probably produce output that the investigator does not really know how to use or interpret anyway.

Sample mock tables were provided in Exhibit 4.1 (Chapter Four). Mock tables should be configured for the analysis to be used to address each study objective (Table 15.4). The table title and headings should clearly identify the study constructs and subgroups for which data are to be reported. The tables should also reflect intended transformations of the data, such as collapsing the original data into categories, constructing summary scales or indexes, or defining the meaning of the special coding of dichotomous variables (as 1 versus 0) in regression analysis (what the categories 1 and 0 represent, such as male versus female or smoker versus nonsmoker). As indicated in Chapter Four (Exhibit 4.1), for cross-sectional analytical designs, the percentages on the dependent variable (being a smoker or not) should sum to 100 percent within each category of the independent variable (friends' smoking behavior). The percentages could then be compared across groups to determine which group, if any, is more likely to fall into a certain category of the dependent variable.

In addition, at the bottom of each mock table, the investigator should indicate the statistical procedure to be used in carrying out the analysis reported in the table (such as frequencies, means, Pearson chi-square, *t*-test, analysis of variance, and so on), as well as the study objective or hypothesis the analysis is intended to address. Researchers are encouraged to review tables in the published literature in their field as a source of examples for how the data for their study would be reported.

Special Considerations for Special Populations

If certain groups are to be a special focus of the study, the implications need to be thought through at the start in planning the design analysis of the survey, not after the data are collected. Particular attention should be paid to whether there will be sufficient cases to carry out key subgroup comparisons of interest, based on the study objectives (see Chapters Six and Seven).

Selected Examples

The findings from the UNICEF Multiple Indicator Surveys are available in country-specific reports. These reports are primarily descriptive in nature. Mock tables, that is, "Tabulation Guidelines," are provided to facilitate the preparation of these reports. In addition, UNICEF makes the data available for secondary analyses by interested investigators (UNICEF, n.d.).

Similarly, reports addressing various state and national policy topics have been generated based on the California Health Interview Survey. The data are also available for public health practitioners, policy professionals, and academic investigators for taking a more analytical look at the rich array of data available through the CHIS core survey and special questionnaire modules (UCLA Center for Health Policy Research, 2005).

The analytical focus of the dentist survey has received considerable attention in this chapter. This survey was, however, part of a larger and much more comprehensive project of research addressing the practice and policy factors that influence dental malpractice experience. In selected analyses of this data set, data on state-level insurance policies and procedures and claims experience were linked to the dentist survey data. This study then serves to demonstrate the utility of linking survey and record data in addressing research questions by drawing on the unique strengths of each data source (Conrad et al., 1995, 1998; Milgrom et al., 1994; Milgrom, Whitney, Conrad, Fiset, & O'Hara, 1995).

Guidelines for Minimizing Survey Errors and Maximizing Survey Quality

Developing an analysis plan means just that! It pays many times over to start with a well-articulated approach for analyzing the data. Other ideas about how to analyze the data will occur once the data-gathering process begins and the distributions on key variables of interest or the results of preliminary analyses are available. However, if one has a basic plan in mind, subsequent departures then can be a further exploration of a rich mine of information. If a plan is not formulated in advance, the process may be more like sifting through a mound of sand and rubble in hopes of finding some gems.

The major types of systematic and variable errors, respectively, that need to be anticipated and addressed in developing the analysis plan are statistical conclusion validity and statistical power or precision (see Table 15.5.) Statistical conclusion validity refers to whether the statistical evidence regarding a relationship between variables is sound. Low statistical power or precision can contribute to poor statistical conclusion validity due to the inability to attest to the statistical significance of important substantive differences that exist (Type II error). Statistical conclusion validity can also be compromised if the assumptions regarding the selection or application of selected statistical procedures are violated. This chapter has provided specific guidance regarding how to best match the choice of analysis procedures to the study design and objectives, level of measurement of study variables, or the underlying population distribution. Chapter Seven elaborated the procedures for ensuring that sufficient cases are obtained to successfully address the study objectives.

Supplementary Sources

Different statistics textbooks focus on the analysis of survey data from different disciplinary perspectives, including, for example, the social sciences (Frankfort-Nachmias & Nachmias, 2000; Knoke, Bohrnstedt, & Mee, 2002), biometry (Pagano & Gauvreau, 2000; Rosner,

TABLE 15.5. SURVEY ERRORS: SOURCES AND SOLUTIONS— PLANNING AND IMPLEMENTING THE ANALYSIS OF THE DATA.

	Systematic Errors: Poor Statistical Conclusion Validity	Variable Errors: Low Statistical Power or Precision
Solutions to Errors	Match the selection of statistical analysis procedures to the study design and objectives, level of measurement of study variables, or the underlying population distribution.	Map out the analysis plan to address each of the study objectives in advance of conducting the study, and estimate the number of cases required to achieve a desired level of power or precision for each objective (also see Chapter Seven).

2000), and epidemiology (Kahn & Sempos, 1989; Kleinbaum, 2003). See Fink (2003) for straightforward guidance regarding how to develop an approach to analyzing survey data in general. Kanji (1999) provides a concise compilation of one hundred commonly used statistical tests. Statistical analysis software is also available on the Internet (American Statistical Association, Section on Survey Research Methods, n.d.-b; Decision Analyst, 2002; University of Texas, M D Anderson Cancer Center, 2003). Huff (1993) importantly points out "how to lie with statistics" and correspondingly how *not* to do so.

CHAPTER SIXTEEN

WRITING THE RESEARCH REPORT

Chapter Highlights

1. The following criteria should be considered in deciding what and how much to say in the final report: (1) the audience, (2) the mode of dissemination, and (3) the replicability of the study's methodology and results.
2. A comprehensive final research report should contain an executive summary, a statement of the problem or research question addressed in the study, a review of relevant literature, and a description of the study design and hypotheses. It should also include a discussion of the survey's methods, its findings, and the implications and relevance of these results. At times, it is appropriate to include a copy of the survey questionnaire as well as additional material on the methods used in conducting the study.
3. The researcher should provide an assessment of the overall strengths and limitations of the study when presenting the final survey results.

The final step in designing and conducting a survey is dissemination of the results to interested audiences. This chapter presents the criteria and guidelines for preparing a final report and points out material in the preceding chapters that will be useful to review when writing it.

Criteria for Writing Research Reports

Criteria for writing reports include the (1) intended audience for the report, (2) appropriate scope and format of the report given the proposed method of disseminating the study results, and (3) replicability of the study from the documentation provided on how it was designed and conducted.

Knowing exactly who the audience for the report will be provides an important point of reference in deciding what to emphasize and how much technical detail to include. A project funder or a dissertation committee might want full documentation of the methods that were used in carrying out the study, as well as a detailed exposition of what was learned. A hospital or health maintenance organization's board of directors might be more interested in a clear and interpretable presentation of the findings and less concerned about documentation of the methodologies used in carrying out the study. Professional colleagues might want to be given enough detail about how the study was designed and conducted to enable them to replicate it or compare some aspects of it with research that they or others have conducted.

In all of these cases, the researcher needs to communicate as clearly as possible the information desired by the respective audiences. Jargon and technical shorthand should be minimized. Examples are often more useful than are long technical descriptions in illustrating complex materials or abstract concepts. Also, failure to understand the material oneself shows in how a report is written. The clarity and readability of reports emanating from survey research projects take on even greater import in the context of trends toward engaging communities and affected populations in the design of studies and interpretation and application of study findings, as well as the wider dissemination of materials over the Internet.

It is useful to have a friend or colleague read an early draft. Even if this person does not fully understand all the technical details of a study, he or she will be able to identify areas that seem unclear or poorly written. If what is written makes sense to the friend or colleague, the author can be assured that he or she is at least on the way to getting the material across to the audience for whom it is ultimately intended. Word processing software such as Microsoft Word also has features for assessing the level or complexity of writing.

A second issue to consider before starting to write the report is the form in which the final results of the study will be disseminated. Table 16.1 presents a suggested outline for a final research report. Sections or appendixes of this kind of

TABLE 16.1. OUTLINE OF THE RESEARCH REPORT.

Sections	Chapter References
Executive Summary	Sixteen
I. Statement of the problem	Two
II. Review of the literature	One
III. Methods	
A. Study design	Two
B. Sample design	Six, Seven
C. Data collection	Five, Thirteen
D. Questionnaire design	Eight through Twelve
E. Measurement	Three
F. Data preparation	Fourteen
G. Analysis plan	Four, Fifteen
IV. Results	Four, Fifteen
V. Conclusions	Sixteen
Appendixes	
Methodological appendix	Three through Seven, Thirteen, Fourteen
Survey questionnaire	Eight through Twelve
References	Sixteen

report will be more or less comprehensive depending on whether the report is a thesis or dissertation, a formal project report to a funder, a research monograph, a book, a working paper, a journal article, a research note, or a nontechnical summary for a lay audience.

The form and format of a thesis or dissertation, a formal project report, or a research monograph generally permit comprehensive exposition and documentation of the study methodology. This means including the survey questionnaire and a detailed methodological appendix in the final research report. If the results of the research are being prepared for publication as a book, some methodological detail will have to be eliminated depending on the projected length and audience for the book. Working papers and journal articles do not generally contain extensive appendix material. Although the basic outline for a research report can be used in drafting such papers, each section should be a much-reduced version of what would appear in a comprehensive final report. Working papers are sometimes considered early drafts of articles that will eventually be submitted for publication. Such papers can be circulated to colleagues for informal review and comment. This provides an opportunity to revise the manuscript before sending it to a journal for formal consideration for publication. Research notes generally report on a very limited aspect of a study's methodology or findings. Articles for a lay audience may focus on the study findings and their implications for issues of particular interest to that audience.

Researchers should also bear in mind that one of the best guarantees of a good final research report is a good initial research proposal (Locke, Spirduso, & Silverman, 2000). The outline in Table 16.1 can also be used as a guide for drafting either a prospectus or a full-blown research proposal for a project. As indicated throughout this book, thinking through the problem to be addressed in the study, identifying related studies and research, figuring out how to design the survey to address the study's main objectives or hypotheses, and specifying the precise methods and procedures for carrying out the study and analyzing the data—*before* beginning to collect them—are critical for ensuring that the study will be carried out as it should be.

Using the prospectus or proposal as a way to specify as many of these aspects as possible beforehand also provides a solid foundation for the first draft of the final report. Documentation of formal specifications for the final report (such as format requirements for theses or government reports) should be obtained before writing the proposal. The investigator will then already have in hand materials that match what should be included in the final report in both form *and* substance.

A third criterion to have in mind when deciding what to include in a final research report is whether other investigators will be able to replicate the methods and results of the study or compare them with those obtained in their own or others' research. Both applied and basic research are best served by building on and extending previous research in the field and by replicating or disconfirming results across studies—provided that there is always a clear understanding of the similarities and differences in the design and methods of the different studies. Of course, full research reports provide a better opportunity to include comprehensive detail on how a survey was carried out than do working papers, articles, or research notes. However, even a short report should contain a clear description of the study's methodology. A useful question to keep in mind throughout the course of study is the following: Can I document and defend not only what I did but also how and why it differs from what was done in similar studies?

Outline of the Research Report

A working outline for a research report, along with references to the chapters in this book that can be useful in preparing it, is presented in Table 16.1. An executive summary of the methods and major findings for the study should appear at the beginning of the report. This summary should be written after all the other sections of the report have been drafted and there has been an opportunity to reflect on and identify the major findings and implications of the study. The summary must be written in a clear and concise manner because many readers will rely heavily or even exclusively on it to get an idea of how the study was carried out and what was learned from it. Executive summaries for books or monographs may be two or three pages in length. For articles, working papers, or theses, these summaries may have to be limited to abstracts of no more than 125 to 250 words.

Section I of the main body of the report should contain the *statement of the problem* to be addressed in the study. Chapter Two in this book provides guidelines for phrasing researchable questions that can serve as the basis for an inquiry into a problem of interest to the investigator. Stating the problem at the beginning of the report aids the reader in understanding why the study was undertaken and what the researchers hoped to learn from it. A clear and concise statement of the problem requires that survey designers identify and read related research on the issue and integrate it into their own inquiry. The study objectives and hypotheses would be stated in this section after a case is made for the importance of addressing the topic.

What has been learned from other studies can be summarized in a formal *review of the literature*, Section II of the report. Chapter One and Resources D and E provide an overview of sources and examples of health surveys that might be useful in compiling such a review. This review should not try to cover everything that has been written about the topic, but it should make clear the current state of the art of research—both methodological and substantive—on the issue and how the question posed in the current study will contribute to fuller understanding of the issue.

Section III of the report should contain a description of the *methods* for the investigation of the problem under study. The methods section should include a description of the study design, sample design, data collection methods, questionnaire design, variable definitions and related measurement issues, the procedures for preparing the data for analysis, and the proposed analysis plan. Chapters Two through Fifteen (and particularly the tables and figures in those chapters) provide useful guidance for what to include in this section of the report.

Chapter Two provides an overview of relevant survey designs. The subsection on *study design* should describe the design and why it is a fitting one for addressing the study's objectives and hypotheses. A discussion of the *sample design* for the study, for instance, should include a description of the target population, sample frame, and sampling elements for the survey; the type of sample and how it was selected, including any procedures for oversampling certain subgroups; the sample size; response rates; procedures for weighting the data; standard errors and design effects for major estimates; and, when appropriate, a discussion of the magnitude of biases due to the noncoverage or nonresponse of certain groups and how these biases were dealt with in the analyses.

Another important subsection of the methods section of the report is a description of the *data collection* procedures employed in the study. This should include an overview of the principal data collection method used (Internet, paper-and-pencil, or computer-assisted personal, telephone, or self-administered approach or some combination of these methods) and the pros and cons of the method for this particular study. The procedures for the pilot study and pretests of the instrument, the results of these trial runs, and how the questionnaire was modified in response to what was learned from them could be summarized in this section. The criteria and procedures for hiring, training, and supervising interviewers or other data collection personnel and following up and monitoring the fieldwork for the study should also be summarized in this section of the report.

A discussion of the *questionnaire design* describes the sources for the questions in the questionnaire and the principles used in modifying them or formulating new ones. A section on *measurement* could present the operational and variable definitions and related summary indicators or scales used in measuring the major concepts of interest in the study, as well as how the validity and reliability of these measures were evaluated.

Another important aspect of the survey to document in this section of the final report is the process of *data preparation,* that is, the procedures for translating the data into numerical codes, entering them into a computerized medium, cleaning and correcting them, and imputing or estimating information on key study variables. The growth of computerized and Internet-based data collection procedures has resulted in the coding and data entry and checking procedures being built into the initial design of the survey questionnaire.

A final subsection of the methods section should include a review of the *analysis plan,* containing a description of the statistical procedures to be used in analyzing the data and why they are appropriate given the study design; the level of measurement of survey variables; the research questions and hypotheses that were addressed in the study; and mock (or blank) data tables that will be used to report the survey findings once the analyses are completed. Researchers may want to incorporate the survey questionnaire and more extensive information on the methods used in carrying out the study into appendixes at the end of the report.

Section IV, the discussion of the *results* of the study, comes next, and here researchers will find it helpful to consult Chapters Four and Fifteen of this book. The order and presentation of the findings in this section should be clearly related to the study objectives and hypotheses presented in Section I. If mock tables were prepared in formulating the analysis plan for the study, they can serve as the basis for selecting the tables to produce and include in the final report. The titles and headings used for the tables should fully describe their content. Conventions for numbering, punctuating, capitalizing, and formatting table titles and headings should be consistent across tables. The data reported in the tables should be double-checked against the computer runs on which they are based.

The text should be written so that readers do not have to refer constantly to the tables to understand the findings. At the same time, it should be clear where the data cited in the text come from in the tables. Tables can be placed either in the body of the text or at the end of the sections of the text in which they are described. Their placement depends on which approach would be more convenient for the reader and on any formal requirements for the format of the final report.

The presentation and discussion of the findings in Section IV of the report should focus principally on describing the empirical results of the study. In the *conclusions* section—Section V—the researcher can be more speculative in discussing what these findings mean: how they relate to or extend previous research in the area; what the limitations and contributions of this particular study are in advancing research on the topic; what further research seems warranted; and what the particular theoretical, policy, or programmatic implications of the study are.

A list of the references cited in the report should follow the appendixes. The format for these references should be based on requirements specified by the funder, publisher, or thesis committee, as appropriate. The author should double-check that all references cited in the text appear in the list of references and that the correct spelling of the authors' names and correct dates of publication are used. Bibliographical software packages such as RefWorks, Reference Manager, or End Notes facilitate the inputting and formatting of sources cited in the proposal or report.

An Overview of Survey Errors

Finally, when interpreting and presenting the final results of their study, health survey researchers should evaluate its overall strengths and limitations through a systematic review of the errors in the survey. (See Table 1.1 and related discussion in Chapter One.)

In the discussion that follows, the systematic and random errors that can be made at each stage of designing and conducting a health survey—all addressed in previous chapters—are summarized in the context of a total survey error approach to evaluating the overall quality of the survey. The various types of survey errors are highlighted in Table 16.2. Guidelines for minimizing the different types of errors appear at the end of the chapters referenced for the respective types of errors in this table. The survey error framework can provide a useful template for identifying the strengths and limitations of a study in the proposal or final report for a survey.

TABLE 16.2. OVERVIEW OF SURVEY ERRORS.

		Types of Errors	
	Systematic Error	Variable Error	Chapter References
Study design	*Poor internal validity.* The study design does not adequately and accurately address the study's hypotheses, particularly with respect to demonstrating a causal relationship between the independent (predictor) and dependent (outcome) variables.	*Design specification ambiguity.* The statement of the study objectives and related concepts to be measured in the survey are not clearly and unambiguously stated, particularly in relationship to the underlying study design and data analysis plan for the study.	Two
	Poor external validity. Findings based on the study design cannot be widely or universally applied to related populations or subgroups.		
Sample design	*Noncoverage bias.* All units of the target population (for example, households, individuals) are not included in the sampling frame (*frame bias*) or the respondent is not selected randomly (*respondent selection bias*).	*Standard errors.* The standard error measures random sampling variation in an estimate (for example, mean or proportion) across all possible random samples of a certain size that could theoretically be drawn from the target population.	Six, Seven
	Weighting errors. Respondents are disproportionately represented in the survey sample by failing to weight each of the cases by the disproportionate probability of their falling into the sample (sampling fraction).	*Design effects.* The design effect, computed as the ratio of the variance of a complex sample to that of a simple random sample, measures the increase in random sampling variation in an estimate due to the complex nature of a sample design.	
Data collection	*Unit nonresponse bias.* Selected units of the study sample (for example, households, individuals) are not included in the final study due to respondent refusals or unavailability during the data collection process.	*Interviewer variability.* Survey interviewers or data collectors vary in how they ask or record answers to the survey questions.	Five, Thirteen

Questionnaire design	*Item nonresponse bias.* Selected questions on the survey questionnaire are not answered due to respondent refusals or interviewer or respondent errors or omissions during the data collection process.	*Mode effects.* The responses to comparable questions by respondents vary across different data collection methods (for example, personal interview, telephone interview, mail self-administered questionnaire, Web survey). (*Note:* If these effects differ in a particular direction across mode, they become systematic errors.)	Eight through Twelve
	Under- or overreporting. An estimate (for example, mean or proportion) across samples differs in a particular (negative or positive) direction from the underlying actual (or true) population value for the estimate, that is, is lower (underreporting) or higher (overreporting).	*Order and context effects.* Answers to selected survey questions vary depending on whether they are asked before or after other questions or appear at the beginning or the end of the survey questionnaire.	
	Yea-saying. Respondents tend to agree rather than disagree with statements as a whole (*acquiescent response set*) or with what are perceived to be socially desirable responses (*social desirability bias*).		
Measurement	*Low or poor validity.* Systematic departures exist in answers to the content of a survey question from the meaning of the concept itself (*content validity*), a criterion for what constitutes an accurate answer based on another data source (*criterion validity*), or hypothesized relationships of the concept being measured with other measures or concepts (*construct validity*).	*Low or poor reliability.* Random variation exists in answers to a survey question due to when it is asked (*test-retest reliability*), who asks it (*inter-rater reliability*), or that it is simply one of a number of questions that could have been asked to obtain the information (*internal consistency reliability*).	Three

TABLE 16.2. OVERVIEW OF SURVEY ERRORS, *continued.*

Survey Design	Systematic Error	Variable Error	Chapter References
		Types of Errors	
Data preparation	*Imputation/estimation errors.* Procedures for assigning values to survey questions for which answers are not available (missing values due to item nonresponse) from data either internal or external to the survey (imputation or estimation, respectively) introduce systematic errors (biases) in estimating or examining relationships between variables.	*Data coding, editing, or data entry errors.* Data coding, editing, or data entry personnel or procedures introduce random errors in producing data files based on the survey questionnaires.	Fourteen
Analysis plan	*Poor statistical conclusion validity.* The accuracy of statistical conclusions is compromised due to the application of statistical procedures that do not meet underlying assumptions related to the study design and objectives, level of measurement of study variables, or the underlying population distribution.	*Low statistical precision or power.* There are insufficient cases in the study sample to estimate population parameters with a reasonable level of precision or to have enough statistical power to detect statistically (and substantively) significant relationships between variables if they do exist.	Four, Seven, Fifteen

Note: See the discussion of "Guidelines for Minimizing Survey Errors and Maximizing Survey Quality" at the end of the chapters referenced for the respective types of errors.

Study Design

Decisions regarding when, with whom, or where the study was done may have major implications for the accuracy and generalizability of study findings. Lack of clarity in the statement of the study objectives and related concepts to be measured in the survey, particularly in relationship to the study design and analysis plan for the study (design specification ambiguity), can mean that there is not a clear road map for how the study should be conducted. The result could be wasted resources or findings that are meaningless at worst and difficult to interpret at best.

Assessments of analytical and experimental designs should consider their internal and external validity in particular. These sources of systematic error are essentially concerned, respectively, with whether factors other than those that were hypothesized or intended account for observed outcomes (internal validity) and to what extent the selectivity or artificiality of the research environment itself might limit the broader applicability of what was learned (external validity). Suggestions could be provided with respect to the types of studies that are needed to address identified weaknesses. These issues are discussed in Chapter Two of this book.

Sample Design

Variable errors are always part of the sampling process for surveys because only a random subset of the entire group of interest for the study is selected. Standard errors are used to estimate the amount of variable (or sampling) error associated with samples of a certain size chosen in particular ways. Complex sample designs, especially those that entail cluster sampling, can yield even higher variable errors, measured through "design effects" (the ratio of the variance of a complex sample to that of a simple random sample).

Biases or systematic errors in sampling result when the basis used for sampling (telephone numbers in a directory, for example) means that certain groups will be left out (people with unlisted numbers or new numbers), so that the statistics based on the sample will always be different from the "true" picture for the population of interest (people with telephones) (noncoverage bias). Weighting errors can result when appropriate weights are not computed and assigned to respondents who are disproportionately sampled initially or under- or overrepresented in a study. These and other sources of errors during the sampling process, as well as the methods for dealing with them, are discussed in Chapters Six and Seven.

Estimates of the standard errors and design effects for the survey, as well as the basis for evaluating the statistical significance of study findings, should be reported. Any problems with noncoverage or nonresponse biases in the data should also be discussed. When possible, comparisons of the distributions should be made with other data sources to estimate the possible magnitude of these biases, and response rate and poststratification weighting procedures should be applied.

Data Collection

Response effects are biases or variable errors that can result from the data collection tasks themselves (problems with the questionnaire or method of data collection chosen) or from certain behaviors on the part of the interviewer or respondent.

For example, interviewers may vary the phrasing of a question for different respondents, or respondents may answer the question the way that they think the interviewer wants them to answer it (interviewer variability). The responses to comparable questions may also vary across different data collection methods (for example, personal interview, telephone interview, mail self-administered questionnaire, Web survey). If these mode effects differ in a particular direction across mode, they take on the character of systematic errors.

Biases in the survey estimates can result when selected units of the study sample (for example, households or individuals) are not included in the final study due to respondent refusals or unavailability during the data collection process (unit nonresponse bias) or selected questions on the survey questionnaire are not answered due to respondent refusals or interviewer or respondent errors or omissions during the data collection process (item nonresponse bias).

These and other errors that can occur during the data collection planning and implementation stages of a survey, as well as ways to minimize them, are discussed in Chapters Five and Thirteen. Researchers should report any problems encountered in carrying out the fieldwork for the study that could give rise to variable or systematic response effects in the data.

Questionnaire Design

Chapters Eight through Twelve provide guidance for the design of survey questions. The development of survey questions should attempt to minimize the likelihood of systematic errors resulting from under- or overreporting as well as yea-saying, in which respondents tend to agree rather than disagree with statements as a whole or with what are perceived to be socially desirable responses (also referred to as an "acquiescent response set").

Survey developers should be aware of likely order and context effects resulting when answers to selected survey questions vary depending on whether they are asked before or after other questions or appear at the beginning or the end of the survey questionnaire.

The discussion of study strengths and limitations in the final report should review any likely errors that may have resulted from the wording of the questions themselves, the response format for answering them, specific instructions, the translation of the survey questionnaire, or the overall organization of the survey instrument.

Measurement

The classic approaches to estimating systematic and variable errors in defining the variables used in a survey are validity and reliability analyses, respectively (see Chapter Three). Measures of validity or bias assume that there is a "true" value (medical records, for example) against which the estimates obtained through the survey (respondent reports of the numbers of visits they made to their physician in the year) can be compared. Indexes of variable error or reliability measure the correspondence between repeated measures of comparable questions or procedures.

Low or poor validity results when there are systematic departures in answers to a survey question from the meaning of the concept itself (*content validity*), a criterion for what constitutes an accurate answer based on another data source (*criterion validity*), or hypothesized relationships of the concept being measured with other measures or concepts (*construct validity*).

Low or poor reliability is reflected in significant random variation in answers to a survey question due to when it is asked (*test-retest reliability*), who asked it (*inter-rater reliability*), or that it is simply one of a number of questions that could have been asked to obtain the information (*internal consistency reliability*).

It may be difficult in some instances to determine whether a particular type of error reflects a bias or a variable error or to estimate bias when it is not clear what the "true" answers to certain types of items, such as attitudinal questions, actually are. However, the final report of the study should contain a thorough discussion of the reliability and validity of the data gathered in the survey.

Data Preparation

Sources of bias and variable errors during the coding and processing of survey data and the ways to reduce them are described in Chapter Fourteen. Random errors can be made during the data coding, editing, or data entry process. The checking procedures used to identify and correct data entry errors should be described. Correspondingly, biases can result if large numbers of certain types of people—those with very low incomes, for example—refuse to report this information when asked. The data imputation or estimation procedures used to reduce these errors and the substantive impact of making up these data should also be reported.

Analysis Plan

Finally, the capstone for the survey undertaking is whether the data that are ultimately gathered adequately and accurately answer the questions that motivated their collection. Chapter Fifteen provides guidance for mapping out an analysis plan guided by survey objectives and hypotheses. Statistical conclusion validity is ensured through the application of statistical procedures that meet underlying assumptions related to the study design and objectives, level of measurement of study variables, or the underlying population distribution.

Chapter Seven outlines the procedures for ensuring that there are sufficient cases in the study sample to estimate population parameters with a reasonable level of precision or to have enough statistical power to detect statistically (and substantively) significant relationships between variables if they do exist. The final report for the study should be firmly grounded in a well-developed plan for the ultimate uses of the data.

The study objectives and hypotheses serve as the compass and the analysis plan as the anchor for a well-designed survey. This book provides a map for undertaking the journey.

Supplementary Sources

Locke, Spirduso, and Silverman (2000) provide specific guidance for developing dissertations and grant proposals. The American Psychological Association's *Publication Manual* (2001) delineates guidelines for preparing manuscripts for publication, and Nicol and Pexman (2003) present useful examples of how to set up tables for presenting study findings.

PERSONAL INTERVIEW SURVEY: UNICEF MULTIPLE INDICATOR CLUSTER SURVEY (MICS-2)— END-DECADE STUDY

Questionnaires for the 1995, 2000, and 2005 UNICEF Multiple Indicator Cluster Surveys may be found on the UNICEF Web site (UNICEF, n.d.). The URL of the Web site for the UNICEF Multiple Indicator Cluster Survey (MICS-2)—End-Decade Study (2000) Survey Questionnaire for which specific questions are referenced in the preceding chapters is http://www.childinfo. org/mics. The files are executable (.EXE) application files and will need to be saved and extracted to be readable in Word. Though the precise procedures may vary by browser, you may use the following general instructions to extract the files:

1. Left-click on the link for the questionnaire component on the files on the Web page.
2. Save the file to a subdirectory.
3. Left-click on the file and open it.
4. The .EXE file will try to extract and save the Word document to a "Temp" folder. To proceed, click the button with the three periods (. . .) to the right of the folder/file display window to choose a place to save it in My Documents and then click on the "Extract" button.

5. The Word document file will be saved to the location specified. A message will be sent when the process is finished: "Finished Extracting File(s)." The file will be placed in the location specified and can be opened as a Word file.

The research for the UNICEF Multiple Indicator Cluster Surveys was conducted by the UNICEF Division of Evaluation, Policy and Planning (Edilberto Loaiza, MICS-2 Coordinator).

RESOURCE B

TELEPHONE INTERVIEW SURVEY: CALIFORNIA HEALTH INTERVIEW SURVEY (CHIS)—2001

Questionnaires for the CHIS 2001, 2003, and 2005 may be found on the CHIS Web site (UCLA Center for Health Policy Research, 2005). The URL of the Web site for the CHIS 2001 Adult Survey Questionnaire for which specific questions are referenced in the preceding chapters is http://www.chis.ucla.edu/pdf/CHIS2001_adult_q.pdf. The California Health Interview Surveys were conducted by the UCLA Center for Health Policy Research (E. Richard Brown, principal investigator).

MAIL QUESTIONNAIRE SURVEY: NATIONAL DENTAL MALPRACTICE SURVEY

R esource C begins on the next page. Pages 409–427 constitute the questionnaire portion. Samples of cover letters and a reminder postcard are reprinted on pages 428–432. All of these materials are typeset, not photographic reproductions of the originals. A copy of the cover page for the survey questionnaire appears in Exhibit 12.1.

For more information on the methodology for the study, see Washington State University, Social and Economic Sciences Research Center (1993).

The research for Resource C was conducted by the University of Washington School of Dentistry (Peter Milgrom, Louis Fiset, principal investigators) and administered by the Social and Economic Sciences Research Center, Washington State University (John Tarnai, principal investigator).

INSTRUCTIONS

Were you in **private practice** as a non-specialist full-time or part-time general dentist during any part of 1991? (*Circle your answer*)

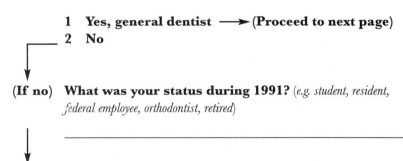

1 Yes, general dentist ⟶ (Proceed to next page)

2 No

(If no) **What was your status during 1991?** (*e.g. student, resident, federal employee, orthodontist, retired*)

_____

(If no) **Even though you were not a practicing general dentist during 1991, and thus are not part of the population under study, we are nevertheless interested in your comments on what you believe to be the greatest malpractice problem facing dentists today, and invite you to turn to the back cover where space is provided.**

Above all, *please return the questionnaire* to us so we'll know what your professional status was in 1991. Thank you.

If you have questions about completing this survey, call the National Dental Malpractice Study at the University of Washington between 8 A.M. and 5 P.M. on the West Coast, and ask for Dr. Fiset or Dr. Milgrom. The phone number is (206)543-2034. Please call collect.

Doctor-Patient Communication

We all know there are visits in which things do not go as well as we would like. This section concerns your interpersonal relationship with your patients.

Q-1 All in all, on a daily basis how satisfied are you with your practice in general? (*Circle your answer*)

1   Extremely satisfied
2   Very satisfied
3   Somewhat satisfied
4   Somewhat dissatisfied
5   Very dissatisfied
6   Extremely dissatisfied

Q-2 What percentage of your patient visits are frustrating in one way or another? (*Circle your answer*)

1   Less than 5%
2   5–10%
3   11–25%
4   26–50%
5   51–75%
6   More than 75%

Q-3 Please indicate the extent to which each of the following statements is typical of your <u>unsatisfactory patient encounters</u>. (*Circle your responses*)

	Very Typical				**Not at All Typical**
	(*Circle one response for each item*)				
1 The patient was trying to manipulate me..................	1	2	3	4	5
2 The patient did not accept responsibility for his/her own dental health.....................................	1	2	3	4	5
3 The patient was telling me what to do to diagnose or treat the problem.....................................	1	2	3	4	5
4 The patient and I could not see eye to eye on the goal of the visit..	1	2	3	4	5
5 There was a lack of trust between us.........................	1	2	3	4	5

	Very Typical			**Not at All Typical**	
	(*Circle one response for each item*)				

6 The patient made inappropriate calls to me...............	1	2	3	4	5
7 The patient had a million complaints........................	1	2	3	4	5
8 The patient had not complied with the treatment I prescribed...	1	2	3	4	5
9 The patient treated me as if I were an impersonal service..	1	2	3	4	5
10 I felt depressed after seeing the patient......................	1	2	3	4	5
11 I felt that the patient didn't believe me......................	1	2	3	4	5
12 I spent more time in the visit than I wanted to..	1	2	3	4	5
13 I felt angry after seeing the patient............................	1	2	3	4	5
14 The visit was interrupted..	1	2	3	4	5
15 I couldn't get the patient to stop talking....................	1	2	3	4	5
16 I felt removed from the patient's problem.................	1	2	3	4	5
17 The patient didn't give me a clear history.................	1	2	3	4	5
18 The patient and I seemed to come from different worlds..	1	2	3	4	5
19 We just didn't hit it off..	1	2	3	4	5
20 The patient was too controlling.................................	1	2	3	4	5
21 Problems in my practice setting interfered with the visit...	1	2	3	4	5
22 The patient didn't follow my instructions..................	1	2	3	4	5

Practice Characteristics

Q-4   Below are a number of clinical problems encountered in everyday practice.
        Please indicate how you typically handle these types of problems, or how you
        would handle them if they occurred. (*Circle one response for each clinical problem*)

	Nearly always	Often	Some-times	Not often	Almost never	Never
	(Circle one response for each item)					

1 When seeing a new patient, I . . .

   a substitute panoramic radiographs
      plus bitewings for full mouth
      periapical films 1   2   3   4   5   6

   b am selective in disclosing
      information to some patients
      about their oral health 1   2   3   4   5   6

   c present all treatment options 1   2   3   4   5   6

   d try to convince the patient to
      accept the recommended treatment
      if he/she is reluctant 1   2   3   4   5   6

   e decline care if the patient rejects
      the recommended treatment plan. 1   2   3   4   5   6

2 If a perforation occurs when using
   an endo post drill in an anterior
   tooth, I . . .

If you do not perform this procedure,
check here ☐

   a tell the patient of the problem. 1   2   3   4   5   6

   b try to repair the hole myself. 1   2   3   4   5   6

   c extract the tooth as unrestorable. 1   2   3   4   5   6

   d refer to a specialist. 1   2   3   4   5   6

   e bill the patient my regular fee
      for the repair. 1   2   3   4   5   6

   f pay for the specialist repair myself. 1   2   3   4   5   6

3 When a patient requests a routine
   tooth extraction, I . . .   If you do not perform this procedure,
                                                            check here ☐

   a refuse to extract it if it is
      restorable.   1   2   3   4   5   6
   b postpone the extraction in the
      presence of swelling/infection.   1   2   3   4   5   6
   c inform the patient of a retained
      root tip following extraction.   1   2   3   4   5   6

Q-5   Below is a list of situations relating to office practice. Please indicate for each
         item the frequency of occurrence in your practice. (*Circle one response for each item*)

	Nearly always	Often	Some-times	Not often	Almost never	Never
	(Circle one response for each item)					
1 If a patient becomes dissatisfied with the esthetics of an anterior crown following cementation, the crown is remade without charge	1	2	3	4	5	6
2 If a dissatisfied patient refuses to pay his/her bill, the amount is written off	1	2	3	4	5	6
3 If a new amalgam restoration fails within the first three months, replacement is made at no cost, regardless of who is responsible	1	2	3	4	5	6
4 A dissatisfied patient who refuses to pay his/her bill is referred to peer review	1	2	3	4	5	6

Q-6   In your practice, how many operatories are fully equipped to treat patients?
         _____ operatories

Q-7   In your practice, what is the average appointment length scheduled for an adult
         prophylaxis (ADA Code 1110)?
              1   Less than 30 minutes
              2   30–45 minutes
              3   46–60 minutes

Q-8   In your practice, what is the average appointment length scheduled for a new
        patient examination (ADA Code 0110)?
        1   Less than 30 minutes
        2   30–45 minutes
        3   46–60 minutes

Q-9   During *your* most recent typical WEEK, how far in advance did you have to
        schedule your average patient for a new patient examination?
        1   One or two days
        2   Three days to a week
        3   One or two weeks
        4   More than two weeks

Q-10   Currently, how long does the average patient have to wait in the reception room
        to see the dentist AFTER the scheduled appointment time? (*Circle the number*)
        1   Less than 5 minutes
        2   About 5–15 minutes
        3   About 16–30 minutes
        4   More than 30 minutes

Q-11   Which *one* of the following *best* describes your employment status during the
        past 12 months? (*Check the one best answer for each practice. If you do not have a
        secondary practice, leave that column blank.*)

		Primary Practice	**Secondary Practice**
a	Sole proprietor (i.e., the only owner in an unincorporated dental practice)	1	1
b	Partner in a complete or limited partnership	2	2
c	Shareholder owner in an incorporated dental practice with *one or more* dentists	3	3
d	Associate in an incorporated dental practice (not a shareholder)	4	4
e	Associate in an unincorporated dental practice	5	5
f	Independent contractor (i.e., a dentist who contracts with an owner dentist to use space and equipment)	6	6
g	Other, _____ (*please specify*)	7	7

Q-12　If you are an associate in an incorporated or unincorporated dental practice (e.g., "d" or "e," above) for either your *primary* or *secondary* practice on which of the following bases do you receive remuneration? (*Circle all that apply*)

　　　1　Salary................................　　Yes　　No　　Does not apply
　　　2　Commission........................　　Yes　　No　　Does not apply

Q-13　Currently, how many hours per week do you personally see patients at chairside in your primary practice? (*Do not include treatment planning, practice management, or lab hours.*)

　　　_____ Hours

Q-14　Excluding yourself, how many *full time* (32 hours or more per week) dentists currently work in the primary clinic in which you practice?

　　　_____ Dentists

Q-15　Excluding yourself, how many *part time* (less than 32 hours per week) dentists currently work in the primary clinic in which you practice?

　　　_____ Dentists

Q-16　How many full- and part-time employees other than dentists currently work in the clinic in which you practice? *Note:* A secretary or receptionist who also provides chairside assistance at least 50% of the time should also be counted as a chairside assistant. (*Write "None" in each space, where appropriate. All blanks should be filled.*)

		Number of Employees	
		Full-time ≥ 32 hrs/wk	Part-time < 32 hrs/wk
a	Dental Hygienists	_____	_____
b	Chairside Assistants	_____	_____
c	Secretary/Receptionists	_____	_____
d	Dental Technicians	_____	_____
e	Business Managers	_____	_____

Q-17　Considering *all* dentists and *all* hygienists working in the clinic in which you practice, including yourself, how many patient visits occurred in your office during the most recent typical *week*? (*Write "none" for hygienist visits if you do not employ a hygienist.*)

　　　a　Dentist visits　　_____
　　　b　Hygienist visits　_____

Q-18   What per hour wage is your *primary* dental assistant paid?
$\underline{\hspace{3em}}$ per hour

Q-19   During a *typical* practice week, what percentage of *your* time is devoted to each of the following procedures? (*Percentages should add up to 100%*)

		Percentage of time per week
a	Diagnostic (exams, x-rays, etc.)	$\underline{\hspace{4em}}$%
b	Preventive (fluoride, prophylaxis, patient education pit & fissure sealants, etc.)	$\underline{\hspace{4em}}$%
c	Restorative (single unit restorations)	$\underline{\hspace{4em}}$%
d	Prosthodontic (fixed and removable multi-unit restorations)	$\underline{\hspace{4em}}$%
e	Endodontics	$\underline{\hspace{4em}}$%
f	Periodontics	$\underline{\hspace{4em}}$%
g	Orthodontics	$\underline{\hspace{4em}}$%
h	Treatment for TMJ	$\underline{\hspace{4em}}$%
i	Oral surgery	$\underline{\hspace{4em}}$%
j	General services (patient management, counseling, miscellaneous)	$\underline{\hspace{4em}}$%
	Total	100%

Q-20   How often do you refer patients to other practitioners for the following categories listed below?

		How often do you make referrals? (*Circle one response for each item*)			
		Never	**Occasionally**	**Often**	**Always**
a	Periodontics	1	2	3	4
b	Prosthodontics-fixed	1	2	3	4
c	Prosthodontics-removable	1	2	3	4
d	Endodontics	1	2	3	4
e	Complex extractions	1	2	3	4
f	Orthodontics	1	2	3	4
g	Medically compromised	1	2	3	4

Q-21   For what proportion of routine hygienist visits do you check the hygiene work, before dismissing the patient? (*Circle one only*)

    1   Less than 50%

    2   50–75%

    3   76–85%

    4   86–100%

    5   No hygienist employed

Q-22   Which of the following best describes your entire practice during the past 12 months?

    1 Provided care to all who requested appointments but the practice was overworked

    2 Provided care to all who requested appointments and the practice was not overworked

    3 Not busy enough—the practice could have treated more patients

Q-23   Please review the dental procedures and their ADA Procedure codes in the following list, then indicate whether or not you perform them in your practice. *Never* indicates you have never performed the procedure in your practice; *Discontinued* means you have stopped performing the procedure; and *Now* implies you presently perform the procedure, even if infrequently. (*Circle one response for each procedure*)

			Never	**Discontinued**	**Now**
			(*Circle one response for each item*)		
a	02952	Cast post & core restoration in addition to crown	1	2	3
b	03330	Root canal therapy—3 canals	1	2	3
c	03410–03430	Surgical endodontia (apicoectomy)	1	2	3
d	04250–04260	Periodontic surgery—mucogingival and/or osseous	1	2	3
e	06030–06050	Surgery for implants	1	2	3
f	06210–06792	Fixed prosthodontics involving replacement of more than one missing tooth	1	2	3

			Never	**Discontinued**	**Now**
g	07240	Surgical extraction of impacted tooth—completely bony	1	2	3
h	08460	Comprehensive orthodontic treatment—transitional dentition: Class I	1	2	3
i	85660	Comprehensive orthodontic treatment—permanent dentition	1	2	3
j	09240	Intravenous sedation	1	2	3
k	09940	Occlusal guards for treatment of TMJ problems	1	2	3

Q-24   Below is a list of items relating to office practice. Please indicate for each item the frequency of occurrence in your practice. If you do not perform the procedure corresponding to the statement then answer "NA." (*Circle one response for each item*)

	Nearly always	**Often**	**Some-times**	**Not often**	**Almost never**	**Never**	**NA**
	(Circle one response for each item)						
1 Blood pressure cuff used at new patient examination	1	2	3	4	5	6	NA
2 When pulp vitality tests are performed, values are recorded in patient's chart	1	2	3	4	5	6	NA
3 Patient receives reminder to take prophylactic antibiotic coverage, when required	1	2	3	4	5	6	NA
4 Written informed consent obtained for treatment	1	2	3	4	5	6	NA
5 *Intra*-operative x-rays taken during endodontic procedures	1	2	3	4	5	6	NA
6 *Post*-operative x-rays taken immediately following endo case completion	1	2	3	4	5	6	NA
7 Follow-up telephone calls made to patients following surgical procedures	1	2	3	4	5	6	NA
8 Study models taken prior to fixed prosthetic procedures	1	2	3	4	5	6	NA
9 Rubber dams used for restorative procedures	1	2	3	4	5	6	NA

| 10 | Throat packs used during extractions | 1 | 2 | 3 | 4 | 5 | 6 | NA |
| 11 | High speed handpieces autoclaved following each treatment visit | 1 | 2 | 3 | 4 | 5 | 6 | NA |

Q-25   Below is a list of items relating to office policies and equipment. Please indicate for each item whether or not the statement is true (i.e., Yes or No) for your practice.

Staff

		Yes	No
1	All staff received Hepatitis-B vaccine series	1	2
2	Written job descriptions exist for auxiliary personnel	1	2
3	Paid employee benefits include:		
	Vacations	1	2
	Sick leave	1	2
	Medical insurance	1	2
	Continuing dental education	1	2

Practice

		Yes	No
4	An established schedule exists for medical history updates	1	2
5	Medical history includes sensitivity to rubber products	1	2
6	Frequent CPR training is required for *all* staff	1	2
7	An emergency phone number is posted	1	2
8	Emergency oxygen is available in the practice	1	2

Q-26   Please indicate the percent of *new patients* in your practice who, prior to initiation of treatment:

a	Receive full mouth periodontal probing	___%
b	Receive full mouth periapical radiographs	___%
c	Have a formal dental history taken	___%
d	Receive a TMJ examination	___%
e	Receive a head and neck examination	___%
f	Receive a separate consultation visit for treatment planning	___%
g	Receive a written treatment plan	___%
h	Receive an outside medical consultation	___%

Practice Finances

Because this is a national survey, practice finances will vary for respondents in different communities. This section concerns the clinic in which *you* practice.

Q-27   Excluding diagnostic and preventive services, how many of your patients know how much their out of pocket dental expenses will be before treatment begins?
   1   Nearly all patients
   2   Most patients
   3   About half the patients
   4   Some patients
   5   Only a few patients, if any

Q-28   Approximately what percentage of patients who visited your practice in 1991 were (*Percentages should add up to 100%*):
   a   Covered by a private fee for service insurance program that pays or partially pays for their dental care?   ____%
   b   Covered by a capitation insurance program that pays or partially pays for their dental care?   ____%
   c   Covered by a government public assistance program that pays or partially pays for their dental care?   ____%
   d   Not covered by an insurance program?   ____%

Q-29   Please indicate the usual and customary fee currently charged for each of the following procedures at the primary clinic in which you practice. Do not indicate capitation fees or insurance co-payments. For procedures that are not performed, write in "NA," or if the procedure is performed free of charge, write in a zero.

		ADA Code	
a	Initial oral examination (excluding radiographs)	(00110)	$_____
b	Four bitewing radiographs	(00274)	$_____
c	3-surface permanent amalgam	(02160)	$_____
d	Gold crown (full cast), single restoration	(02790)	$_____
e	Cast post and core	(02952)	$_____
f	Anterior root canal therapy (1 canal)	(03310)	$_____
g	Molar root canal therapy (3 canal)	(03330)	$_____
h	Surgical endodontia (apicoectomy anterior tooth)	(03410)	$_____
i	Periodontal curettage and root planing (per quadrant)	(04220)	$_____
j	Periodontic osseous surgery (per quadrant)	(04260)	$_____

k	Complete upper denture	(05110) $_____
l	Endosseous implant surgery	(06030) $_____
m	Fixed prosthodontics, per unit—high noble metal	(06700) $_____
n	Simple extraction, single tooth	(07110) $_____
o	Surgical extraction of impacted tooth, fully bony	(07240) $_____

Malpractice Insurance

Before answering the first 4 questions in this section please review your current malpractice policy where you will find the answers.

Q-30   What type of malpractice insurance coverage do you *presently* carry?
1   Occurrence
2   Claims made
3   None within the past 1–4 years (Skip to Q-35)
4   None within the past 5 years (Skip to Q-53)

Q-31   Who writes your current malpractice insurance coverage? (e.g., Safeco, CNA, Farmers)

_____   _____
Insurance Company   Insurance Broker (Agent)

Q-32   What are the policy limits of your current malpractice coverage? (*Circle one response in each column*)

	PER INCIDENT		PER YEAR (aggregate)
1	$100,000	1	$200,000
2	$200,000	2	$300,000
3	$300,000	3	$600,000
4	$400,000	4	$1,000,000
5	$500,000	5	$1,500,000
6	$1,000,000	6	$2,000,000
7	$2,000,000 or more	7	$3,000,000 or more

Q-33   Does your malpractice policy provide premium adjustments based upon claims experience or individual behavior? (*Circle all that apply*)
1   No
2   Yes, surcharge for past claims
3   Yes, discount for claims-free experience
4   Yes, discount for participation in specific loss prevention programs
5   Don't know

Q-34 For your most recent policy period what premium did you pay for malpractice coverage?

    1   Less than $1,000

    2   $1,000–$1,499

    3   $1,500–$1,999

    4   $2,000–$2,499

    5   $2,500–$2,999

    6   More than $3,000

Q-35 How many times over the past five years have you reported to your agent, your broker, or your insurance carrier a potential or an actual complaint against you, even if no formal claim was ever filed, or no attorney was involved?

    1   Never (Skip to Q-53)

    2   Once

    3   Twice   (Proceed to Q-36)

    4   Three or more times

Most Recent Incident Report

Q-36 When did you report your most recent incident?

    1   During 1992   4   During 1988 or 1989

    2   During 1991   5   Before 1988

    3   During 1990

Q-37 Did this most recent incident report result in having a claim filed against you with your insurance company?

    1   Yes

    2   No (Skip to Q-44)

Q-38 Which area of dentistry was involved?

    1   Oral surgery   4   Periodontics

    2   Endodontic post   5   Endodontics

    3   Fixed prosthetics   6   Other: _____

Q-39   Did the allegations involve

		Yes	No
1	Diagnosis	1	2
2	Treatment process/outcome	1	2
3	Therapeutic drugs	1	2
4	Lack of informed consent	1	2
5	Failure to refer/consult	1	2
6	Lack of follow-up treatment	1	2
7	Other: (*Please specify*) _____	1	2

Q-40   Has this insurance claim been finally resolved, with or without payment to the patient?

1   Yes
2   No   ⎤ (Skip to Q-42)
3   Don't know ⎦

Q-41   What dollar amount, if any, was paid by the insurance company to the patient?
$_____ (*If nothing was paid, write in "none"*)

Q-42   Did you sign an "agreement to settle" statement requested by your insurance carrier?

1   Yes
2   No

Q-43   Please write in the name of the insurance company or companies involved in this claim.

a. _____   b. _____

Second Most Recent Incident Report

Q-44   Did you make a second, but less recent incident report?

1   Yes
2   No (Skip to Q-53)

Q-45   When did this occur?

1   During 1992   4   During 1988 or 1989
2   During 1991   5   Before 1988
3   During 1990

Q-46 Did this second most recent incident report result in having a claim filed against you with your insurance company?

1 Yes

2 No (Skip to Q-53)

Q-47 Which area of dentistry was involved?

1 Oral surgery   4 Periodontics

2 Endodontic post   5 Endodontics

3 Fixed prosthetics   6 Other: _____

Q-48 Did the allegations involve

	Yes	No
1 Diagnosis	1	2
2 Treatment process/outcome	1	2
3 Therapeutic drugs	1	2
4 Lack of informed consent	1	2
5 Failure to refer/consult	1	2
6 Lack of follow-up treatment	1	2
7 Other: (*Please specify*) _____	1	2

Q-49 Has this insurance claim been finally resolved, with or without payment to the patient?

1 Yes

2 No   ⎤ (Skip to Q-51)

3 Don't know ⎦

Q-50 What amount, if any, was paid by the insurance company to the patient?

$_____ (*If nothing was paid, write in "none"*)

Q-51 Did you sign an "agreement to settle" statement requested by your insurance carrier?

1 Yes

2 No

Q-52 Please write in the name of the insurance company or companies involved in this claim.

a. _____   b. _____

Demographics

Finally, we would like to ask a few questions about yourself for statistical purposes. This section will help us determine how representative the dentists are who complete this questionnaire.

Q-53   How old were you on your last birthday?
____ years old

Q-54   What is your gender?
1 Male
2 Female

Q-55   Which of the following best describes your racial or ethnic identification?
1 African American
2 Hispanic
3 White (Caucasian)
4 Native American (American Indian, Aleut or Eskimo)
5 Asian or Pacific Islander
6 Other: (*please specify*)

Q-56   At how many dental office locations do you practice?
____ offices

Q-57   How many years have you been practicing dentistry at your primary practice location?
____ years

Q-58   Please give the Zip code and county of your primary practice.
Zip code   _____
County   _____

Q-59   From which Dental School did you receive your principal dental degree?
School: _____
State: _____
Country: _____
Year of Graduation: _____

CONTINUE   ⟶

Q-60   Have you completed any clock hours of continuing education during the past
        12 months?
        1   Yes
        2   No (Go to back cover)

Q-61   For the past 12 month period please estimate *the number of clock hours* of
        continuing education you accumulated in *each* of the following areas. (*Fill in the
        number of hours in each space.*)

a ___ Practice Management   f ___ Treatment Planning
b ___ Oral Medicine/Pathology   g ___ Pedodontics
c ___ Infection Control   h ___ Malpractice
d ___ Radiology   i ___ TMJ
e ___ Medical Emergencies   j ___ Implants (Surgical or
                                                Prosthetic)

Periodontics   Orthodontics
k ___ Non Surgical Therapy   n ___ Minor Tooth Movement
l ___ Mucogingival Surgery   o ___ Interceptive Orthodontics
m ___ Osseous Surgery   p ___ Comprehensive Orthodontics

Restorative Dentistry   Endodontics
q ___ Cast Post & Core   u ___ Molar Root Canal Therapy
r ___ Prefabricated Post & Core   v ___ Surgical Endodontia
s ___ Cosmetic/esthetic Dentistry   w ___ Special Problems in
t ___ Dental Materials   Endodontics

Removable Prosthetics   Anesthesia
x ___ Full Dentures   z ___ Local Anesthesia
y ___ Partial Dentures   aa ___ Nitrous oxide
                                         bb ___ IV Sedation

Fixed Prosthetics   Exodontia
cc ___ Resin Bonded Bridges   ff ___ Simple Extractions
        (e.g. Maryland Bridge)   gg ___ Bony Impactions
dd ___ Long Span Bridges (>3 units)
ee ___ Other, (*please specify*) _____

Your Opinion

What do you believe to be the greatest malpractice problem facing dentists today?

<hr />

Thank you for your participation. If you wish a copy of the results of this study, please provide your name and address on the *back side* of the return envelope and write "copy of results requested."

Please return your completed questionnaire in the enclosed envelope to:

National Dental Malpractice Study
Social and Economic Sciences Research Center
Washington State University
Pullman, WA 99164-4014

National Dental Malpractice Survey
Data Report (#93–10): By SESRC—April, 1993
Survey Instruments—Advance Letter

November 5, 1992

Dr. First Name Last Name
Street
City, State Zip

Dear Dr. Last Name:

Recent years have seen a crisis in the availability and cost of dental malpractice insurance. Even though the crisis has leveled off for the time being malpractice claims and the sizes of awards are on the rise because of the increasing complexities of modern dentistry. Our research team at the University of Washington has been federally funded by the National Institutes of Health to examine the problem. This is the first dental malpractice study of its kind and the results may ultimately influence the availability and cost of malpractice insurance.

With the assistance of the American Dental Association we are currently mailing a questionnaire to a representative sample of practicing general dentists throughout the U.S. in order to learn more about their patient experiences during the past several years. Your practice was selected from the ADA's member and non-member directory. Approximately five percent of clinicians throughout the country are being asked to participate. The questionnaire should be arriving in about a week.

In order that the results of this study be truly representative of the experiences of general dentists in the country it is important that all individuals in the sample return their questionnaire, *including those who have never had a malpractice claim filed against them.* If you have questions about the study I will be happy to talk to you. Please call me collect at (206) 543–2034, between 8 a.m. and 5 p.m. on the West Coast.

I look forward to your participation in this important research topic.

Sincerely yours,

Louis Fiset, DDS
Research Associate Professor

National Dental Malpractice Survey
Data Report (#93–10): By SESRC—April, 1993
Survey Instruments—Cover Letter

November 12, 1992

Dr. First Name Last Name
Street
City, State Zip

Dear Dr. Last Name:

Last week I wrote to you about our federally funded nationwide survey of dentists' experiences with their patients. This survey, entitled *National Dental Malpractice Survey,* is enclosed.

Recent years have seen a crisis in the availability and cost of dental malpractice insurance. Claims have grown in number and award sizes continue to rise. Despite the temporary stability in insurance premiums the future is uncertain because little is known about the determinants of malpractice problems in dentistry. No nationwide study of dental malpractice has ever been undertaken until now, which is being made possible by funding from the National Institutes of Health.

Your practice is one of a small number nationwide being asked to provide information about their malpractice experiences during the past five years. With the assistance of the American Dental Association your name was drawn in a random sampling of practicing non-specialists throughout the United States. In order that the results truly represent the experience of general dentists it is important that each questionnaire be completed and returned. *We are interested in your response regardless of whether you have ever had a malpractice claim against you.*

You may be assured of complete confidentiality. The questionnaire has an identification number for mailing purposes only. This is so that we may check your name off the mailing list when it is returned. Your name will never be placed on the questionnaire. While your participation is voluntary, we hope you will complete and return the questionnaire so that we can know about your experiences with patients.

We will send you a summary of results if you write, "Copy of results requested" on the back of the return envelope and print your name and address below it. Please *do not* put this information on the questionnaire, itself. I am also enclosing a token of appreciation for taking the time to complete the survey.

I will be happy to answer any questions you might have. Please call collect, (206) 543–2034, between 8 a.m. and 5 p.m. on the West Coast.

Thank you for your assistance

Sincerely yours,

Louis Fiset, DDS
Research Associate Professor

National Dental Malpractice Survey
Data Report —(#93–10): By SESRC—April, 1993
Survey Instruments—Postcard

November 23, 1992

Last week I mailed you a questionnaire requesting information about your dental experiences
with patients. If you have already completed and returned the survey please accept our sincere
thanks. If not, we ask that you do so today.

   We are especially grateful for your help. The results of this study will help influence the
future availability and cost of dental malpractice insurance.

   Because it has been sent to only a small, but representative, sample of U.S. non-specialist
clinicians, it is extremely important that yours also be included in the study if the results are to
accurately represent the experiences of general dentists. *We are interested in your response even if you
have never had a malpractice claim against you.*

   If by some chance you did not receive the questionnaire, or it was misplaced, please call me
collect at (206) 543–2034 between 8 a.m. and 5 p.m. on the West Coast, and I will get another
one in the mail to you right away.

Sincerely,

Louis Fiset, DDS
Research Associate Professor

National Dental Malpractice Survey
Data Report (#93–10): By SESRC—April, 1993
Survey Instruments—Second Follow-Up

December 3, 1992

Dr. First Name Last Name
Street
City, State Zip

Dear Dr. Last Name:

About three weeks ago I wrote to you seeking information about your dental malpractice experience. As of today we have not yet received your completed questionnaire.

The National Institutes of Health funded this study, with the cooperation of the American Dental Association, because of the future uncertainty in the availability and cost of dental malpractice insurance. This study is the first of its kind to examine malpractice in dentistry, nationwide.

I am writing to you again because of the significance each questionnaire has to the usefulness of this study. *We are interested in your response even if you have never had a malpractice claim brought against you.* Your name was drawn through a specific sampling process in which every non-specialist clinical practice in the United States had an equal chance of being selected. Less than five percent of practicing dentists are being asked to complete this questionnaire. In order that the results be truly representative of the experiences of all general dentists it is essential that each person in the sample return his or her questionnaire.

All the information you provide will remain strictly confidential. Please do not write your name or provide any other identifying information anywhere on the questionnaire booklet. Your participation is voluntary. However, because of the importance each individual has to the success of the study we hope that you will complete and return this questionnaire.

In the event that your questionnaire has been misplaced, a replacement is enclosed.

Your cooperation is greatly appreciated.

Cordially,

Louis Fiset, DDS
Research Associate Professor

National Dental Malpractice Survey
Data Report (#93–10): By SESRC—April, 1993
Survey Instruments—Third Follow-Up

December 31, 1992

Dr. First Name Last Name
Street
City, State Zip

Dear Dr. Last Name:

I am writing you about our federally funded, nationwide study of dentists' malpractice experiences. We have not yet received your completed questionnaire.

The large number of questionnaires returned is very encouraging. But whether we will be able to describe accurately the malpractice experiences of dentists in the U.S. depends upon you and the others who have not yet responded. This is because our past experiences suggest that those who have not yet sent in their questionnaire may have had different experiences than those who have.

This research is the first nationwide study of dental malpractice ever to be conducted. The results will be important to all general dentists and clinicians who face an uncertain future fueled by increasing claims and sizes of awards. It is for these reasons that I am sending this by certified mail to ensure delivery.

All information you provide will be kept strictly confidential. Although your participation is voluntary, I urge you to complete and return the questionnaire as quickly as possible. Your response is important to the success of this study. In case our other correspondence did not reach you I am enclosing a replacement questionnaire.

I will be happy to send you a copy of the results when they become available. Simply put your name, address, and "Copy of results requested" on the back of the return envelope.

Your contribution to the study is greatly appreciated.

Sincerely,

Louis Fiset, DDS
Research Associate Professor

SELECTED SOURCES
ON HEALTH SURVEYS

Journals such as the *American Journal of Epidemiology*, the *American Journal of Public Health*, the *Journal of Health and Social Behavior*, and *Medical Care* routinely publish research articles based on data collected from health surveys. A number of journals published in the United States and elsewhere also report studies of methodological research on surveys in general and health surveys in particular. These include the *International Journal of Public Opinion Research*, the *Journal of the American Statistical Association*, the *Journal of Marketing Research*, the *Journal of Official Statistics*, *Public Opinion Quarterly*, and *Survey Methodology*.

The advent of indexes of periodical literature in a variety of areas and the computerization of databases of this literature have greatly facilitated researchers' access to previous studies in these areas. These databases are generally available at research and university libraries through online access. The databases produced by the National Library of Medicine (NLM) are based on indexes to literature in medicine and the health professions (see the selected list that follows). They are a particularly valuable source of bibliographical information on health survey methods and applications. MEDLINE, for example, is a widely used database for identifying relevant biomedical literature. Terms that might be used in combination with other descriptors for identifying health-related surveys in MEDLINE include *data collection, dental health surveys, diet surveys, health surveys, interviews, questionnaires,* and *sampling studies.* Databases in related fields (nursing and allied health, education, psychology, and sociology) are also useful sources of information on methodological research or applications of surveys on related topics. Databases such as CRISP and HSRProj provide inventories of funded research projects for which published results are not yet available.

The information highway that has been opened up through the Internet provides a wide network of places to search for information on health surveys. World Wide Web addresses for selected agencies or sources are provided in this resource. Selected databases provide the full text of the survey questionnaires and extensive methodological reports on survey procedures and results.

The American Statistical Association, the Agency for Healthcare Research and Quality, the National Center for Health Statistics, and the U.S. Bureau of the Census also periodically hold conferences or proceedings devoted to methodological issues in the design and conduct of surveys. Many of the papers or presentations at those conferences report on studies of techniques developed and tested in health surveys, which can be used to guide decision making about the utility of these or related approaches. The U.S. Office of Management and Budget also periodically publishes instructive papers on survey methodology, with particular reference to federally sponsored surveys, in its Statistical Policy Working Paper Series.

University-based and other private and public data archives contain extensive data sets from national, state, and local health surveys. A selected list of these data archives also appears at the end of this resource. The Area Resource File, compiled by the Bureau of Health Professions in the U.S. Department of Health Resources and Services Administration, is a rich source of information on health care services and resources from surveys for each county in the United States. CDC WONDER, a menu-driven online program available from the Centers for Disease Control and Prevention (CDC), provides access to CDC reports and data sets. A number of schools of public health also serve as repositories for National Center for Health Statistics data disks and tapes. Potential users may request catalogues of the data sets available in these or other national or regional archives or consult university-based survey research organizations in their areas about health surveys that they have conducted.

Selected Sources on Health Surveys

Journals

Studies Using Health Surveys

American Journal of Clinical Nutrition

American Journal of Epidemiology

American Journal of Public Health

Annual Review of Public Health

Epidemiologic Reviews

Evaluation and the Health Professions

Health Affairs

Health Care Financing Review

Health Care Management Review

Health Education Quarterly

Health Marketing Quarterly

Health Services Research

Hospitals

Inquiry

International Journal of Epidemiology

International Journal of Health Services

Journal of Chronic Diseases

Journal of Community Health

Journal of Epidemiology and Community Health

Journal of Health Administration Education

Journal of Health Care Marketing

Journal of Health Politics, Policy, and Law

Journal of Health and Social Behavior

Journal of Public Health Policy

Medical Care

Medical Care Research and Review

Milbank Memorial Fund Quarterly

New England Journal of Medicine

Nursing Research

Public Health Nursing

Public Health Reports

Quality Review Bulletin

Social Science and Medicine

World Health Statistics Quarterly

Methodological Studies on Surveys

Advances in Consumer Research

Annual Review of Sociology

Applied Cognitive Psychology

Behavior Research Methods, Instruments, and Computers

Evaluation Review

International Journal of Public Opinion Research

Journal of the American Statistical Association

Journal of Economic and Social Measurement

Journal of Marketing Research

Journal of Official Statistics

Public Opinion Quarterly

Quality and Quantity

Social Science Computer Review

Sociological Methods and Research

Survey Methodology

Computerized Bibliographic Databases

Alcohol Studies Database

CINAHL (Cumulative Index to Nursing and Allied Health Literature)

Cochrane Library of The Cochrane Collaboration

CRISP (Computer Retrieval of Information on Scientific Projects)

ERIC (Educational Resources Information Center)

ETOH (Alcohol and Alcohol Problems Science Database)

HaPI (Health and Psychosocial Instruments)

HSSR (Health Services and Sciences Research Resources)

HSTAT (Health Services/Technology Assessment Text)

HSRProj (Health Services Research Projects in Progress)

MEDLINE/PubMed (biomedical journal literature from
MEDLINE/PubMed, as well as AIDS, bioethics, cancer, complementary

health, dental journals, nursing journals, selected meeting abstracts, and systematic reviews)

Mental Measurements Yearbook

OSHLINE with NIOSHTIC Database (international coverage of documents on occupational health and safety, as well as related fields)

PapersFirst

POPLINE (POPulation information onLINE)

Population Index—on the Web

ProceedingsFirst

PsycARTICLES

PsycINFO (PSYChological literature INFOrmation database)

Web of Science

WorldCat

Major Government Information Sources

Agency for Healthcare Research and Quality (http://www.ahrq.gov/)

Centers for Disease Control and Prevention (http://www.cdc.gov/)

USA Services: the "front door" to the U.S. government (http://www.info.gov/)

National Center for Health Statistics (http://www.cdc.gov/nchs/)

National Institutes of Health (http://www.nih.gov/)

National Library of Medicine (http://www.nlm.nih.gov/)

United Nations Children's Fund (http://www.unicef.org/)

U.S. Department of Health and Human Services (http://www.hhs.gov/)

World Health Organization (http://www.who.int/en/)

Conference Proceedings

American Statistical Association

  Section on Social Statistics

  Section on Survey Research Methods

Agency for Healthcare Research and Quality (AHRQ) and National Center for Health Statistics (NCHS)

  Conferences on Health Survey Research Methods

National Center for Health Statistics

Conferences on Public Health Records and Statistics

U.S. Bureau of the Census

Annual Research Conferences

Data Archives

Agency for Healthcare Research and Quality
Office of Communications and Knowledge Transfer
540 Gaither Road, Suite 2000
Rockville, MD 20850
(301)427-1364
http://www.ahrq.gov/data/

CDC WONDER
Centers for Disease Control and Prevention
1600 Clifton Road
Atlanta, GA 30333
(888)496-8347
http://wonder.cdc.gov/wonder/help/main.html#DataSets

Inter-University Consortium for Political and Social Research
Institute for Social Research
University of Michigan
P.O. Box 1248
Ann Arbor, MI 48106-1248
(734)647-5000
http://www.icpsr.umich.edu/index.html

Lou Harris Data Center (and) Social Science Data Library
Odum Institute for Research in Social Science
Manning Hall, CB#3355
University of North Carolina at Chapel Hill
Chapel Hill, NC 27599-3355
(919)962-3061
http://www2.irss.unc.edu/irss/dataservices/dataservicesindex.asp

Medical Outcomes Trust
235 Wyman Street, Suite 130
Waltham, MA 02451
(781)890-4884
http://www.outcomes-trust.org/instruments.htm

National Center for Health Statistics
3311 Toledo Road
Hyattsville, MD 20782
(301)458-4000
1-(866)441-NCHS
http://www.cdc.gov/nchs/datawh/ftpserv/ftpdata/ftpdata.htm

National Institute on Drug Abuse
National Institutes of Health
6001 Executive Boulevard, Room 5213
Bethesda, MD 20892-9561
Data archives are available through the Substance Abuse and Mental Health Data
Archives managed by the Inter-University Consortium for Political and Social Re-
search at the University of Michigan.
http://www.icpsr.umich.edu/SAMHDA/index.html

National Opinion Research Center
University of Chicago
1155 East Sixtieth Street
Chicago, IL 60637
(773)256-6000
http://www.norc.uchicago.edu/

National Technical Information Service
U.S. Department of Commerce
5285 Port Royal Road
Springfield, VA 22161
(703)605-6000
http://www.ntis.gov/

RAND Corporation
Computer Services Department Data Facility
1776 Main Street
P.O. Box 2138
Santa Monica, CA 90407-2138
(310)393-0411
http://www.rand.org/services/databases.html

Roper Center for Public Opinion Research
341 Mansfield Road, Unit 1164
University of Connecticut
Storrs, CT 06269-1164
(860)486-4440
http://www.ropercenter.uconn.edu/

Substance Abuse and Mental Health Services Administration,
Office of Applied Studies
Data archives are available through the Substance Abuse and Mental Health Data
Archives managed by the Inter-University Consortium for Political and Social Re-
search at the University of Michigan.
http://www.icpsr.umich.edu/SAMHDA/index.html

UNICEF—Multiple Indicator Cluster Surveys
3 United Nations Plaza
New York, NY 10017
(212)326-7243
http://www.childinfo.org/mics/

UCLA Center for Health Policy Research
California Health Interview Survey
10911 Weyburn Avenue, Suite 300
Los Angeles, CA 90024
(310)794-0925
http://www.chis.ucla.edu/default.asp

University of Michigan
Gerald R. Ford School of Public Policy—Poverty Research Centers
1015 East Huron Street
Ann Arbor, MI 48104-1689
(734)615-4326
http://www.fordschool.umich.edu/research/poverty/research_proj.html

U.S. Census Bureau
4700 Silver Hill Road
Washington DC 20233-0001
(301)763-INFO (4636)
http://www.census.gov/acs/www/Products/PUMS/index.htm (data from the
American Community Survey)
http://www.census.gov/main/www/cen2000.html (Census 2000)

U.S. National Archives and Records Administration
Electronic and Special Media Records Services Division
National Archives at College Park
8601 Adelphi Road, Room 5320
College Park, MD 20740-6001
(301)837-0470
http://www.archives.gov/research_room/center_for_electronic_records/info_for_
researchers.html

SELECTED EXAMPLES
OF HEALTH SURVEYS

Selected examples of international, national, and state surveys are highlighted here and in Table E.1. A fuller description of the surveys and related informational sources on the studies discussed are also provided in Table E.1. The surveys presented are intended to be illustrative, but obviously not fully encompassing, of the multitude of health surveys conducted across countries, states, or localities or with special target populations or subgroups. The classification of topics addressed in the studies is based on Figure 1.1.

International

The World Health Organization (WHO) has had a major role in encouraging cross-national comparative surveys in both developed and Third World countries. It and other international health agencies (such as UNICEF) have designed standardized survey design and sampling methodologies to make it easier to conduct such studies. WHO has also encouraged nations throughout the world to develop their own national health survey capacities. Many developing and developed countries, such as Canada, Great Britain, and Switzerland, have conducted their own surveys to measure their populations' health and health care practices. Normal problems of data comparability, collection, and quality in health surveys become even more of an issue in trying to carry out surveys in developing countries or in comparing data from countries with widely varying political, cultural, social, economic, and physical environments.

National: United States

The Agency for Healthcare Research and Quality, formerly the Agency for Health Care Policy and Research, has funded a number of surveys on the health care utilization and expenditures of the American public. AHCPR conducted the large-scale National Medical Care Expenditure Survey (NMCES) in 1977 and initiated an even more comprehensive study that oversampled a number of policy-relevant subgroups of interest (the poor, elderly, disabled, and others) in the 1987 National Medical Expenditure Survey (NMES). The Medical Expenditure Panel Survey (MEPS), launched in 1996, was designed to gather data on the health care coverage and expenditures of the U.S. population that could be used directly in formulating health policy in this area. The AHCPR HIV Cost and Services Utilization Study (HCSUS) provided national estimates on the utilization and costs of care for persons with HIV/AIDS in particular.

The growth of the managed care industry in health care has been accompanied by a growing interest in finding out from consumers what they want and how satisfied they are with the care they receive. Patient surveys are an important component of the resultant report cards issued on plan performance. The Consumer Assessment of Health Plans Study (CAHPS) provides a protocol for plans to use in eliciting and comparing participants' evaluation of the plans in which they are enrolled.

The American Hospital Association and the American Medical Association routinely gather information on U.S. hospitals and physicians, respectively. Similarly, professional associations of physician specialty groups, dentists, nurses, and so on may periodically survey their members to gather a variety of demographic and practice data.

The Current Population Survey (CPS), a monthly survey of approximately sixty thousand households conducted by the U.S. Bureau of the Census for the Bureau of Labor Statistics, provides longitudinal data on health insurance coverage, disability, and utilization. The CPS has been particularly important in monitoring trends in health insurance coverage in the United States.

The National Center for Health Statistics (NCHS) is the major health survey data-gathering agency of the U.S. government. It conducts its National Health Interview Survey continuously to gather (1) a core set of data on the health status and health care utilization of the American people each year and (2) supplementary information on a variable set of topics (such as disability, smoking behavior, vitamin use, exercise patterns, and knowledge and attitudes regarding HIV/AIDS).

The National Immunization Survey (NIS) is a joint project of NCHS and the Centers for Disease Control and Prevention National Immunization Program to gather data on the immunization coverage of children nineteen months to thirty-five months of age. The National Health and Nutrition Examination Survey (NHANES) program of NCHS and the Hispanic NHANES (HHANES) study of Hispanics in selected states collect direct clinical examination and laboratory data on study participants.

The NCHS National Employer Health Insurance Survey, launched in 1994, is a national survey of businesses in both the private and public sectors regarding employer provision of health insurance and spending for health care.

In the early 1990s, four NCHS record-based surveys (the National Hospital Discharge Survey, National Ambulatory Medical Care Survey, National Nursing Home Survey, and National Health Provider Inventory) were merged and expanded into one integrated survey of health care providers: the National Health Care Survey (NHCS). In addition, three new surveys were added and incorporated into the NHCS: the National Survey of Ambulatory Surgery, the National Hospital Ambulatory Medical Care Survey, and the National Home and Hospice Care Survey. This series of NHCS surveys gathers data on the characteristics of the patients seen and services provided in the respective health care settings.

The Centers for Medicare and Medicaid Services sponsors the Medicare Current Beneficiary Survey (MCBS), which gathers data on health care utilization and expenditures from a representative panel of Medicare enrollees.

As documented in Resource D and throughout the rest of this book, a number of federal agencies periodically collect survey data or sponsor surveys on health-related topics. These include the Bureau of Labor Statistics, the Centers for Disease Control and Prevention, the Census Bureau, the National Cancer Institute, the National Institute of Mental Health, the National Institute on Drug Abuse, the Social Security Administration, and the Veterans Administration, among others.

In addition, the Robert Wood Johnson Foundation, the Commonwealth Fund, the Kaiser Family Foundation, and other private philanthropies have sponsored national or statewide surveys dealing with various aspects of health and health care system performance. Concerns with the growing numbers of uninsured in many states, as well as the dominance of managed care arrangements in both the private and public sectors, have given rise to an array of studies to assess the impact of these emerging trends and innovations, such as the Center for Studying Health System Change project, the Commonwealth Fund Health Care Quality Survey, and the Urban Institute Survey of America's Families survey.

States: United States

Since 1981, the Centers for Disease Control and Prevention have sponsored Behavioral Risk Factor Surveys, using telephone interview designs in almost all the states and the District of Columbia, to gather information on residents' health practices that could put them at risk of developing serious illness (such as obesity, lack of exercise, uncontrolled hypertension, smoking, heavy drinking).

The State Health Access Data Assistance Center sponsors the Coordinated State Coverage Survey (CSCS), which helps states in monitoring insurance coverage status and related access statewide and for selected subgroups. The California Health Interview Survey, used as an example throughout this book, represents a major commitment to examining these issues across the diverse racial/ethnic subgroups and localities in California.

TABLE E.1. SELECTED EXAMPLES OF HEALTH SURVEYS.

Study, Years (References)	Topics	Research Design	Population/Samples	Data Collection
International				
World Health Organization				
• World Health Survey (WHS), 2002 and ongoing (WHO, n.d.), http://www3.who.int/whs/	Health care system Population Health status Utilization Expenditures	Cross-sectional, group comparison	Nationally representative household-based sample of adult population in participating countries	Personal interviews, telephone interviews
• Global School-Based Student Health Survey (GSHS), 2003 and ongoing (WHO, 2005), http://www.who.int/school_youth_health/assessment/gshs/en/	Population Health status Utilization	Cross-sectional, group comparison	Nationally representative school-based sample of 13- to 15-year-olds in participating countries	Self-administered questionnaires
• WHO Multicountry Survey on Health and Responsiveness, 2000–2001 (WHO, 2001, November 30), http://www3.who.int/whs/P/gpediscpaper37.pdf	Health care system Population Health status Utilization Expenditures	Cross-sectional, group comparison	Nationally representative household-based sample of adult population in participating countries	Personal interviews (90 minutes, 30 minutes), telephone interviews, mail questionnaires
United Nations International Children's Education Fund (UNICEF)	Environment Population Health status Utilization	Cross-sectional, group comparison	Nationally representative household-based sample of mothers and children in participating countries	Personal interviews
• Multiple Indicator Cluster Survey (MICS), 1995, 2000, 2005 (UNICEF, n.d.), http://www.childinfo.org/mics/				
Binational				
• Joint Canada/United States Survey of Health, 2002–2003 (Statistics Canada, 2003), http://www.cdc.gov/nchs/data/nhis/jcush_analyticalreport.pdf	Population Health status Utilization	Cross-sectional, group comparison	Nationally representative household-based sample of adults residing in the United States and Canada residing in households with a telephone (i.e., landline)	Telephone interviews
National—United States				
Agency for Healthcare Research and Quality				
• HIV Cost and Services Utilization Study, 1994–2000 (AHRQ, 1998, December), http://www.ahrq.gov/data/hcsus.htm	Population Health status Utilization Expenditures	Cross-sectional	Nationally representative sample of persons in care for HIV-infection	Personal interviews; clinical exams; medical, cost, and pharmaceutical records

Source	Focus	Design	Sample	Data Collection
• Medical Expenditure Panel Survey (MEPS), Household Component, 1996–present (AHRQ, n.d.-c), http://www.meps.ahrq.gov/	Health care system Population Health status Utilization Expenditures	Longitudinal—panel	Nationally representative sample of civilian, household-based population	Personal interviews
• Consumer Assessment of Health Plans, (Health Plan CAHPS), 1997–present (AHRQ, n.d.-b), http://www.ahrq.gov/qual/cahpsix.htm	Health care system Population Health status Utilization	Cross-sectional, group comparison	Samples of individuals enrolled in health plans, public and private	Telephone interviews, mail questionnaires, combination of telephone and mail
American Hospital Association • Annual Survey of Hospitals, 1946–present (AHA, n.d.), http://www.ahaonlinestore.com/ProductDisplay.asp?ProductID=637&cartID=2921104&PCatID=16	Health care system—hospitals	Longitudinal—trend	Sample of all (6,000+) U.S. hospitals	Mail questionnaires, Web-based surveys
American Medical Association • Socioeconomic Monitoring System (SMS), 1982–1999 (AMA, 2005, February 24), http://www.ama-assn.org/ama/pub/category/7801.html	Health care system—physicians Practice characteristics	Longitudinal—trend	Nationally representative sample of nonfederal patient-care physicians	Telephone interviews
Bureau of Labor Statistics • Current Population Survey (CPS), 1940–present (U.S. Department of Labor, Bureau of Labor Statistics, n.d.), http://www.bls.gov/cps/home.htm	Population	Longitudinal—trend	Nationally representative sample of households and civilian, non-institutionalized individuals, age 15+	Personal interviews, telephone interviews
National Center for Health Statistics • National Health Interview Survey (NHIS), 1957–present (NCHS, 2005i, May 11), http://www.cdc.gov/nchs/nhis.htm	Population Health status Utilization	Longitudinal—trend	Nationally representative sample of households and civilian, non-institutionalized individuals	Personal interviews
• National Immunization Survey (NIS), 1994–present (NCHS, 2005i; May 26), http://www.cdc.gov/nis/	Population Health status Utilization	Longitudinal—trend	Nationally representative sample of children 19–35 months in households with telephones and their vaccination providers	Telephone interviews (households), mail questionnaires (providers)
• National Health and Nutrition Examination Survey (NHANES), 1970–1975, 1976–1980, 1988–1994, 1999–2004 (NCHS, 2005l, June 2), http://www.cdc.gov/nchs/nhanes.htm	Health care system Population Health status Utilization	Longitudinal—trend	Nationally representative sample of households and civilian, non-institutionalized individuals	Personal interviews, ACASI, clinical exams

TABLE E.1. SELECTED EXAMPLES OF HEALTH SURVEYS, *continued.*

Study, Years (References)	Topics	Research Design	Population/Samples	Data Collection
National—United States National Center for Health Statistics (cont.)				
• National Employer Health Insurance Survey (NEHIS), 1994 (NCHS, 2004d, December 16), http://www.cdc.gov/nchs/about/major/nehis/about_nehis.htm	Health care system	Cross-sectional	Nationally representative sample of employers, in the public and private sectors and including the self-employed	Telephone interviews
National Health Care Survey (includes NAMCS, NHAMCS, NSAS, NHDS, NNHS, NHHCS, described below) (NCHS, 2005f, February 25), http://www.cdc.gov/nchs/nhcs.htm				
• National Ambulatory Medical Care Survey (NAMCS), 1973–1981, 1985, 1989–present (NCHS, 2004c, December 16), http://www.cdc.gov/nchs/about/major/ahcd/namcsdes.htm	Health care system Population Health status Utilization	Longitudinal—trend	Sample of visits to nonfederal office-based physicians in direct patient care	Logs, records of patient visits
• National Hospital Ambulatory Medical Care Survey (NHAMCS), 1992–present (NCHS, 2005a, February 1), http://www.cdc.gov/nchs/about/major/ahcd/nhamcsds.htm	Health care system Population Health status Utilization Expenditures	Longitudinal—trend	National sample of visits to emergency rooms and out-patient departments of nonfederal general and short-stay hospitals	Record abstraction
• National Survey of Ambulatory Surgery (NSAS), 1994–1996 (NCHS, 2005c, February 1), http://www.cdc.gov/nchs/about/major/hdasd/nsasdes.htm	Health care system Population Health status Utilization Expenditures	Longitudinal—trend	National sample of visits to nonfederal free-standing and ambulatory surgery centers	Record abstraction
• National Hospital Discharge Survey (NHDS), 1965–present (NCHS, 2005b, February 1), http://www.cdc.gov/nchs/about/major/hdasd/nhdsdes.htm	Health care system Population Health status Utilization Expenditures	Longitudinal—trend	National sample of discharges from short-stay, nonfederal general and children's general hospitals	Record abstraction

Survey	Content	Design	Sample	Data Collection
National Nursing Home Survey (NNHS), 1973–1974, 1977, 1985, 1995, 1997, 1999 (NCHS, 2004f, December 16), http://www.cdc.gov/nchs/about/major/nnhsd/nnhsdesc.htm	Health care system Population Health status Utilization Expenditures	Longitudinal—trend	Sample of nursing homes—staff and residents	Personal interviews, self-administered questionnaires
National Home and Hospice Care Survey (NHHCS), 1992, 1994, 1996, 1998, 2000 (NCHS, 2004e, December 16), http://www.cdc.gov/nchs/about/major/nhhcsd/nhhcsdes.htm	Health care system Population Health status Utilization Expenditures	Longitudinal—trend	Sample of agencies that provide home and hospice care—administrators and staff	Personal interviews
Centers for Medicare & Medicaid Services				
Medicare Current Beneficiary Survey (MCBS), 1991–present (CMMS, 2004, September 23), http://www.cms.hhs.gov/mcbs/	Health care system Population Health status Utilization Expenditures	Longitudinal—trend	Nationally representative sample of Medicare beneficiaries (aged, disabled, community-dwelling and institutionalized)	Personal interviews, administrative data
Center for Studying Health System Change				
Community Tracking Study (CTS)/Household Survey, 1996–1997, 1998–1999, 2000–2001, 2003 (Center for Studying Health System Change, 2005, May 27), http://www.hschange.org/index.cgi?data=02	Health care system Population Health status Utilization	Longitudinal—trend, cross-sectional	Nationally representative sample of the civilian, noninstitutionalized population	Telephone interviews; families without telephones visited by interviewers who provide cell phone
Commonwealth Fund				
Commonwealth Fund Health Care Quality Survey, 2001 (Commonwealth Fund, 2005), http://www.cmwf.org/surveys/surveys_show.htm?doc_id=228171	Health care system Population Health status Utilization	Cross-sectional	Nationally representative sample of adults ages 18 and older	Telephone interviews

TABLE E.1. SELECTED EXAMPLES OF HEALTH SURVEYS, *continued*.

Study, Years (References)	Topics	Research Design	Population/Samples	Data Collection
National—United States				
Urban Institute				
• National Survey of America's Families (NSAF), 1997, 1999, 2002 (Urban Institute, 2001), http://www.urban.org/Content/Research/NewFederalism/NSAF/Overview/NSAFOverview.htm	Health care system Population Health status Utilization	Longitudinal—trend, cross-sectional	Noninstitutionalized, civilian population under age 65, representing United States and selected states, and families with children	Telephone interviews; families without telephones visited by interviewers who provide cell phone
States—United States				
Centers for Disease Control and Prevention, National Center for Chronic Disease Prevention and Health Promotion				
• Behavioral Risk Factor Surveillance System (BRFSS), 1984–present (CDC, 2005, May 2), http://www.cdc.gov/brfss/index.htm	Population Health status	Cross-sectional, group comparison	Sample of adults aged 18 years or older in the states and District of Columbia	Telephone interview
State Health Access Data Assistance Center (SHADAC)				
• Coordinated State Coverage Survey (CSCS) (University of Minnesota, State Health Access Data Assistance Center, 2004), http://www.shadac.umn.edu/collecting/cscs.asp	Health care system Population Utilization	Cross-sectional	Varies by state; typically a stratified random sample of the noninstitutionalized, civilian population with oversamples of subpopulations of interest (for example, blacks, Hispanics, low-income families)	Telephone interviews
UCLA Center for Health Policy Research				
• California Health Interview Survey (CHIS), 2001, 2003, 2005 (UCLA Center for Health Policy Research, 2005), http://www.chis.ucla.edu/	Health care system Population Health status Utilization	Cross-sectional, longitudinal–trend	Representative sample of California residents; adults, adolescents 12–17 years, and children under 12	Telephone interviews

REFERENCES

Abramson, J. H., & Abramson, Z. H. (1999). *Survey methods in community medicine: Epidemiological research, programme evaluation, clinical trials* (5th ed.). New York: Churchill Livingstone.

Abramson, J. H., & Abramson, Z. H. (2001). *Making sense of data: A self-instruction manual on the interpretation of epidemiological data* (3rd ed.). New York: Oxford University Press.

Adams-Esquivel, H., & Lang, D. A. (1987). The reliability of telephone penetration estimates in specialized target groups: The Hispanic case. *Journal of Data Collection, 27,* 35–39.

Aday, L. A. (1996). *Designing and conducting health surveys: A comprehensive guide* (2nd ed.). San Francisco: Jossey-Bass.

Aday, L. A. (2001). *At risk in America: The health and health care needs of vulnerable populations in the United States* (2nd ed.). San Francisco: Jossey-Bass.

Aday, L. A., & Awe, W. C. (1997). Health services utilization models. In D. S. Gochman (Ed.), *Handbook of health behavior research I: Personal and social determinants* (pp. 153–172). New York: Plenum Press.

Adler, M. C., Clark, R. F., DeMaio, T. J., Miller, L. F., & Saluter, A. F. (1999). Collecting information on disability in the 2000 Census: An example of interagency cooperation. *Social Security Bulletin, 62,* 21–30.

Agency for Healthcare Research and Quality. (1998, December). *HIV Cost and Services Utilization Study (HCSUS).* Retrieved June 1, 2005, from http://www.ahrq.gov/data/hcsus.htm.

Agency for Healthcare Research and Quality. (1999). *The outcome of outcomes research at AHCPR: Final report* (ed. S. Tunis & D. Stryer). (Publication No. AHCPR 99-R044). Rockville, MD: Author.

Agency for Healthcare Research and Quality. (2000, March). *Outcomes research fact sheet: What is outcomes research?* Retrieved July 15, 2004, from http://www.ahrq.gov/clinic/outfact.htm.

Agency for Healthcare Research and Quality. (2003). *Fact sheet: CAHPS and the National CAHPS Benchmarking Database.* (AHRQ Publication No. 03-P001). Rockville, MD.

Agency for Healthcare Research and Quality. (2005, May 23). *National quality measures clearinghouse.* Retrieved May 26, 2005, from http://www.qualitymeasures.ahrq.gov.

Agency for Healthcare Research and Quality. (n.d.-a). *AHRQ homepage.* Retrieved May 29, 2005, from http://www.ahrq.gov.

Agency for Healthcare Research and Quality. (n.d.-b). *Consumer Assessment of Health Plans Study (CAHPS).* Retrieved June 1, 2005, from http://www.ahrq.gov/qual/cahpsix.htm.

Agency for Healthcare Research and Quality. (n.d.-c). *Medical Expenditure Panel Survey (MEPS).* Retrieved June 1, 2005, from http://www.meps.ahrq.gov/.

Albrecht, G. L., Levy, J. A., Sugrue, N. M., Prohaska, T. R., & Ostrow, D. G. (1989). Who hasn't heard about AIDS? *AIDS Education and Prevention, 1,* 261–267.

Alonso, J., Ferrer, M., Gandek, B., Ware, J. E., Aaronson, N. K., Mosconi, P., et al. (2004). Health-related quality of life associated with chronic conditions in eight countries: Results from the International Quality of Life Assessment (IQOLA) Project. *Quality of Life Research, 13,* 283–298.

Alreck, P. L., & Settle, R. B. (2004). *The survey research handbook* (3rd ed.). New York: McGraw-Hill.

Alwin, D. F., & Krosnick, J. A. (1985). The measurement of values in surveys: A comparison of ratings and rankings. *Public Opinion Quarterly, 49,* 535–552.

Amaya-Jackson, L., Socolar, R. R., Hunter, W., Runyan, D. K., & Colindres, R. (2000). Directly questioning children and adolescents about maltreatment: A review of survey measures used. *Journal of Interpersonal Violence, 15,* 725–759.

American Association for Public Opinion Research. (2004). *Standard definitions: Final dispositions of case codes and outcome rates for surveys* (4th major ed.). Ann Arbor, MI.

American Hospital Association. (n.d.). *AHA Annual Survey Database.* Retrieved June 16, 2005, from http://www.ahaonlinestore.com/ProductDisplay.asp?ProductID=637&cartID= 2921104&PCatID=16.

American Medical Association. (2005, February 24). *Socioeconomic Monitoring System (SMS).* Retrieved June 1, 2005, from http://www.ama-assn.org/ama/pub/category/7801.html.

American Psychiatric Association. (2000). *Diagnostic and statistical manual of mental disorders: DSM-IV-TR* (4th, text revision). Washington, DC: Author.

American Psychological Association. (1999). *Standards for educational and psychological testing.* Washington, DC: Author.

American Psychological Association. (2001). *Publication manual of the American Psychological Association* (5th ed.). Washington, DC: Author.

American Statistical Association, Section on Survey Research Methods. (1998a). *Judging the quality of a survey.* Retrieved December 8, 2003, from http://www.amstat.org/sections/ srms/whatsurvey.html.

American Statistical Association, Section on Survey Research Methods. (1998b). *What is a margin of error?* Retrieved December 8, 2003, from http://www.amstat.org/sections/srms/ whatsurvey.html.

American Statistical Association, Section on Survey Research Methods. (n.d.-a). *Summary of survey analysis software* (comp. A. Zaslavsky). Retrieved March 23, 2005, from http://www.hcp.med.harvard.edu/statistics/survey-soft/.

American Statistical Association, Section on Survey Research Methods. (n.d.-b). *Survey research methods section: Links and resources.* Retrieved April 1, 2005, from http://www.amstat.org/ sections/SRMS/links.html.

Andersen, R. M., Kasper, J., Frankel, M. R., & Associates. (1979). *Total survey error.* San Francisco: Jossey-Bass.

Andersen, R. M. (1995). Revisiting the behavioral model and access to medical care: Does it matter? *Journal of Health and Social Behavior, 36,* 1–10.

Anderson, M., & Fienberg, S. E. (2000). Race and ethnicity and the controversy over the U.S. Census. *Current Sociology, 48,* 87–110.

Andresen, E. M., Diehr, P. H., & Luke, D. A. (2004). Public health surveillance of low-frequency populations. *Annual Review of Public Health, 25,* 25–52.

Andresen, E. M., Fitch, C. A., McLendon, P. M., & Meyers, A. R. (2000). Reliability and validity of disability questions for U.S. Census 2000. *American Journal of Public Health, 90,* 1297–1299.

Andresen, E. M., & Meyers, A. R. (2000). Health-related quality of life outcomes measures. *Archives of Physical Medicine and Rehabilitation, 81*(Suppl. 2), S30–S45.

Andrews, F. M. (1984). Construct validity and error components of survey measures: A structural modeling approach. *Public Opinion Quarterly, 48,* 409–442.

Andrich, D. (1988). *Rasch models for measurement.* Thousand Oaks, CA: Sage.

Aquilino, W. S. (1994). Interview mode effects in surveys of drug and alcohol use: A field experiment. *Public Opinion Quarterly, 58,* 210–240.

Aquilino, W. S., & Lo Sciuto, L. A. (1990). Effects of interview mode on self-reported drug use. *Public Opinion Quarterly, 54,* 362–395.

Areni, C. S., Ferrell, M. E., & Wilcox, J. B. (1999). The effects of need for cognition and topic importance on the latency and extremity of responses to attitudinal inquiries. *Advances in Consumer Research, 26,* 63–68.

Armstrong, A. M., MacDonald, A., Booth, I. W., Platts, R. G., Knibb, R. C., & Booth, D. A. (2000). Errors in memory for dietary intake and their reduction. *Applied Cognitive Psychology, 14,* 183–191.

Armstrong, J. S., & Lusk, E. J. (1987). Return postage in mail surveys: A meta-analysis. *Public Opinion Quarterly, 51,* 233–248.

Arzheimer, K., & Klein, M. (1999). The effect of material incentives on return rate, panel attrition and sample composition of a mail panel survey. *International Journal of Public Opinion Research, 11,* 368–377.

Axinn, W. G., Fricke, T. E., & Thornton, A. (1991). The microdemographic community-study approach: Improving survey data by integrating the ethnographic method. *Sociological Methods and Research, 20,* 187–217.

Ayidiya, S. A., & McClendon, M. J. (1990). Response effects in mail surveys. *Public Opinion Quarterly, 54,* 229–247.

Babbie, E. R. (2004). *The practice of social research* (10th ed.). Belmont, CA: Thomson/Wadsworth.

Bachman, J. G., & O'Malley, P. M. (1984). Yea-saying, nay-saying, and going to extremes: Black-white differences in response styles. *Public Opinion Quarterly, 48,* 491–509.

Bailar, B. A., & Lanphier, C. M. (1978). *Development of survey methods to assess survey practices.* Washington, DC: American Statistical Association.

Baker, R., Zahs, D., & Popa, G. (2004). Health surveys in the 21st century: Telephone vs. Web. In National Center for Health Statistics, *Eighth Conference on Health Survey Research Methods* (ed. S. B. Cohen & J. M. Lepkowski) (pp. 143–148). (DHHS Publication No. (PHS) 04-1013). Hyattsville, MD: National Center for Health Statistics.

Ball, L. A. (1996). A paradigm shift for data editing. In Federal Committee on Statistical Methodology (Ed.), *Data Editing Workshop and Exposition, 1996: Conference Proceedings* (pp. 3–15). (Statistical Policy Working Paper No. 25). Washington, DC: Office of Management and Budget, Office of Information and Regulatory Affairs, Statistical Policy Office.

Bardwell, W. A., Ancoli-Israel, S., & Dimsdale, J. E. (2001). Response bias influences mental health symptom reporting in patients with obstructive sleep apnea. *Annals of Behavioral Medicine, 23,* 313–317.

Bardwell, W. A., Major, J. M., Rock, C. L., Newman, V. A., Thomson, C. A., Chilton, J. A., et al. (2004). Health-related quality of life in women previously treated for early-stage breast cancer. *Psycho-Oncology, 13,* 595–604.

Bartman, B. A., Rosen, M. J., Bradham, D. D., Weissman, J., Hochberg, M., & Revicki, D. A. (1998). Relationship between health status and utility measures in older claudicants. *Quality of Life Research, 7,* 67–73.

Bassili, J. N., & Scott, B. S. (1996). Response latency as a signal to question problems in survey research. *Public Opinion Quarterly, 60,* 390–399.

Bauman, L. J., & Adair, E. G. (1992). The use of ethnographic interviewing to inform questionnaire construction. *Health Education Quarterly, 19,* 9–23.

Beals, J., Manson, S. M., Mitchell, C. M., Spicer, P., & AI-SUPERPFP Team. (2003). Cultural specificity and comparison in psychiatric epidemiology: Walking the tightrope in American Indian research. *Culture Medicine and Psychiatry, 27,* 259–289.

Beatty, P. (1995). Understanding the standardized/nonstandardized interviewing controversy. *Journal of Official Statistics, 11,* 147–160.

Beatty, P., Herrmann, D., Puskar, C., & Kerwin, J. (1998). "Don't know" responses in surveys: Is what I know what you want to know and do I want you to know it? *Memory, 6,* 407–426.

Beaufait, D. W., Nelson, E. C., Landgraf, J. M., Hayes, R. D., Kirk, J. W., Wasson, J. H., et al. (1992). COOP measures of functional status. In M. Stewart, F. Tudiver, M. J. Bass, E. V. Dunn, & P. G. Norton (Eds.), *Tools for primary care research* (pp. 151–167). Thousand Oaks, CA: Sage.

Becker, G., Gates, R. J., & Newsom, E. (2004). Self-care among chronically ill African Americans: Culture, health disparities, and health insurance status. *American Journal of Public Health, 94,* 2066–2073.

Beldt, S. F., Daniel, W. W., & Garcha, B. S. (1982). The Takahasi-Sakasegawa randomized response technique: A field test. *Sociological Methods and Research, 11,* 101–111.

Belli, R. F., Shay, W. L., & Stafford, F. P. (2001). Event history calendars and question list surveys: A direct comparison of interviewing methods. *Public Opinion Quarterly, 65,* 45–74.

Bennett, S., Woods, T., Liyanage, W. M., & Smith, D. L. (1991). A simplified general method for cluster-sample surveys of health in developing countries. *World Health Statistics Quarterly, 44,* 98–106.

Bergner, M., Bobbitt, R. A., Carter, W. B., & Gilson, B. S. (1981). The Sickness Impact Profile: Development and final revision of a health status measure. *Medical Care, 19,* 787–805.

Bergner, M., Bobbitt, R. A., Kressel, S., Pollard, W. E., Gilson, B. S., & Morris, J. R. (1976). Sickness Impact Profile: Conceptual formulation and methodology for development of a health status measure. *International Journal of Health Services, 6,* 393–415.

Berk, M. L., & Bernstein, A. B. (1988). Interviewer characteristics and performance on a complex health survey. *Social Science Research, 17,* 239–251.

Bertrand, M., & Mullainathan, S. (2001). *Do people mean what they say? Implications for subjective survey data.* (Working Paper Series, Massachusetts Institute of Technology, Department of Economics, 01-04). Cambridge, MA: Massachusetts Institute of Technology, Department of Economics.

Bickart, B. A., Blair, J., Menon, G., & Sudman, S. (1990). Cognitive aspects of proxy reporting of behavior. *Advances in Consumer Research, 17,* 198–206.

Bickart, B. A., Menon, G., Sudman, S., & Blair, J. (1992). Context effects in proxy judgments. *Advances in Consumer Research, 19,* 64–71.

Bickman, L. (Ed.). (2000). *Validity and social experimentation: Donald Campbell's legacy.* Thousand Oaks, CA: Sage.

Biemer, P. P., & Caspar, R. (1994). Continuous quality improvement for survey operations: Some general principles and applications. *Journal of Official Statistics, 10,* 307–326.

Biemer, P. P., Groves, R. M., Lyberg, L. E., Mathiowetz, N. A., & Sudman, S. (Eds). (1991). *Measurement errors in surveys.* Hoboken, NJ: Wiley.

Biemer, P. P., & Lyberg, L. E. (2003). *Introduction to survey quality.* Hoboken, NJ: Wiley.

Billiet, J., & Loosveldt, G. (1988). Improvement of the quality of responses to factual survey questions by interviewer training. *Public Opinion Quarterly, 52,* 190–211.

Binder, D. A. (1998). Longitudinal surveys: Why are these surveys different from all other surveys? *Survey Methodology, 24,* 101–108.

Binson, D., Canchola, J. A., & Catania, J. A. (2000). Random selection in a national telephone survey: A comparison of the Kish, next-birthday, and last-birthday methods. *Journal of Official Statistics, 16,* 53–59.

Binson, D., & Catania, J. A. (1998). Respondents' understanding of the words used in sexual behavior questions. *Public Opinion Quarterly, 62,* 190–208.

Bishop, G. F. (1987). Experiments with the middle response alternative in survey questions. *Public Opinion Quarterly, 51,* 220–232.

Bishop, G. F. (1990). Issue involvement and response effects in public opinion surveys. *Public Opinion Quarterly, 54,* 209–218.

Bishop, G. F., Oldendick, R. W., & Tuchfarber, A. J. (1982). Effects of presenting one versus two sides of an issue in survey questions. *Public Opinion Quarterly, 46,* 69–85.

Bishop, G. F., & Smith, A. (2001). Response-order effects and the early Gallup split-ballots. *Public Opinion Quarterly, 65,* 479–505.

Bishop, G. F., Tuchfarber, A. J., & Oldendick, R. W. (1986). Opinions on fictitious issues: The pressure to answer survey questions. *Public Opinion Quarterly, 50,* 240–250.

Blair, E., & Burton, S. (1987). Cognitive processes used by survey respondents to answer behavioral frequency questions. *Journal of Consumer Research, 14,* 280–288.

Blair, J., & Czaja, R. (1982). Locating a special population using random digit dialing. *Public Opinion Quarterly, 46,* 585–590.

Bland, J. M., & Altman, D. G. (1995). Calculating correlation coefficients with repeated observations: Part 1—Correlation within subjects. *British Medical Journal, 310,* 446.

Bless, H., Bohner, G., Hild, T., & Schwarz, N. (1992). Asking difficult questions: Task complexity increases the impact of response alternatives. *European Journal of Social Psychology, 22,* 309–312.

Blumberg, S. J., Luke, J. V., & Cynamon, M. L. (2004). Has cord-cutting cut into random-digit-dialed health surveys? The prevalence and impact of wireless substitution. In National Center for Health Statistics, *Eighth Conference on Health Survey Research Methods* (ed. S. B. Cohen & J. M. Lepkowski) (pp. 137–142). (DHHS Publication No. (PHS) 04-1013). Hyattsville, MD: National Center for Health Statistics.

Blyth, B., & Piper, H. (1994). Speech recognition: A new dimension in survey research. *Journal of the Market Research Society, 36,* 183–203.

Borenstein, M., Cohen, J., & Rothstein, H. (2000). *Power and precision, version 2: A computer program for statistical power analysis and confidence intervals* [Computer software]. St. Paul, MN: Assessment Systems Corporation.

Boruch, R., May, H., Turner, H., Lavenberg, J., Petrosino, A., De Moya, D., et al. (2004). Estimating the effects of interventions that are deployed in many places: Place-randomized trials. *American Behavioral Scientist, 47,* 608–633.

Bosch, A. M., Grootenhuis, M. A., Bakker, H. D., Heijmans, H.S.A., Wijburg, F. A., & Last, B. F. (2004). Living with classical galactosemia: Health-related quality of life consequences. *Pediatrics, 113,* 423–428.

Bourque, L. B., & Clark, V. A. (1992). *Processing data: The survey example.* Thousand Oaks, CA: Sage.

Bourque, L. B., & Fielder, E. P. (2003). *The survey kit: Vol. 3. How to conduct self-administered and mail surveys* (2nd ed.). Thousand Oaks, CA: Sage.

Bowling, A. (2005). *Measuring health: A review of quality of life measurement scales* (3rd ed.). New York: Open University Press.

Bowman, J. A., Redman, S., Dickinson, J. A., Gibberd, R., & Sanson-Fisher, R. W. (1991). The accuracy of pap smear utilization self-report: A methodological consideration in cervical screening research. *Health Services Research, 26,* 97–107.

Boyle, M. H., Furlong, W., Feeny, D., Torrance, G. W., & Hatcher, J. (1995). Reliability of the Health Utilities Index—Mark-III used in the 1991 Cycle-6 Canadian General Social Survey Health Questionnaire. *Quality of Life Research, 4,* 249–257.

Bradburn, N. (1999). Models of the survey process. In National Center for Health Statistics, *A new agenda for interdisciplinary survey research methods: Proceedings of the CASM II Seminar* (ed. M. G. Sirken, T. Jabine, G. Willis, E. Martin, & C. Tucker) (pp. 79–83). Hyattsville, MD: National Center for Health Statistics.

Bradburn, N., & Danis, C. (1984). Potential contributions of cognitive research to survey questionnaire design. In National Research Council Committee on National Statistics, *Cognitive aspects of survey methodology: Building a bridge between disciplines* (ed. T. B. Jabine, M. L. Straf, J. M. Tanur, & R. Tourangeau) (pp. 101–129). Washington, DC: National Academies Press.

Bradburn, N. M., Sudman, S., Blair, E., et al. (1979). *Improving interview method and questionnaire design.* San Francisco: Jossey-Bass.

Bradburn, N. M., Sudman, S., & Wansink, B. (2004). *Asking questions: The definitive guide to questionnaire design: For market research, political polls, and social and health questionnaires* (Rev. ed.). San Francisco: Jossey-Bass.

Brand, J.P.L., van Buuren, S., Groothuis-Oudshoorn, K., & Gelsema, E. S. (2003). A toolkit in SAS for the evaluation of multiple imputation methods. *Statistica Neerlandica, 57,* 36–45.

Brook, R. H., Ware, J. E., Davies-Avery, A., Stewart, A. L., Donald, C. A., Rogers, W. H., et al. (1979). Overview of adult health status measures fielded in Rand's Health Insurance Study [Entire issue]. *Medical Care, 17*(Suppl. 7).

Brown, E. R. (2004). Community participation and community benefit in large surveys: Enhancing quality, relevance, and use of the California Health Interview Survey. In National Center for Health Statistics, *Eighth Conference on Health Survey Research Methods* (ed.

S. B. Cohen & J. M. Lepkowski) (pp. 49–54). (DHHS Publication No. (PHS) 04-1013). Hyattsville, MD: National Center for Health Statistics.

Bulmer, M. (1998). The problem of exporting social survey research: Introduction. *American Behavioral Scientist, 42,* 153–167.

Bulmer, M., Bales, K., & Sklar, K. K. (Eds). (1991). *The social survey in historical perspective, 1880–1940.* Cambridge: Cambridge University Press.

Burgos, A. E., Schetzina, K. E., Dixon, L. B., & Mendoza, F. S. (2005). Importance of generational status in examining access to and utilization of health care services by Mexican American children. *Pediatrics, 115,* 322–330.

Burton, S., & Blair, E. (1991). Task conditions, response formulation processes, and response accuracy for behavioral frequency questions in surveys. *Public Opinion Quarterly, 55,* 50–79.

Bush, J. W. (1984). General Health Policy Model/Quality of Well-Being (QWB) Scale. In N. K. Wenger, M. E. Mattson, C. D. Furberg, & J. Elinson (Eds.), *Assessment of quality of life in clinical trials of cardiovascular therapies* (pp. 189–199). New York: LeJacq.

Buzzard, I. M., & Sievert, Y. A. (1994). Research priorities and recommendations for dietary assessment methodology. *American Journal of Clinical Nutrition, 59*(Suppl.), S275–S280.

Call, K. T., McAlpine, D., Britt, H., Cha, V., Osman, S., Suarez, W., & Beebe, T. (2004). Partnering with communities in survey design and implementation. In National Center for Health Statistics, *Eighth Conference on Health Survey Research Methods* (ed. S. B. Cohen & J. M. Lepkowski) (pp. 61–66). (DHHS Publication No. (PHS) 04-1013). Hyattsville, MD: National Center for Health Statistics.

Campbell, D. T., & Russo, M. J. (1999). *Social experimentation.* Thousand Oaks, CA: Sage.

Cameron, S. (2002). Drug databases for users of hand-held computers. *Canadian Family Physician, 48,* 752–753.

Cannell, C., Miller, P. V., & Oksenberg, L. (1982). Research on interviewing techniques. In S. Leinhardt (Ed.), *Sociological methodology 1982* (pp. 389–437). San Francisco: Jossey-Bass.

Carmines, E. G., & Zeller, R. A. (1979). *Reliability and validity assessment.* Thousand Oaks, CA: Sage.

Casady, R. J., & Lepkowski, J. M. (1998). Telephone sampling. In P. Armitage & T. Colton (Eds.), *Encyclopedia of biostatistics* (pp. 4498–4511). Hoboken, NJ: Wiley.

Cassidy, C. M. (1994). Walk a mile in my shoes: Culturally sensitive food-habit research. *American Journal of Clinical Nutrition, 59*(Suppl.), S190-S197.

Catania, J. A., Binson, D., Canchola, J., Pollack, L. M., Hauck, W., & Coates, T. J. (1996). Effects of interviewer gender, interviewer choice, and item wording on responses to questions concerning sexual behavior. *Public Opinion Quarterly, 60,* 345–375.

Cella, D. F. (1995). Methods and problems in measuring quality of life. *Supportive Care in Cancer, 3,* 11–22.

Center for Studying Health System Change. (2005, May 27). *Community Tracking Study (CTS)/ Household Survey.* Retrieved June 1, 2005, from http://www.hschange.org/index.cgi?data=02.

Centers for Disease Control and Prevention, Division of Public Health Surveillance and Informatics. (2004, April 7). *EpiInfo.* Retrieved June 8, 2005, from http://www.cdc.gov/epiinfo/.

Centers for Disease Control and Prevention, National Center for Chronic Disease Prevention and Health Promotion. (2005, May 2). *Behavioral Risk Factor Surveillance System.* Retrieved June 13, 2005, from http://www.cdc.gov/brfss/.

Centers for Medicare and Medicaid Services. (2004, September 23). *Medicare Current Beneficiary Survey (MCBS) homepage.* Retrieved May 31, 2005, from http://www.cms.hhs.gov/mcbs/.

Chambers, R. L., & Skinner, C. J. (Eds). (2003). *Analysis of survey data.* Hoboken, NJ: Wiley.

Characteristics of community report cards: United States, 1996. (1997). *Morbidity and Mortality Weekly Report, 46,* 647–648, 655.

Chen, J., & Shao, J. (2000). Nearest neighbor imputation for survey data. *Journal of Official Statistics, 16,* 113–131.

Church, A. H. (1993). Estimating the effect of incentives on mail survey response rates: A meta-analysis. *Public Opinion Quarterly, 57,* 62–79.

Cohen, J. (1988). *Statistical power analysis for the behavioral sciences* (2nd ed.). Mahwah, NJ: Erlbaum.

Cohen, S. B. (1997). An evaluation of alternative PC-based software packages developed for the analysis of complex survey data. *American Statistician, 51,* 285–292.

Cohen, S. B. (2003). Design strategies and innovations in the Medical Expenditure Panel Survey. *Medical Care, 41* (7 Suppl.), III5–III12.

Collins, D. (2003). Pretesting survey instruments: An overview of cognitive methods. *Quality of Life Research, 12,* 229–238.

Collins, M., & Sykes, W. (1999). Extending the definition of survey quality. *Journal of Official Statistics, 15,* 57–66.

Commonwealth Fund. (2005). *Commonwealth Fund Health Care Quality Survey.* Retrieved June 1, 2005, from http://www.cmwf.org/surveys/surveys_show.htm?doc_id=228171.

Connelly, N. A., Brown, T. L., & Decker, D. J. (2003). Factors affecting response rates to natural resource: Focused mail surveys: Empirical evidence of declining rates over time. *Society and Natural Resources, 16,* 541–549.

Conover, W. J. (1999). *Practical nonparametric statistics* (3rd ed.). Hoboken, NJ: Wiley.

Conrad, D. A., Milgrom, P., Whitney, C., O'Hara, D., & Fiset, L. (1998). The incentive effects of malpractice liability rules on dental practice behavior. *Medical Care, 36,* 706–719.

Conrad, D. A., Whitney, C., Milgrom, P., O'Hara, D., Ammons, R., Fiset, L., et al. (1995). Malpractice premiums in 1992: Results of a national survey of dentists. *Journal of the American Dental Association, 126,* 1045–1056.

Conrad, F. G., & Schober, M. F. (2000). Clarifying question meaning in a household telephone survey. *Public Opinion Quarterly, 64,* 1–28.

Conrad, K. D., & Smith, E. V., Jr. (Eds.). (2004). *Applications of Rasch analysis in health care.* Hagerstown, MD: Lippincott Williams & Wilkins.

Converse, J. M., & Presser, S. (1986). *Survey questions: Handcrafting the standardized questionnaire.* Thousand Oaks, CA: Sage.

Coons, S. J., Rao, S., Keininger, D. L., & Hays, R. D. (2000). A comparative review of generic quality-of-life instruments. *Pharmacoeconomics, 17,* 13–35.

Corel. (2005). *Word Perfect Office 12.* Retrieved May 23, 2005, from http://www.corel.com/servlet/Satellite?pagename=Corel3/Products/Display&pfid=1047024307359&pid=1047022958453.

Corey, C. R., & Freeman, H. E. (1990). Use of telephone interviewing in health care research. *Health Services Research, 25,* 129–144.

Corkrey, R., & Parkinson, L. (2002). A comparison of four computer-based telephone interviewing methods: Getting answers to sensitive questions. *Behavior Research Methods, Instruments, and Computers, 34,* 354–363.

Cornelius, L. J., Booker, N. C., Arthur, T. E., Reeves, I., & Morgan, O. (2004). The validity and reliability testing of a consumer-based cultural competency inventory. *Research on Social Work Practice, 14,* 201–209.

Cornelius, L. J., Lloyd, J. L., Bishai, D., Latkin, C. A., Huettner, S., Brown, M. I., et al. (2006). *The Treatment Retention Intervention: A case study of an evaluation of a case management intervention to improve treatment outcomes for injection drug users.* Manuscript submitted for publication.

Council of American Survey Research Organizations. (1982). *On the definition of response rates: A special report of the CASRO Task Force on Completion Rates.* Port Jefferson, NY: Author.

Couper, M. P. (2000). Web surveys: A review of issues and approaches. *Public Opinion Quarterly, 64,* 464–494.

Couper, M. P. (2004). Of frames and nonresponse: Issues related to nonobservation. In National Center for Health Statistics, *Eighth Conference on Health Survey Research Methods* (ed. S. B. Cohen & J. M. Lepkowski) (pp. 159–164). (DHHS Publication No. (PHS) 04-1013). Hyattsville, MD: National Center for Health Statistics.

Couper, M. P., Baker, R. P., Bethlehem, J., Clark, C.Z.F., Martin, J., Nicholls, W. L., II, et al. (Eds.). (1998). *Computer assisted survey information collection.* Hoboken, NJ: Wiley.

Couper, M. P., Blair, J., & Triplett, T. (1999). A comparison of mail and e-mail for a survey of employees in U.S. statistical agencies. *Journal of Official Statistics, 15,* 39–56.

Couper, M. P., & Groves, R. M. (1996). Social environmental impacts on survey cooperation. *Quality and Quantity, 30,* 173–188.

Couper, M. P., Singer, E., & Tourangeau, R. (2003). Understanding the effects of audio-CASI on self-reports of sensitive behavior. *Public Opinion Quarterly, 67,* 385–395.

Cox, B. G., & Cohen, S. B. (1985). *Methodological issues for health care surveys.* New York: Dekker.

Cox, C. E., Donohue, J. F., Brown, C. D., Kataria, Y. P., & Judson, M. A. (2004). Health-related quality of life of persons with sarcoidosis. *Chest, 125,* 997–1004.

Coyle, J., & Williams, B. (1999). Seeing the wood for the trees: Defining the forgotten concept of patient dissatisfaction in the light of patient satisfaction research. *International Journal of Health Care Quality Assurance Incorporating Leadership in Health Services, 12,* i–ix.

Crabb, P. B. (1999). The use of answering machines and caller ID to regulate home privacy. *Environment and Behavior, 31,* 657–670.

Crawford, C. M., Caputo, L. A., & Littlejohn, G. O. (2000). Back to basics . . . . Clinical assessment in rheumatic disease. *Topics in Clinical Chiropractic, 7,* 1–12, 66, 68–70.

Crawford, L. E., Huttenlocher, J., & Engebretson, P. H. (2000). Category effects on estimates of stimuli: Perception or reconstruction? *Psychological Science, 11,* 280–284.

Creative Research Systems. (2004). *The survey system.* Retrieved June 8, 2005, from http://www.surveysystem.com/.

Criswell, D. F., & Parchman, M. L. (2002). Handheld computer use in U.S. family practice residency programs. *Journal of the American Medical Informatics Association, 9,* 80–86.

Crowne, D. P., & Marlowe, D. (1960). A new scale of social desirability independent of psychopathology. *Journal of Consulting Psychology, 24,* 349–354.

Czaja, R. F., & Blair, J. (1990). Using network sampling in crime victimization surveys. *Quantitative Criminology, 6,* 185–206.

Czaja, R. F., Blair, J., Bickart, B., & Eastman, E. (1994). Respondent strategies for recall of crime victimization incidents. *Journal of Official Statistics, 10,* 257–276.

Czaja, R. F., Blair, J., & Sebestik, J. P. (1982). Respondent selection in a telephone survey: A comparison of three techniques. *Journal of Marketing Research, 19,* 381–385.

Czaja, R. F., Snowden, C. B., & Casady, R. J. (1986). Reporting bias and sampling errors in a survey of a rare population using multiplicity counting rules. *Journal of the American Statistical Association, 81,* 411–419.

Czaja, R. F., Trunzo, D. H., & Royston, P. N. (1992). Response effects in a network survey. *Sociological Methods and Research, 20,* 340–366.

Czaja, R. F., Warnecke, R. B., Eastman, E., Royston, P., Sirken, M., and & Tuteur, D. (1984). Locating patients with rare diseases using network sampling: Frequency and quality of reporting. In National Center for Health Statistics, *Health Survey Research Methods: Proceedings of the Fourth Conference on Health Survey Research Methods* (ed. C. F. Cannell & R. M. Groves) (pp. 311–324). (DHHS Publication No. (PHS) 84-3346). Rockville, MD: National Center for Health Services Research.

Davies, A. R., & Ware, J. E. (1988). *GHAA's consumer satisfaction survey and user's manual.* Washington, DC: Group Health Association of America.

Davies, A. R., & Ware, J. E. (1991). *GHAA's consumer satisfaction survey and user's manual* (2nd ed.). Washington, DC: Group Health Association of America.

Davies, A. R., Ware, J. E., & Kosinski, M. (1995). Standardizing health care evaluations. *Medical Outcomes Trust Bulletin, 3,* 2–3.

Davis, D. W. (1997). Nonrandom measurement error and race of interviewer effects among African Americans. *Public Opinion Quarterly, 61,* 183–207.

de Leeuw, E. D., & Hox, J. J. (1988). The effects of response-stimulating factors on response rates and data quality in mail surveys: A test of Dillman's Total Design Method. *Journal of Official Statistics, 4,* 241–249.

de Vaus, D. A. (Ed.). (2002). *Social surveys.* Thousand Oaks, CA: Sage.

Decision Analyst. (2002). *Free statistical software.* Retrieved April 1, 2005, from http://www.decisionanalyst.com/download.asp.

DeGraaf, D., & Jordan, D. (2003, December). Social capital: How parks and recreation help to build community. *Parks and Recreation, 38.* Retrieved May 25, 2005, from http://www.nrpa.org/content/default.aspx?documentId=783.

DeVellis, R. F. (2003). *Scale development: Theory and applications* (2nd ed.). Thousand Oaks, CA: Sage.

Di Palo, M. T. (1997). Rating satisfaction research: Is it square poor, square fair, square good, square very good, or square excellent? *Arthritis Care and Research, 10,* 422–430.

Dielman, T. E., & Couper, M. P. (1995). Data quality in a CAPI survey: Keying errors. *Journal of Official Statistics, 11,* 141–146.

Dijkstra, W., Smit, J. H., & Comijs, H. C. (2001). Using social desirability scales in research among the elderly. *Quality and Quantity, 35,* 107–115.

Dillman, D. A. (1978). *Mail and telephone surveys: The total design method.* Hoboken, NJ: Wiley.

Dillman, D. A. (1991). The design and administration of mail surveys. *Annual Review of Sociology, 17,* 225–249.

Dillman, D. A. (1998, March). *Mail and other self-administered surveys in the 21st century: The beginning of a new era.* Retrieved May 30, 2005, from http://survey.sesrc.wsu.edu/dillman/papers/svys21st.pdf.

Dillman, D. A. (2000). *Mail and Internet surveys: The tailored design method* (2nd ed.). Hoboken, NJ: Wiley.

Dillman, D. A. (2002). Navigating the rapids of change: Some observations on survey methodology in the early twenty-first century. *Public Opinion Quarterly, 66,* 473–494.

Dillman, D. A. (2004). The conundrum of mixed-mode surveys in the 21st century. In National Center for Health Statistics, *Eighth Conference on Health Survey Research Methods* (ed. S. B. Cohen & J. M. Lepkowski) (pp. 165–170). (DHHS Publication No. (PHS) 04-1013). Hyattsville, MD: National Center for Health Statistics.

Dillman, D. A., Brown, T. L., Carlson, J. E., Carpenter, E. H., Lorenz, F. O., Mason, R., et al. (1995). Effects of category order on answers in mail and telephone surveys. *Rural Sociology, 60,* 674–687.

Dillman, D. A., Eltinge, J. L., Groves, R. M., & Little, R.J.A. (2002). Survey nonresponse in design, data collection, and analysis. In R. M. Groves, D. A. Dillman, J. L. Eltinge, & R.J.A. Little (Eds.), *Survey nonresponse* (pp. 3–26). Hoboken, NJ: Wiley.

Dillman, D. A., & Miller, K. J. (1998). Response rates, data quality, and cost feasibility for optically scannable mail surveys by small research centers. In M. P. Couper, R. P. Baker, J. Bethlehem, C.Z.F. Clark, J. Martin, W. L. Nicholls II, & J. M. O'Reilly (Eds.), *Computer assisted survey information collection* (pp. 475–497). Hoboken, NJ: Wiley.

Dillman, D. A., Tortora, R. D., & Bowker, D. (1999, March 5). *Principles for constructing Web surveys.* Retrieved June 6, 2005, from http://survey.sesrc.wsu.edu/dillman/papers/ websurveyppr.pdf.

Dilorio, C., Dudley, W. N., Soet, J., Watkins, J., & Maibach, E. (2000). A social cognitive-based model for condom use among college students. *Nursing Research, 49,* 208–214.

Dobrez, D. G., & Calhoun, E. A. (2004). Testing subject comprehension of utility questionnaires. *Quality of Life Research, 13,* 369–376.

Donenberg, G. R., Lyons, J. S., & Howard, K. I. (1999). Clinical trials versus mental health services research: Contributions and connections. *Journal of Clinical Psychology, 55,* 1135–1146.

Donovan, R. J., Holman, C.D.J., Corti, B., & Jalleh, G. (1997). Face-to-face household interviews versus telephone interviews for health surveys. *Australian and New Zealand Journal of Public Health, 21,* 134–140.

Doornbos, M. M. (1996). The strengths of families coping with serious mental illness. *Archives of Psychiatric Nursing, 10,* 214–220.

Drukker, M., & van Os, J. (2003). Mediators of neighbourhood socioeconomic deprivation and quality of life. *Social Psychiatry and Psychiatric Epidemiology, 38,* 698–706.

Ebel, R. L. (1951). Estimation of the reliability of ratings. *Psychometrika, 16,* 407–424.

Edwards, S., Slattery, M. L., Mori, M., Berry, T. D., Caan, B. J., Palmer, P., et al. (1994). Objective system for interviewer performance evaluation for use in epidemiologic studies. *American Journal of Epidemiology, 140,* 1020–1028.

EpiData Association. (2000). *EpiData—freeware.* Retrieved June 8, 2005, from http://www. epidata.dk/.

Ersser, S. J., Surridge, H., & Wiles, A. (2002). What criteria do patients use when judging the effectiveness of psoriasis management? *Journal of Evaluation in Clinical Practice, 8,* 367–376.

EuroQol Group. (1990). EuroQol: A new facility for the measurement of health-related quality of life. *Health Policy, 16,* 199–208.

EuroQol Group. (n.d.). *EQ-5D: An instrument to describe and value health.* Retrieved May 31, 2005, from http://www.euroqol.org/web/.

Evans, R. G., Barer, M. L., & Marmor, T. R. (Eds). (1994). *Why are some people healthy and others not? The determinants of health of populations.* New York: Aldine de Gruyter.

Evans, R. G., & Stoddart, G. L. (1990). Producing health, consuming health care. *Social Science and Medicine, 31,* 1347–1363.

Ezzati-Rice, T., & Cohen, S. B. (2004). Design and estimation strategies in the Medical Expenditure Panel Survey for investigation of trends in health expenditures. In National Center for Health Statistics, *Eighth Conference on Health Survey Research Methods* (ed.

S. B. Cohen & J. M. Lepkowski) (pp. 23–28). (DHHS Publication No. (PHS) 04-1013). Hyattsville, MD: National Center for Health Statistics.

Fagerberg, T., Rekkedal, T., & Russell, J. (2002, January). *Designing and trying out a learning environment for mobile learners and teachers: Sub-project of the EU Leonardo Project. From e-learning to m-learning?* Retrieved May 25, 2005, from http://www.nettskolen.com/pub/artikkel.xsql?artid=115.

Feeny, D. H., & Torrance, G. W. (1989). Incorporating utility-based quality-of-life assessment measures in clinical trials: Two examples. *Medical Care, 27*(Suppl. 3), S190–S204.

Feinstein, A. R. (1987). *Clinimetrics.* New Haven, CT: Yale University Press.

Fendrich, M., & Vaughn, C. M. (1994). Diminished lifetime substance use over time: An inquiry into differential underreporting. *Public Opinion Quarterly, 58,* 96–123.

Field, A. E., Taylor, C. B., Celio, A., & Colditz, G. A. (2004). Comparison of self-report to interview assessment of bulimic behaviors among preadolescent and adolescent girls and boys. *International Journal of Eating Disorders, 35,* 86–92.

Fienberg, S. E., & Tanur, J. M. (1989). Combining cognitive and statistical approaches to survey design. *Science, 243,* 1017–1022.

Fikar, C. R., & Keith, L. (2004). Information needs of gay, lesbian, bisexual, and transgendered health care professionals: Results of an Internet survey. *Journal of the Medical Library Association, 92,* 56–65.

Fink, A. (2003). *The survey kit* (2nd ed.). Thousand Oaks, CA: Sage.

Fink, J. C. (1983). CATI's first decade: The Chilton experience. *Sociological Methods and Research, 12,* 153–168.

Finney, L. J., & Iannotti, R. J. (2001). The impact of family history of breast cancer on women's health beliefs, salience of breast cancer family history, and degree of involvement in breast cancer issues. *Women and Health, 33,* 15–28.

Foddy, W. H. (1993). *Constructing questions for interviews and questionnaires: Theory and practice in social research.* Cambridge: Cambridge University Press.

Foddy, W. H. (1998). An empirical evaluation of in-depth probes used to pretest survey questions. *Sociological Methods and Research, 27,* 103–133.

Ford, K., & Norris, A. (1991). Methodological considerations for survey research on sexual behavior: Urban African American and Hispanic youth. *Journal of Sex Research, 28,* 539–555.

Fowler, F. J. (1989). Coding behavior in pretests to identify unclear questions. In National Center for Health Services Research, *Health Survey Research Methods: Conference Proceedings* (ed. F. J. Fowler) (pp. 8–12). (DHHS Publication No. (PHS) 89-3447). Rockville, MD: National Center for Health Services Research.

Fowler, F. J. (1995). *Improving survey questions: Design and evaluation.* Thousand Oaks: Sage.

Fowler, F. J. (2002). *Survey research methods* (3rd ed.). Thousand Oaks, CA: Sage.

Fowler, F. J., Gallagher, P. M., Stringfellow, V. L., Zaslavsky, A. M., Thompson, J. W., & Cleary, P. D. (2002). Using telephone interviews to reduce nonresponse bias to mail surveys of health plan members. *Medical Care, 40,* 190–200.

Fowler, F. J., & Mangione, T. W. (1990). *Standardized survey interviewing: Minimizing interviewer-related error.* Thousand Oaks, CA: Sage.

Fowler, F. J., Roman, A. M., & Di, Z. X. (1998). Mode effects in a survey of Medicare prostate surgery patients. *Public Opinion Quarterly, 62,* 29–46.

Fowler, F. J., & Stringfellow, V. L. (2001). Learning from experience: Estimating teen use of alcohol, cigarettes, and marijuana from three survey protocols. *Journal of Drug Issues, 31,* 643–664.

Fox, J. A., & Tracy, P. E. (1986). *Randomized response: A method for sensitive surveys*. Thousand Oaks, CA: Sage.

Framingham.com. (1995). *The Framingham Heart Study*. Retrieved March 23, 2005, from http://www.framingham.com/heart/.

Frankel, M. R. (2004). RDD surveys: Past and future. In National Center for Health Statistics, *Eighth Conference on Health Survey Research Methods* (ed. S. B. Cohen & J. M. Lepkowski) (pp. 131–136). (DHHS Publication No. (PHS) 04-1013). Hyattsville, MD: National Center for Health Statistics.

Frankfort-Nachmias, C., & Nachmias, D. (2000). *Research methods in the social sciences* (6th ed.). New York: Worth.

Fremont, A. M., Bierman, A., Wickstrom, S. L., Bird, C. E., Shah, M., Escarce, J. J., et al. (2005). Use of geocoding in managed care settings to identify quality disparities: How indirect measures of race/ethnicity and socioeconomic status can be used by the nation's health plans to demonstrate disparities. *Health Affairs, 24*(2), 516–526.

Frey, J. H., & Fontana, A. (1991). The group interview in social research. *Social Science Journal, 28,* 175–187.

Frey, J. H., & Oishi, S. M. (1995). *How to conduct interviews by telephone and in person*. Thousand Oaks, CA: Sage.

Froberg, D. G., & Kane, R. L. (1989a). Methodology for measuring health-state preferences—1: Measurement strategies. *Journal of Clinical Epidemiology, 42,* 345–354.

Froberg, D. G., & Kane, R. L. (1989b). Methodology for measuring health-state preferences—2: Scaling methods. *Journal of Clinical Epidemiology, 42,* 459–471.

Froberg, D. G., & Kane, R. L. (1989c). Methodology for measuring health-state preferences—3: Population and context effects. *Journal of Clinical Epidemiology, 42,* 585–592.

Froberg, D. G., & Kane, R. L. (1989d). Methodology for measuring health-state preferences—4: Progress and a research agenda. *Journal of Clinical Epidemiology, 42,* 675–685.

Fuchs, M., Couper, M. P., & Hansen, S. E. (2000). Technology effects: Do CAPI or PAPI interviews take longer? *Journal of Official Statistics, 16,* 273–286.

Gallagher, P. M., & Fowler, F. J. (2004). Don't forget about personal interviewing. In National Center for Health Statistics, *Eighth Conference on Health Survey Research Methods* (ed. S. B. Cohen & J. M. Lepkowski) (pp. 155–158). (DHHS Publication No. (PHS) 04-1013). Hyattsville, MD: National Center for Health Statistics.

Gandek, B., & Ware, J. E. (1998). Methods for validating and norming translations of health status questionnaires: The IQOLA Project approach. International Quality of Life Assessment. *Journal of Clinical Epidemiology, 51,* 953–959.

Ganley, B. J., Young, M., Denny, G., & Wood, E. (1998). Fourth graders: Tobacco attitudes, behaviors, and knowledge. *American Journal of Health Behavior, 22,* 39–45.

Garry, M., Sharman, S. J., Feldman, J., Marlatt, G. A., & Loftus, E. F. (2002). Examining memory for heterosexual college students' sexual experiences using an electronic mail diary. *Health Psychology, 21,* 629–634.

Gaskell, G. D., O'Muircheartaigh, C. A., & Wright, D. B. (1994). Survey questions about the frequency of vaguely defined events: The effects of response alternatives. *Public Opinion Quarterly, 58,* 241–254.

Geer, J. G. (1991). Do open-ended questions measure "salient" issues? *Public Opinion Quarterly, 55,* 360–370.

Ghaderi, A. & Scott, B. (2002). The preliminary reliability and validity of the Survey for Eating Disorders (SEDs): A self-report questionnaire for diagnosing eating disorders. *European Eating Disorders Review, 10,* 61–76.

Giammattei, F. P. (2003). Implementing a total joint registry using personal digital assistants: A proof of concept. *Orthopaedic Nursing, 22,* 284–288.

Gill, T. M., & Feinstein, A. R. (1994). A critical appraisal of the quality of quality-of-life measurements. *Journal of the American Medical Association, 272,* 619–626.

Gilljam, M., & Granberg, D. (1993). Should we take don't know for an answer? *Public Opinion Quarterly, 57,* 348–357.

Glynn, C. J., Hayes, A. F., & Shanahan, J. (1997). Perceived support for one's opinions and willingness to speak out: A meta-analysis of survey studies on the "spiral of silence." *Public Opinion Quarterly, 61,* 452–463.

Gold, M., & Wooldridge, J. (1995). Plan-based surveys of satisfaction with access and quality of care: Review and critique. In Agency for Healthcare Policy and Research, *Consumer survey information in a reforming health care system* (pp. 75–109). (AHCPR Publication No. 95-0083). Rockville, MD: Agency for Healthcare Policy and Research.

Goldstein, M. S., Elliott, S. D., & Guccione, A. A. (2000). The development of an instrument to measure satisfaction with physical therapy. *Physical Therapy, 80,* 853–863.

Gordis, L. (2004). *Epidemiology* (3rd ed.). Philadelphia: Saunders.

Goyder, J. (1985). Face-to-face interviews and mailed questionnaires: The net difference in response rate. *Public Opinion Quarterly, 49,* 234–252.

Graesser, A. C., Kennedy, T., Wiemer-Hastings, P., & Ottati, V. (1999). The use of computational cogitative models to improve questions on surveys and questionnaires. In National Center for Health Statistics, *A new agenda for interdisciplinary survey research methods: Proceedings of the CASM II Seminar* (ed. M.G. Sirken, T. Jabine, G. Willis, E. Martin, & C. Tucker) (p. 28). Hyattsville, MD: National Center for Health Statistics.

Graham, C. A., Catania, J. A., Brand, R., Duong, B., & Canchola, J. A. (2003). Recalling sexual behavior: A methodological analysis of memory recall bias via interview using the diary as the gold standard. *Journal of Sex Research, 40,* 325–332.

Grembowski, D. (2001). *The practice of health program evaluation.* Thousand Oaks, CA: Sage.

Grembowski, D., Milgrom, P., & Fiset, L. (1990). Factors influencing variation in dentist service rates. *Journal of Public Health Dentistry, 50,* 244–250.

Groves, R. M. (1987). Research on survey data quality. *Public Opinion Quarterly, 51,* S156–S172.

Groves, R. M. (1989). *Survey errors and survey costs.* Hoboken, NJ: Wiley.

Groves, R. M. (1990). Theories and methods of telephone surveys. *Annual Review of Sociology, 16,* 221–240.

Groves, R. M., Biemer, P. P., Lyberg, L. E., Massey, J. T., Nicholls, W. L., & Waksberg, J. (Eds). (1988). *Telephone survey methodology.* Hoboken, NJ: Wiley.

Groves, R. M., Cialdini, R. B., & Couper, M. P. (1992). Understanding the decision to participate in a survey. *Public Opinion Quarterly, 56,* 475–495.

Groves, R. M., & Couper, M. P. (1998). *Nonresponse in household interview surveys.* Hoboken, NJ: Wiley.

Groves, R. M., Dillman, D. A., Eltinge, J. L., & Little, R.J.A. (Eds). (2002). *Survey nonresponse.* Hoboken, NJ: Wiley.

Groves, R. M., & Kahn, R. L. (1979). *Surveys by telephone: A national comparison with personal interviews.* New York: Academic Press.

Groves, R. M., & Nicholls, W. L., II (1986). Computer-assisted telephone interviewing: Part II—Data quality issues. *Journal of Official Statistics, 2,* 117–134.

Groves, R. M., Singer, E., & Corning, A. (2000). Leverage-saliency theory of survey participation: Description and an illustration. *Public Opinion Quarterly, 64,* 299–308.

Gubrium, J. F., & Holstein, J. A. (Eds). (2002). *Handbook of interview research: Context and method.* Thousand Oaks, CA: Sage.

Gunn, H. (2002, December). Web-based surveys: Changing the survey process. *First Monday, 7*(12). Retrieved July 25, 2004, from http://www.firstmonday.dk/issues/issue7_12/gunn/.

Gwiasda, V., Taluc, N., & Popkin, S. J. (1997). Data collection in dangerous neighborhoods: Lessons from a survey of public housing residents in Chicago. *Evaluation Review, 21,* 77–93.

Gwyer, P., & Clifford, B. R. (1997). The effects of the cognitive interview on recall, identification, confidence and the confidence/accuracy relationship. *Applied Cognitive Psychology, 11,* 121–145.

Hagan, D. E., & Collier, C. M. (1983). Must respondent selection procedures for telephone surveys be invasive? *Public Opinion Quarterly, 47,* 547–556.

Haley, S. M., McHorney, C. A., & Ware, J. E. (1994). Evaluation of the MOS SF-36 physical functioning scale (PF10): I. Unidimensionality and reproducibility of the Rasch Item Scale. *Journal of Clinical Epidemiology, 47,* 671–684.

Hambleton, R. K., Swaminathan, H., & Rogers, H. J. (1991). *Fundamentals of item response theory.* Thousand Oaks, CA: Sage.

Hanley, J. A. (1983). Appropriate uses of multivariate analysis. *Annual Review of Public Health, 4,* 155–180.

Harkness, J. A. (2004). Problems in establishing conceptually equivalent health definitions across multiple cultural groups. In National Center for Health Statistics, *Eighth Conference on Health Survey Research Methods* (ed. S. B. Cohen & J. M. Lepkowski) (pp. 85–90). (DHHS Publication No. (PHS) 04-1013). Hyattsville, MD: National Center for Health Statistics.

Harkness, J. A., van de Vijver, F.J.R., & Mohler, P. P. (Eds.). (2003). *Cross-cultural survey methods.* Hoboken, NJ: Wiley.

Harpole, L. H., Samsa, G. P., Jurgelski, A. E., Shipley, J. L., Bernstein, A., & Matchar, D. B. (2003). Headache management program improves outcome for chronic headache. *Headache, 43,* 715–724.

Harris, K. W. (1996). Data editing at the National Center for Health Statistics. In Federal Committee on Statistical Methodology (Ed.), *Data Editing Workshop and Exposition* (pp. 24–38). Washington, DC: Statistical Policy Office.

Harris-Kojetin, L. D., Fowler, F. J., Brown, J. A., Schnaier, J. A., & Sweeny, S. F. (1999). The use of cognitive testing to develop and evaluate CAHPS 1.0 core survey items. *Medical Care, 37,* MS10–MS21.

Hatfield, A. B. (1997). Families of adults with severe mental illness: New directions in research. *American Journal of Orthopsychiatry, 67,* 254–260.

Hay, D. A. (1990). Does the method matter on sensitive survey topics? *Survey Methodology, 16,* 131–136.

Hays, R. D., Larson, C., Nelson, E. C., & Batalden, P. B. (1991). Hospital quality trends: A short-form patient-based measure. *Medical Care, 29,* 661–668.

Health Utilities Group. (2005, January 12). *Health Utilities Index.* Retrieved May 31, 2005, from http://www.fhs.mcmaster.ca/hug/.

Heckathorn, D. D. (1997). Respondent-driven sampling: A new approach to the study of hidden populations. *Social Problems, 44,* 174–199.

Heckathorn, D. D. (2002). Respondent-driven sampling II: Deriving valid population estimates from chain-referral samples of hidden populations. *Social Problems, 49,* 11–34.

Hennekens, C. H., & Buring, J. E. (1987). *Epidemiology in medicine.* New York: Little, Brown.

Hennigan, K. M., Maxson, C. L., Sloane, D., & Ranney, M. (2002). Community views on crime, and policing: Survey mode effects on bias in community surveys. *Justice Quarterly, 19,* 565–587.

Hernandez, B., Keys, C., & Balcazar, F. (2003). The Americans with Disabilities Act Knowledge Survey: Strong psychometrics and weak knowledge. *Rehabilitation Psychology, 48,* 93–99.

Highland, K. B., Strange, C., Mazur, J., & Simpson, K. N. (2003). Treatment of pulmonary arterial hypertension: A preliminary decision analysis. *Chest, 124,* 2087–2092.

Hippler, H.-J., & Hippler, G. (1986). Reducing refusal rates in the case of threatening questions: The "door-in-the-face" technique. *Journal of Official Statistics, 2,* 25–33.

Hippler, H.-J., & Schwarz, N. (1986). Not forbidding isn't allowing: The cognitive basis of the forbid-allow asymmetry. *Public Opinion Quarterly, 50,* 87–96.

Hippler, H.-J., & Schwarz, N. (1989). "No opinion" filters: A cognitive perspective. *International Journal of Public Opinion Research, 1,* 77–87.

Hippler, H.-J., Schwarz, N., & Sudman, S. (Eds). (1987). *Social information processing and survey methodology.* New York: Springer-Verlag.

Hirschi, T., & Selvin, H. C. (1996). *Delinquency research: An appraisal of analytic methods* (New ed.). New Brunswick, NJ: Transaction Publishers.

Holbrook, A. L., Green, M. C., & Krosnick, J. A. (2003). Telephone versus face-to-face interviewing of national probability samples with long questionnaires: Comparisons of respondent satisficing and social desirability response bias. *Public Opinion Quarterly, 67,* 79–125.

Hornik, J., Zaig, T., Shadmon, D., & Barbash, G. I. (1990). Comparison of three inducement techniques to improve compliance in a health survey conducted by telephone. *Public Health Reports, 105,* 524–529.

Hosmer, D. W., & Lemeshow, S. (2000). *Applied logistic regression* (2nd ed.). Hoboken, NJ: Wiley.

House, C. C. (1985). Questionnaire design with computer-assisted telephone interviewing. *Journal of Official Statistics, 1,* 219.

Houtkoop-Steenstra, H. (2000). *Interaction and the standardized survey interview: The living questionnaire.* Cambridge: Cambridge University Press.

Hox, J., & de Leeuw, E. (2002). The influence of interviewers' attitude and behavior on household survey nonresponse: An international comparison. In R. M. Groves, D. A. Dillman, J. L. Eltinge, & R.J.A. Little (Eds.), *Survey nonresponse* (pp. 103–120). Hoboken, NJ: Wiley.

Hudak, P. L., & Wright, J. G. (2000). The characteristics of patient satisfaction measures. *Spine, 25,* 3167–3177.

Huff, D. (1993). *How to lie with statistics.* New York: Norton.

Hulka, B. S., Zyzanski, S. J., Cassel, J. C., & Thompson, S. J. (1970). Scale for the measurement of attitudes toward physicians and primary medical care. *Medical Care, 8,* 429–436.

Hulley, S. B., Cummings, S. R., Browner, W. S., Grady, D., Hearst, N., & Newman, T. B. (2001). *Designing clinical research: An epidemiological approach* (2nd ed.). Philadelphia: Lippincott Williams & Wilkins.

Hung, K., & Heeler, R. (1998). Bilinguals' brand perceptions reported on different-language questionnaires. *Advances in Consumer Research, 25,* 246–251.

Hunt, S. D., Sparkman, R. D., & Wilcox, J. B. (1982). The pretest in survey research: Issues and preliminary findings. *Journal of Marketing Research, 19,* 269–273.

Hunt, S. M., & McEwen, J. (1980). The development of a subjective health indicator. *Sociology of Health and Illness, 2,* 231–246.

Hunt, S. M., McEwen, J., & McKenna, S. P. (1992). Nottingham Health Profile: "English." In D. Wilkin, L. Hallam, & M.-A. Doggett (Eds.), *Measures of need and outcome for primary health care* (pp. 142–146). New York: Oxford University Press.

Hunt, S. M., McKenna, S. P., McEwen, J., Williams, J., & Papp, E. (1981). The Nottingham health profile: Subjective health-status and medical consultations. *Social Science and Medicine Part A—Medical Sociology, 15,* 221–229.

Hurst, N. P., Ruta, D. A., & Kind, P. (1998). Comparison of the MOS Short Form-12 (SF12) health status questionnaire with the SF36 in patients with rheumatoid arthritis. *British Journal of Rheumatology, 37,* 862–869.

Hurtado, A. (1994). Does similarity breed respect? Interviewer evaluations of Mexican-descent respondents in a bilingual survey. *Public Opinion Quarterly, 58,* 77–95.

Huttenlocher, J., Hedges, L. V., & Bradburn, N. M. (1990). Reports of elapsed time: Bounding and rounding processes in estimation. *Journal of Experimental Psychology: Learning Memory and Cognition, 16,* 196–213.

Hyman, H. H. (1955). *Survey design and analysis: Principles, cases, and procedures.* New York: Free Press.

Hyman, H. H. (1991). *Taking society's measure: A personal history of survey research.* New York: Russell Sage Foundation.

Im, E. O., & Chee, W. (2004). Issues in an Internet survey among midlife Asian women. *Health Care for Women International, 25,* 150–164.

Imperial College London. (2004). *MRC National Survey of Health and Development NSHD.* Retrieved May 29, 2005, from http://www1.imperial.ac.uk/medicine/about/divisions/pcphs/eph/projects/cdel/euroblcs/cohorts/nshd.html.

Institute of Medicine, Committee on Understanding and Eliminating Racial and Ethnic Disparities in Health Care. (2003). *Unequal treatment: Confronting racial and ethnic disparities in health care* (ed. B. D. Smedley, A. Y. Stith, & A. R. Nelson). Washington, DC: National Academies Press.

Inter-University Corsortium for Political and Social Research. (n.d.). *Search results: Alameda County [California] Health and Ways of Living Panels.* Retrieved May 29, 2005, from http://search.icpsr.umich.edu/ICPSR/query.html?nh=25&rf=0&ws=0&ty0=w&tx0=alameda+county+ways+of+living+study&fl0=&col=website&col=abstract&col=series&col=uncat&op0=%2B&tx1=ICPSR&op1=%2B&fl1=archive%3A&ty1=w&tx2=restricted&op2=-&fl2=availability%3A&ty2=w.

Israel, B. A., Schulz, A. J., Parker, E. A., & Becker, A. B. (1998). Review of community-based research: Assessing partnership approaches to improve public health. *Annual Review of Public Health, 19,* 173–202.

Ivanov, L. L. (2000). Use of a Western theoretical model to investigate the relationships among characteristics of pregnant women, utilization, and satisfaction with prenatal care services in St. Petersburg, Russia. *Public Health Nursing, 17,* 111–120.

Jackson, J. L., & Kroenke, K. (1997). Patient satisfaction and quality of care. *Military Medicine, 162,* 273–277.

James, J. M., & Bolstein, R. (1990). The effect of monetary incentives and follow-up mailings on the response rate and response quality in mail surveys. *Public Opinion Quarterly, 54,* 346–361.

Janda, L. H., Janda, M., & Tedford, E. (2001). IVR Test and Survey: A computer program to collect data via computerized telephonic applications. *Behavior Research Methods Instruments & Computers, 33,* 513–516.

Jobe, J. B. (2003). Cognitive psychology and self-reports: Models and methods. *Quality of Life Research, 12,* 219–227.

Jobe, J. B., Tourangeau, R., & Smith, A. F. (1993). Contributions of survey research to the understanding of memory. *Applied Cognitive Psychology, 7,* 567–584.

Jobe, J. B., White, A. A., Kelley, C. L., Mingay, D. J., Sanchez, M. J., & Loftus, E. F. (1990). Recall strategies and memory for health care visits. *Milbank Quarterly, 68,* 171–189.

Johnson, M. F., Sallis, J. F., & Hovell, M. F. (2000). Self-report assessment of walking: Effects of aided recall instructions and item order. *Measurement in Physical Education and Exercise Science, 4,* 141–155.

Johnson, T. P., Jobe, J. B., O'Rourke, D., Sudman, S., Warnecke, R. B., Chavez, N. et al. (1997). Dimensions of self-identification among multiracial and multiethnic respondents in survey interviews. *Evaluation Review, 21,* 671–687.

Jones, C. P., LaVeist, T. A., & Lillie-Blanton, M. (1991). Race in the epidemiologic literature: An examination of the American Journal of Epidemiology, 1921–1990. *American Journal of Epidemiology, 134,* 1079–1084.

Jones, S. G. (Ed). (1999). *Doing Internet research: Critical issues and methods for examining the Net.* Thousand Oaks, CA: Sage.

Jones, S. L. (1996). The association between objective and subjective caregiver burden. *Archives of Psychiatric Nursing, 10,* 77–84.

Jöreskog, K. G. (2000). *LISREL 8: New statistical features.* Lincolnwood, IL: Scientific Software International.

Jöreskog, K. G., Cudeck, R., du Toit, S., & Sörbom, D. (Eds.). (2001). *Structural equation modelling, present and future: A festschrift in honor of Karl J. Jöreskog.* Lincolnwood, IL: Scientific Software International.

Jöreskog, K. G., & Sörbom, D. (1996). *LISREL 8 user's reference guide* (2nd ed.). Chicago: Scientific Software International.

Jorgensen, D. L. (1989). *Participant observation: A methodology for human studies.* Thousand Oaks, CA: Sage.

Kahn, H. A., & Sempos, C. T. (1989). *Statistical methods in epidemiology.* New York: Oxford University Press.

Kahn, R. L., & Cannell, C. F. (1957). *The dynamics of interviewing: Theory, technique, and cases.* Hoboken, NJ: Wiley.

Kalsbeek, W. D. (2003). Sampling minority groups in health surveys. *Statistics in Medicine, 22,* 1527–1549.

Kalton, G. (1983). *Introduction to survey sampling.* Thousand Oaks, CA: Sage.

Kalton, G., & Anderson, D. W. (1986). Sampling rare populations. *Journal of the Royal Statistical Society Series A-Statistics in Society, 149,* 65–82.

Kalton, G., & Kasprzyk, D. (1986). The treatment of missing survey data. *Survey Methodology, 12,* 1–16.

Kane, R. L. (Ed.). (2004). *Understanding health care outcomes research* (2nd ed.). Boston: Jones and Bartlett.

Kanji, G. K. (1999). *100 statistical tests* (New ed.). Thousand Oaks, CA: Sage.

Kanouse, D. E., Berry, S. H., Duan, N., Lever, J., Carson, S., Perlman, J. F., et al. (1999). Drawing a probability sample of female street prostitutes in Los Angeles County. *Journal of Sex Research, 36,* 45–51.

Kaplan, R. M. (1989). Health outcome models for policy analysis. *Health Psychology, 8,* 723–735.

Kaplan, R. M., & Anderson, J. P. (1988). A general health policy model: Update and applications. *Health Services Research, 23,* 203–235.

Katz, S., Ford, A. B., Moskowitz, R. W., Jackson, B. A., & Jaffe, M. W. (1963). Studies of illness in the aged. The Index of ADL: A standardized measure of biological and psychosocial function. *Journal of the American Medical Association, 185,* 914–919.

Keeter, S. (1995). Estimating telephone noncoverage bias with a telephone survey. *Public Opinion Quarterly, 59,* 196–217.

Keeter, S., Miller, C., Kohut, A., Groves, R. M., & Presser, S. (2000). Consequences of reducing nonresponse in a national telephone survey. *Public Opinion Quarterly, 64,* 125–148.

Kehoe, C. M., & Pitkow, J. E. (1996). Surveying the territory: GVU's five WWW user surveys. *World Wide Web Journal, 1*(3), 77–84. Retrieved July 16, 2004, from http://www.cc.gatech.edu/gvu/user_surveys/papers/w3j.pdf.

Keith, R. A. (1994). Functional status and health status. *Archives of Physical Medicine and Rehabilitation, 75,* 478–483.

Kenagy, G. P. (2005). Transgender health: Findings from two needs assessment studies in Philadelphia. *Health and Social Work, 30,* 19–26.

Kiecolt, K. J., & Nathan, L. E. (1985). *Secondary analysis of survey data.* Thousand Oaks, CA: Sage.

Kiesler, S., & Sproull, L. S. (1986). Response effects in the electronic survey. *Public Opinion Quarterly, 50,* 402–413.

Kindig, D., & Stoddart, G. (2003). What is population health? *American Journal of Public Health, 93,* 380–383.

Kirshner, B., & Guyatt, G. (1985). A methodological framework for assessing health indexes. *Journal of Chronic Diseases, 38,* 27–36.

Kirsner, R. S., & Federman, D. G. (1997). Patient satisfaction: Quality of care from the patients' perspective. *Archives of Dermatology, 133,* 1427–1431.

Kish, L. (1965). *Survey sampling.* Hoboken, NJ: Wiley.

Kleinbaum, D. G. (2003). *ActivEpi* [CD-ROM]. New York: Springer.

Kleinbaum, D. G., Klein, M., & Pryor, E. R. (2002). *Logistic regression: A self-learning text* (2nd ed.). New York: Springer.

Kluegel, J. R. (1990). Trends in whites' explanations of the black-white gap in socioeconomic status, 1977–1989. *American Sociological Review, 55,* 512–525.

Knäuper, B. (1999). The impact of age and education on response order effects in attitude measurement. *Public Opinion Quarterly, 63,* 347–370.

Kneipp, S. M., & Yarandi, H. N. (2002). Complex sampling designs and statistical issues in secondary analysis. *Western Journal of Nursing Research, 24,* 552–566.

Knoke, D., Bohrnstedt, G. W., & Mee, A. P. (2002). *Statistics for social data analysis* (4th ed.). Itasca, IL: F. E. Peacock.

Kohlmeier, L. (1994). Gaps in dietary assessment methodology: Meal-based versus list-based methods. *American Journal of Clinical Nutrition, 59* (Suppl.), S175–S179.

Korn, E. L., & Graubard, B. I. (1991). Epidemiologic studies utilizing surveys: Accounting for the sampling design. *American Journal of Public Health, 81,* 1166–1173.

Korn, E. L., & Graubard, B. I. (1995). Analysis of large health surveys: Accounting for the sampling design. *Journal of the Royal Statistical Society: Series A. Statistics in Society, 158*(Pt. 2), 263–295.

Kosinski, M., Bjorner, J. B., Ware, J. E., Batenhorst, A., & Cady, R. K. (2003). The responsiveness of headache impact scales scored using "classical" and "modern" psychometric methods: A re-analysis of three clinical trials. *Quality of Life Research, 12,* 903–912.

Kraemer, H. C., & Thiemann, S. (1987). *How many subjects? Statistical power analysis in research.* Thousand Oaks, CA: Sage.

Kreft, I.G.G. (1995). Hierarchical linear models: Problems and prospects. *Journal of Educational and Behavioral Statistics, 20,* 109–113.

Krieger, N., Chen, J. T., Waterman, P. D., Rehkopf, D. H., & Subramanian, S. V. (2003). Race/ethnicity, gender, and monitoring socioeconomic gradients in health: A comparison of area-based socioeconomic measures—The Public Health Disparities Geocoding Project. *American Journal of Public Health, 93,* 1655–1671.

Kristal, A. R., White, E., Davis, J. R., Corycell, G., Raghunathan, T., Kinne, S., et al. (1993). Effects of enhanced calling efforts on response rates, estimates of health behavior, and costs in a telephone health survey using random-digit dialing. *Public Health Reports, 108,* 372–379.

Krosnick, J. A. (1991). Response strategies for coping with the cognitive demands of attitude measures in surveys. *Applied Cognitive Psychology, 5,* 213–236.

Krosnick, J. A. (2002). The causes of no-opinion responses to attitude measures in surveys: They are rarely what they appear to be. In R. M. Groves, D. A. Dillman, J. L. Eltinge, & R.J.A. Little (Eds.), *Survey nonresponse* (pp. 87–100). Hoboken, NJ: Wiley.

Krosnick, J. A., & Alwin, D. F. (1987). An evaluation of a cognitive theory of response-order effects in survey measurement. *Public Opinion Quarterly, 51,* 201–219.

Krosnick, J. A., Holbrook, A. L., Berent, M. K., Carson, R. T., Hanemann, W. M., Kopp, R. J., et al. (2002). The impact of "no opinion" response options on data quality: Non-attitude reduction or an invitation to satisfice? *Public Opinion Quarterly, 66,* 371–403.

Krueger, R. A., & Casey, M. A. (2000). *Focus groups: A practical guide for applied research* (3rd ed.). Thousand Oaks, CA: Sage.

Ksobiech, K., Somlai, A. M., Kelly, J. A., Benotsch, E., Gore-Felton, C., McAuliffe, T., et al. (2004). Characteristics and HIV risk behaviors among injection drug users in St. Petersburg, Russia: A comparison of needle exchange program attenders and nonattenders. *Journal of Drug Issues, 34,* 787–803.

Kuechler, M. (1998). The survey method: An indispensable tool for social science research everywhere? *American Behavioral Scientist, 42,* 178–200.

Kukulska-Hulme, A. (2002). *Cognitive, ergonomic and affective aspects of PDA use for learning.* Retrieved July 25, 2004, from http://iet.open.ac.uk/pp/a.m.kukulska-hulme/PDAsBirmingham.htm.

Kurbat, M. A., Shevell, S. K., & Rips, L. J. (1998). A year's memories: The calendar effect in autobiographical recall. *Memory and Cognition, 26,* 532–552.

Kutner, M. H., Nachtsheim, C. J., Neter, J., & Li, W. (2005). *Applied linear statistical models* (5th ed.). New York: McGraw-Hill Irwin.

Kuusela, V., & Simpanen, M. (2005, March). *Effects of mobile phones on telephone survey practices and results.* Retrieved May 30, 2005, from http://icis.dk/ICIS_papers/A_2_3.pdf.

Landsheer, J. A., van der Heijden, P., & van Gils, G. (1999). Trust and understanding, two psychological aspects of randomized response: A study of a method for improving the estimate of social security fraud. *Quality and Quantity, 33,* 1–12.

Laroche, M., Kim, C., & Tomiuk, M. A. (1998). Translation fidelity: An IRT analysis of Likert-type scale items from a culture change measure for Italian-Canadians. *Advances in Consumer Research, 25,* 240–245.

Laroche, M., Kim, C., & Tomiuk, M. A. (1999). IRT-based item level analysis: An additional diagnostic tool for scale purification. *Advances in Consumer Research, 26,* 141–149.

Larson, J. S. (1991). *The measurement of health: Concepts and indicators.* Westport, CT: Greenwood Press.

Last, J. M., Spasoff, R. A., Harris, S. S., & Thuriaux, M. C. (Eds.). (2001). *A dictionary of epidemiology* (4th ed.). New York: Oxford University Press.

Lavine, H., Huff, J. W., Wagner, S. H., & Sweeney, D. (1998). The moderating influence of attitude strength on the susceptibility to context effects in attitude surveys. *Journal of Personality and Social Psychology, 75,* 359–373.

Lavizzo-Mourey, R. J., Zinn, J., & Taylor, L. (1992). Ability of surrogates to represent satisfaction of nursing home residents with quality of care. *Journal of the American Geriatrics Society, 40,* 39–47.

Lavrakas, P. J. (1993). *Telephone survey methods: Sampling, selection, and supervision* (2nd ed.). Thousand Oaks, CA: Sage.

Lavrakas, P. J., Stasny, E. A., & Harpuder, B. (2000). A further investigation of the last-birthday respondent selection method and within-unit coverage error. *Proceedings of the American Statistical Association Section on Survey Research Methods.* Retrieved May 30, 2005, from http://www.amstat.org/sections/SRMS/Proceedings/papers/2000_152.pdf.

Leal, D. L., & Hess, F. M. (1999). Survey bias on the front porch: Are all subjects interviewed equally? *American Politics Quarterly, 27,* 468–487.

Lee, E. S., Forthofer, R. N., & Lorimor, R. J. (1986). Analysis of complex sample survey data: Problems and strategies. *Sociological Methods and Research, 15,* 69–100.

Lee, E. S., Forthofer, R. N., & Lorimor, R. J. (1989). *Analyzing complex survey data.* Thousand Oaks, CA: Sage.

Lee, L., Brittingham, A., Tourangeau, R., Willis, G., Ching, P., Jobe, J., et al. (1999). Are reporting errors due to encoding limitations or retrieval failure? Surveys of child vaccination as a case study. *Applied Cognitive Psychology, 13,* 43–63.

Lee, R. M. (1993). *Doing research on sensitive topics.* Thousand Oaks, CA: Sage.

Lemeshow, S., Hosmer, D. W., Jr., Klar, J., & Lwanga, S. K. (1990). *Adequacy of sample size in health studies.* Hoboken, NJ: Wiley.

Lepkowski, J. M. (1988). Telephone sampling methods in the United States. In R. M. Groves, P. P. Biemer, L. E. Lyberg, W. L. Massey, W. L. Nicholls II, & J. Waksberg (Eds.), *Telephone survey methodology* (pp. 73–98). Hoboken, NJ: Wiley.

Lessler, J. T. (1995). Choosing questions that people can understand and answer. *Medical Care, 33*(Suppl. 4), AS203–AS208.

Lessler, J. T., & Kalsbeek, W. D. (1992). *Nonsampling error in surveys.* Hoboken, NJ: Wiley.

Levy, P. S., & Lemeshow, S. (1999). *Sampling of populations: Methods and applications* (3rd ed.). Hoboken, NJ: Wiley.

Lewis, C. E., Freeman, H. E., & Corey, C. R. (1987). AIDS-related competence of California primary care physicians. *American Journal of Public Health, 77,* 795–799.

Lewis, J. R. (1994). Patient views on quality care in general practice: Literature review. *Social Science and Medicine, 39*, 655–670.

Lindley, L. L., Nicholson, T. J., Kerby, M. B., & Lu, N. (2003). HIV/STI-associated risk behaviors among self-identified lesbian, gay, bisexual, and transgender college students in the United States. *AIDS Education and Prevention, 15*, 413–429.

Link, B. G., & Phelan, J. (1995). Social conditions as fundamental causes of disease. *Journal of Health and Social Behavior* [Special issue], 80–94.

Link, M. W., & Mokdad, A. (2004). Are Web and mail modes feasible options for the Behavioral Risk Factor Surveillance System? In National Center for Health Statistics, *Eighth Conference on Health Survey Research Methods* (ed. S. B. Cohen & J. M. Lepkowski) (pp. 149–154). (DHHS Publication No. (PHS) 04-1013). Hyattsville, MD: National Center for Health Statistics.

Link, M. W., & Oldendick, R. W. (1999). Call screening: Is it really a problem for survey research? *Public Opinion Quarterly, 63*, 577–589.

Lipsey, M. W. (1990). *Design sensitivity: Statistical power for experimental research.* Thousand Oaks, CA: Sage.

Little, R.J.A., & Rubin, D. B. (1989). The analysis of social science data with missing values. *Sociological Methods and Research, 18*, 292–326.

Little, R.J.A., & Rubin, D. B. (2002). *Statistical analysis with missing data* (2nd ed.). Hoboken, NJ: Wiley.

Locander, W. B., & Burton, J. P. (1976). Effect of question form on gathering income data by telephone. *Journal of Marketing Research, 13*, 189–192.

Locke, L. F., Spirduso, W. W., & Silverman, S. J. (2000). *Proposals that work: A guide for planning dissertations and grant proposals* (4th ed.). Thousand Oaks, CA: Sage.

Loftus, E. F., Klinger, M. R., Smith, K. D., & Fiedler, J. (1990). A tale of two questions: Benefits of asking more than one question. *Public Opinion Quarterly, 54*, 330–345.

Loo, R., & Thorpe, K. (2000). Confirmatory factor analyses of the full and short versions of the Marlowe-Crowne Social Desirability Scale. *Journal of Social Psychology, 140*, 628–635.

Losch, M. E., Maitland, A., Lutz, G., Mariolis, P., & Gleason, S. C. (2002). The effect of time of year of data collection on sample efficiency: An analysis of behavioral risk factor surveillance survey data. *Public Opinion Quarterly, 66*, 594–607.

Luna, D., & Peracchio, L. A. (1999). What's in a bilingual's mind? How bilingual consumers process information. *Advances in Consumer Research, 26*, 306–311.

Lwanga, S. K., & Lemeshow, S. (1991). *Sample size determination in health studies: A practical manual.* Geneva, Switzerland: World Health Organization.

Lyberg, L. E., Biemer, P., Collins, M., de Leeuw, E., Dippo, C., Schwarz, N., et al. (Eds.). (1997). *Survey measurement and process quality.* Hoboken, NJ: Wiley.

Ma, G. X., Yajia, L., Edwards, R. L., Shive, S. E., & Chau, T. (2004). Evaluation of a culturally tailored smoking prevention program for Asian American youth. *Journal of Alcohol and Drug Education, 48*, 17–38.

Madow, W. G., Nisselson, H., Olkin, I., & Rubin, D. B. (Eds.). (1983). *Incomplete data in sample surveys.* Orlando, FL: Academic Press.

Magaziner, J., Bassett, S. S., Hebel, J. R., & Gruber-Baldini, A. (1996). Use of proxies to measure health and functional status in epidemiologic studies of community-dwelling women aged 65 years and older. *American Journal of Epidemiology, 143*, 283–292.

Magaziner, J., Simonsick, E. M., Kashner, T. M., & Hebel, J. R. (1988). Patient proxy response comparability on measures of patient health and functional status. *Journal of Clinical Epidemiology, 41,* 1065–1074.

Magaziner, J., Zimmerman, S. I., Gruber-Baldini, A. L., Hebel, J. R., & Fox, K. M. (1997). Proxy reporting in five areas of functional status: Comparison with self-reports and observations of performance. *American Journal of Epidemiology, 146,* 418–428.

Malec, D. (1995). Model-based state estimates from the National Health Interview Survey. In W. Schaible (Ed.), *Indirect estimators in U.S. federal programs* (pp. 145–167). New York: Springer.

Mangione, T. W. (1995). *Mail surveys: Improving the quality.* Thousand Oaks, CA: Sage.

Marcus, A. C., & Crane, L. A. (1986). Telephone surveys in public health research. *Medical Care, 24,* 97–112.

Marín, G., & Marín, B. V. (1991). *Research with Hispanic populations.* Thousand Oaks, CA: Sage.

Marín, G., Vanoss, B., & Perez-Stable, E. J. (1990). Feasibility of a telephone survey to study a minority community: Hispanics in San Francisco. *American Journal of Public Health, 80,* 323–326.

Marker, D. A., Judkins, D. R., & Winglee, M. (2002). Large-scale imputation for complex surveys. In R. M. Groves, D. A. Dillman, J. L. Eltinge, & R.J.A. Little (Eds.), *Survey nonresponse* (pp. 329–342). Hoboken, NJ: Wiley.

MarketTools. (1999). *Zoomerang homepage.* Retrieved June 15, 2005, from http://info.zoomerang.com.

Marks, R. G. (1982). *Designing a research project: The basics of biomedical research methodology.* New York: Van Nostrand.

Markus, H., & Zajonc, R. B. (1985). The cognitive perspective in social psychology. In G. Lindzey & E. Aronson (Eds.), *Handbook of social psychology* (3rd ed., pp. 137–230). New York: Random House.

Marshall, G. N., Hays, R. D., Sherbourne, C. D., & Wells, K. B. (1993). The structure of patient satisfaction with outpatient medical care. *Psychological Assessment, 5,* 477–483.

Martin, D., & Moore, J. (1999). Income measurement. In National Center for Health Statistics, *A New Agenda for Interdisciplinary Survey Research Methods: Proceedings of the CASM II Seminar* (ed. M. G. Sirken, T. Jabine, G. Willis, E. Martin, & C. Tucker) (pp. 62–66). Hyattsville, MD: National Center for Health Statistics.

Martin, J., Anderson, J., Romans, S., Mullen, P., & O'Shea, M. (1993). Asking about child sexual abuse: Methodological implications of a two-stage survey. *Child Abuse and Neglect, 17,* 383–392.

Martin, J., O'Muircheartaigh, C., & Curtice, J. (1993). The use of CAPI for attitude surveys: An experimental comparison with traditional methods. *Journal of Official Statistics, 9,* 641–661.

Mason, R., Carlson, J. E., & Tourangeau, R. (1994). Contrast effects and subtraction in part-whole questions. *Public Opinion Quarterly, 58,* 569–578.

Mays, V. M., & Jackson, J. S. (1991). AIDS survey methodology with black Americans. *Social Science and Medicine, 33,* 47–54.

McCarthy, J. S., & Safer, M. A. (2000). Remembering heads and bushels: Cognitive processes involved in agricultural establishments' reports of inventories. *Journal of Official Statistics, 16,* 419–434.

McDonald, R. P. (1999). *Test theory: A unified treatment.* Mahwah, NJ: Erlbaum.

McDowell, I., & Newell, C. (1996). *Measuring health: A guide to rating scales and questionnaires* (2nd ed.). New York: Oxford University Press.

McEwan, R. T., Harrington, B. E., Bhopal, R. S., Madhok, R., & McCallum, A. (1992). Social surveys in HIV/AIDS: Telling or writing? A comparison of interview and postal methods. *Health Education Research, 7,* 195–202.

McGovern, P. D., & Bushery, J. M. (1999). Data mining the CPS reinterview: Digging into response error. In Federal Committee on Statistical Methodology (Ed.), *Federal Committee on Statistical Methodology Research Conference [Proceedings—Monday B sessions]* (pp. 76–85). Washington, DC: Statistical Policy Office.

McGraw, S. A., McKinlay, J. B., Crawford, S. A., Costa, L. A., & Cohen, D. L. (1992). Health survey methods with minority populations: Some lessons from recent experience. *Ethnicity and Disease, 2,* 273–287.

McHorney, C. A., & Cohen, A. S. (2000). Equating health status measures with item response theory: Illustrations with functional status items. *Medical Care, 38*(Suppl. 2), 43–59.

McHorney, C. A., Haley, S. M., & Ware, J. E. (1997). Evaluation of the MOS SF-36 physical functioning scale (PF-10): II. Comparison of relative precision using Likert and Rasch scoring methods. *Journal of Clinical Epidemiology, 50,* 451–461.

McHorney, C. A., Ware, J. E., Lu, J.F.R., & Sherbourne, C. D. (1994). The MOS 36-item short-form health survey (SF-36): III. Tests of data quality, scaling assumptions, and reliability across diverse patient groups. *Medical Care, 32,* 40–66.

McHorney, C. A., Ware, J. E., & Raczek, A. E. (1993). The MOS 36-item short-form health survey (SF-36): II. Psychometric and clinical tests of validity in measuring physical and mental health constructs. *Medical Care, 31,* 247–263.

Means, B., & Loftus, E. F. (1991). When personal history repeats itself: Decomposing memories for recurring events. *Applied Cognitive Psychology, 5,* 297–318.

Measurement Excellence and Training Resource Information Center. (n.d.). *Patient Judgment System (PJS).* Retrieved June 6, 2005, from http://www.measurementexperts.org/instrument/instrument_reviews.asp?detail=31.

Medical Outcomes Trust. (2001, July). *Instruments.* Retrieved May 31, 2005, from http://www.outcomes-trust.org/instruments.htm.

Mellor, A. C., & Milgrom, P. (1995). Dentists' attitudes toward frustrating patient visits: Relationship to satisfaction and malpractice complaints. *Community Dentistry and Oral Epidemiology, 23,* 15–19.

Menon, G., Bickart, B., Sudman, S., & Blair, J. (1995). How well do you know your partner? Strategies for formulating proxy-reports and their effects on convergence to self-reports. *Journal of Marketing Research, 32,* 75–84.

Mercator Research Group. (2005). *SnapSurveys.* Retrieved June 8, 2005, from http://www.snapsurveys.com/software/.

Mertler, C. (2002). Demonstrating the potential for Web-based survey methodology with a case study. *American Secondary Education, 30,* 49–61.

Merton, R. K., Fiske, M., & Kendall, P. L. (1990). *The focused interview: A manual of problems and procedures* (2nd ed.). New York: Free Press.

Meterko, M., Nelson, E. C., & Rubin, H. R. (1990). Patient judgments of hospital quality: Report of a pilot study [Entire issue]. *Medical Care, 28*(Suppl.).

Michaels, S., & Giami, A. (1999). The polls—Review sexual acts and sexual relationships: Asking about sex in surveys. *Public Opinion Quarterly, 63,* 401–420.

Microsoft Corporation. (2005). *Word 2003*. Retrieved May 23, 2005, from http://office. microsoft.com/en-us/FX010857991033.aspx.

Milgrom, P., Fiset, L., Whitney, C., Conrad, D., Cullen, T., & O'Hara, D. (1994). Malpractice claims during 1988–1992: A national survey of dentists. *Journal of the American Dental Association, 125*, 462–469.

Milgrom, P., Whitney, C., Conrad, D., Fiset, L., & O'Hara, D. (1995). Tort reform and malpractice liability insurance. *Medical Care, 33*, 755–764.

Milligan, P., Njie, A., & Bennett, S. (2004). Comparison of two cluster sampling methods for health surveys in developing countries. *International Journal of Epidemiology, 33*, 469–476.

Mishler, E. G. (1986). *Research interviewing: Context and narrative.* Cambridge, MA: Harvard University Press.

Mishra, S. I., Dooley, D., Catalano, R., & Serxner, S. (1993). Telephone health surveys: Potential bias from noncompletion. *American Journal of Public Health, 83*, 94–99.

Mohadjer, L. (1988). Stratification of prefix areas for sampling rare populations. In R. M. Groves, P. P. Biemer, L. E. Lyberg, W. L. Massey, W. L. Nicholls II, & J. Waksberg (Eds.), *Telephone survey methodology.* Hoboken, NJ: Wiley.

Mokdad, A. H., Stroup, D. F., Giles, W. H., & Behavioral Risk Factor Surveillance Team. (2003). Public health surveillance for behavioral risk factors in a changing environment: Recommendations from the Behavioral Risk Factor Surveillance Team. *Morbidity and Mortality Weekly Report: Recommendations and Reports, 52(RR-9)*, 1–12.

Molenaar, N. J., & Smit, J. H. (1996). Asking and answering yes/no-questions in survey interviews: A conversational approach. *Quality and Quantity, 30*, 115–136.

Mondak, J. J. (2001). Developing valid knowledge scales. *American Journal of Political Science, 45*, 224–238.

Mondak, J. J., & Davis, B. C. (2001). Asked and answered: Knowledge levels when we will not take "don't know" for an answer. *Political Behavior, 23*, 199–224.

Mooney, L. A., & Gramling, R. (1991). Asking threatening questions and situational framing: The effects of decomposing survey items. *Sociological Quarterly, 32*, 289–300.

Moore, J. C. (1988). Self/proxy response status and survey response quality: A review of the literature. *Journal of Official Statistics, 4*, 155–172.

Moore, J. C., Stinson, L. L., & Welniak, E. J., Jr. (2000). Income measurement error in surveys: A review. *Journal of Official Statistics, 16*, 331–361.

Moore, K. A., Halle, T. G., Vandivere, S., & Mariner, C. L. (2002). Scaling back survey scales: How short is too short? *Sociological Methods and Research, 30*, 530–567.

Morales, L. S., Weidmer, B. O., & Hays, R. D. (2001). Readability of CAHPS 2.0 child and adult core surveys. In National Center for Health Statistics, *Seventh Conference on Health Survey Research Methods* (ed. M. L. Cynamon & R. A. Kulka) (pp. 83–90). (DHHS Publication No. (PHS) 01-1013). Hyattsville, MD: National Center for Health Statistics.

Morgan, D. L. (1997). *Focus groups as qualitative research.* (2nd ed.). Thousand Oaks, CA: Sage.

Moriarty, H. J., Deatrick, J. A., Mahon, M. M., Feetham, S. L., Carroll, R. M., Shepard, M. P., et al. (1999). Issues to consider when choosing and using large national databases for research of families. *Western Journal of Nursing Research, 21*, 143–153.

Morrel-Samuels, P. (2003). Web surveys' hidden hazards. *Harvard Business Review, 81*, 16–17.

Morris, M. C., Colditz, G. A., & Evans, D. A. (1998). Response to a mail nutritional survey in an older bi-racial community population. *Annals of Epidemiology, 8*, 342–346.

Morrow, R. H., & Bryant, J. H. (1995). Health policy approaches to measuring and valuing human life: Conceptual and ethical issues. *American Journal of Public Health, 85*, 1356–1360.

Mosely, R. R., & Wolinsky, F. D. (1986). The use of proxies in health surveys: Substantive and policy implications. *Medical Care, 24,* 496–510.

Moxey, L. M., & Sanford, A. J. (2000). Communicating quantities: A review of psycholinguistic evidence of how expressions determine perspectives. *Applied Cognitive Psychology, 14,* 237–255.

Muhib, F. B., Lin, L. S., Stueve, A., Miller, R. L., Ford, W. L., Johnson, W. D., et al. (2001). A venue-based method for sampling hard-to-reach populations. *Public Health Reports, 116*(Suppl. 1), 216–222.

Murphy, E., Marquis, K., Hoffman, R., III, Saner, L., Tedesco, H., Harris, C., & Roske-Hofstrand, R. (1999). Improving electronic data collection and dissemination through usability testing. *Federal Committee on Statistical Methodology Research Conference, 1999.* Washington, DC: Statistical Policy Office.

Murray, D. M., Moskowitz, J. M., & Dent, C. W. (1996). Design and analysis issues in community-based drug abuse prevention. *American Behavioral Scientist, 39,* 853–867.

Narayan, S., & Krosnick, J. A. (1996). Education moderates some response effects in attitude measurement. *Public Opinion Quarterly, 60,* 58–88.

National Center for Health Services Research. (1977). *Advances in Health Survey Methods: Proceedings of a National Invitational Conference.* (DHEW Publication No. (HRA) 77-3154). Rockville, MD: Author.

National Center for Health Services Research. (1978). *Health Survey Research Methods: Second Biennial Conference.* (DHEW Publication No. (PHS) 79-3207). Hyattsville, MD: Author.

National Center for Health Services Research. (1981). *Health Survey Research Methods: Third Biennial Conference.* (DHHS Publication No. (PHS) 81-3268). Hyattsville, MD.

National Center for Health Services Research. (1984). *Health Survey Research Methods: Proceedings of the Fourth Conference on Health Survey Research Methods* (ed. C. F. Cannell & R. M. Groves). (DHHS Publication No. (PHS) 84-3346). Rockville, MD: Author.

National Center for Health Services Research. (1989). *Health Survey Research Methods: Conference Proceedings* (ed. F. J. Fowler). (DHHS Publication No. (PHS) 89-3447). Rockville, MD: Author.

National Center for Health Statistics. (1985). *The National Health Interview Survey design, 1973–84, and procedures, 1975–83* (ed. P. Salovey, W. J. Sieber, A. F. Smith, D. C. Turk, J. B. Jobe, & G. B. Willis). (DHHS Publication No. (PHS) 85-1320). Hyattsville, MD: Author.

National Center for Health Statistics. (1987). *An experimental comparison of telephone and personal health interview surveys* (ed. O. T. Thornberry Jr.). (DHHS Publication No. (PHS) 87-1380). Vital and Health Statistics Series 2, No. 106. Hyattsville, MD: Author.

National Center for Health Statistics. (1989a). *Autobiographical memory for health-related events* (ed. B. Means et al.). (DHHS Publication No. (PHS) 89-1077). Vital and Health Statistics Series 6, No. 2. Hyattsville, MD: Author.

National Center for Health Statistics. (1989b). *Social cognition approach to reporting chronic conditions in health surveys* (ed. M. B. Brewer, V. T. Dull, & J. B. Jobe). (DHHS Publication No. (PHS) 89-1078). Vital and Health Statistics Series 6, No. 3. Hyattsville, MD: Author.

National Center for Health Statistics. (1991). *Cognitive processes in long-term dietary recall* (ed. A. F. Smith). (DHHS Publication No. (PHS) 91-1079). Vital and Health Statistics Series 6, No. 4. Hyattsville, MD: Author.

National Center for Health Statistics. (1992a). *Cognitive research on response error in survey questions on smoking* (ed. B. Means). (DHHS Publication No. (PHS) 92-1080). Vital and Health Statistics Series 6, No. 5. Hyattsville, MD: Author.

National Center for Health Statistics. (1992b). *Reporting chronic pain episodes on health surveys* (ed. P. Salovey, W. J. Sieber, A. F. Smith, D. C. Turk, J. B. Jobe, & G. B. Willis). DHHS Publication No. (PHS) 92-1081). Vital and Health Statistics Series 6, No. 6. Hyattsville, MD: Author.

National Center for Health Statistics. (1994a). *Cognitive aspects of reporting cancer prevention examinations and tests* (ed. S. Sudman). (DHHS Publication No. (PHS) 94-1082). Vital and Health Statistics Series 6, No. 7. Hyattsville, MD: Author.

National Center for Health Statistics. (1994b). *Cognitive interviewing and survey design: A training manual* (ed. G. Willis). (Cognitive Methods Staff Working Paper Series Report No. 7). Hyattsville, MD: Author.

National Center for Health Statistics. (1994c). *The contributions of the NCHS Collaborative Research Program to memory research* (ed. D. Hermann). (Cognitive Methods Staff Working Paper Series Report No. 14). Hyattsville, MD: Author.

National Center for Health Statistics. (1996). *Health Survey Research Methods: Conference Proceedings* (ed. R. B. Warnecke). (DHHS Publication No. (PHS) 96-1013). Hyattsville, MD: Author.

National Center for Health Statistics. (1999). *A New Agenda for Interdisciplinary Survey Research Methods: Proceedings of the CASM II Seminar* (ed. M. G. Sirken, T. Jabine, G. Willis, E. Martin, & C. Tucker). Hyattsville, MD: Author.

National Center for Health Statistics. (2001). *Seventh Conference on Health Survey Research Methods* (ed. M. L. Cynamon & R. A. Kulka). (DHHS Publication No. (PHS) 01-1013). Hyattsville, MD: Author.

National Center for Health Statistics. (2004a). *2003 National Health Interview Survey (NHIS) public use data release: NHIS survey description.* Hyattsville, MD: Author.

National Center for Health Statistics. (2004b). *Eighth Conference on Health Survey Research Methods* (ed. S. B. Cohen & J. M. Lepkowski). (DHHS Publication No. (PHS) 04-1013). Hyattsville, MD: National Center for Health Statistics.

National Center for Health Statistics. (2004c, December 16). *National Ambulatory Medical Care Survey (NAMCS)*. Retrieved June 1, 2005, from http://www.cdc.gov/nchs/about/major/ahcd/namcsdes.htm.

National Center for Health Statistics. (2004d, December 16). *National Employer Health Insurance Survey (NEHIS)*. Retrieved June 1, 2005, from http://www.cdc.gov/nchs/about/major/nehis/about_nehis.htm.

National Center for Health Statistics. (2004e, December 16). *National Home and Hospice Care Survey (NHHCS)*. Retrieved June 1, 2005, from http://www.cdc.gov/nchs/about/major/nhhcsd/nhhcsdes.htm.

National Center for Health Statistics. (2004f, December 16). *National Nursing Home Survey (NNHS)*. Retrieved June 1, 2005, from http://www.cdc.gov/nchs/about/major/nnhsd/nnhsdesc.htm.

National Center for Health Statistics. (2004g, December 30). *CDC Wonder: DATA2010 . . . the Healthy People 2010 database.* Retrieved May 9, 2005, from http://wonder.cdc.gov/data2010/

National Center for Health Statistics. (2005a, February 1). *National Hospital Ambulatory Medical Care Survey (NHAMCS)*. Retrieved June 1, 2005, from http://www.cdc.gov/nchs/about/major/ahcd/nhamcsds.htm.

National Center for Health Statistics. (2005b, February 1). *National Hospital Discharge Survey (NHDS)*. Retrieved June 1, 2005, from http://www.cdc.gov/nchs/about/major/hdasd/nhdsdes.htm.

National Center for Health Statistics. (2005c, February 1). *National Survey of Ambulatory Surgery (NSAS)*. Retrieved June 1, 2005, from http://www.cdc.gov/nchs/about/major/hdasd/nsasdes.htm.

National Center for Health Statistics. (2005d, February 11). *NCHS vital and health statistics series number 6: Cognition and survey measurement*. Retrieved May 23, 2005, from http://www.cdc.gov/nchs/products/pubs/pubd/series/sr06/ser6.htm.

National Center for Health Statistics. (2005e, February 14). *NCHS cognitive methods working paper series*. Retrieved May 23, 2005, from http://www.cdc.gov/nchs/products/pubs/workpap/workpap.htm.

National Center for Health Statistics. (2005f, February 25). *National Health Care Survey*. Retrieved June 16, 2005, from http://www.cdc.gov/nchs/nhcs.htm.

National Center for Health Statistics. (2005g, March 23). *National Health Interview Survey (NHIS) homepage*. Retrieved April 9, 2005, from http://www.cdc.gov/nchs/nhis.htm.

National Center for Health Statistics. (2005h, April 13). *Healthy people: Tracking the nation's health*. Retrieved June 13, 2005, from http://www.cdc.gov/nchs/hphome.htm#healthy%20people%202010.

National Center for Health Statistics. (2005i, May 11). *National Health Interview Survey (NHIS) homepage*. Retrieved June 16, 2005, from http://www.cdc.gov/nchs/nhis.htm.

National Center for Health Statistics. (2005j, May 26). *National Immunization Survey (NIS)*. Retrieved June 1, 2005, from http://www.cdc.gov/nis/

National Center for Health Statistics. (2005k, June 1). *National Center for Health Statistics homepage*. Retrieved June 1, 2005, from http://www.cdc.gov/nchs.

National Center for Health Statistics. (2005l, June 2). *National Health and Nutrition Examination Survey (NHANES)*. Retrieved June 16, 2005, from http://www.cdc.gov/nchs/nhanes.htm.

National Center for Health Statistics. (n.d.). *2004 NHIS: Survey questionnaires (draft), flashcards, field representative manual*. Retrieved May 26, 2005, from ftp://ftp.cdc.gov/pub/Health_Statistics/NCHS/Survey_Questionnaires/NHIS/2004/.

National Committee for Quality Assurance. (2004). *The state of health care quality 2004* Washington, DC: Author.

National Committee for Quality Assurance. (2005, June 13). *HEDIS 2005: Vol. 1. Narrative: What's in it and why it matters*. Washington, DC: Author.

National Committee for Quality Assurance. (n.d.). *Health Plan Employer Data and Information Set (HEDIS)*. Retrieved June 16, 2005, from http://www.ncqa.org/Programs/HEDIS/.

National Institutes of Health. (2004, July 13). *Protecting personal health information in research: Understanding the HIPAA privacy rule*. Retrieved May 9, 2005, from http://privacyruleandresearch.nih.gov/pr_02.asp.

National Partnership for Reinventing Government. (1998, July). *"Conversations with America": Frequently asked questions about customer survey clearance and the Paperwork Reduction Act*. Retrieved April 24, 2005, from http://govinfo.library.unt.edu/npr/library/misc/pra-qa.html.

National Research Council, Committee on National Statistics. (1984). *Cognitive aspects of survey methodology: Building a bridge between disciplines* (ed. T. B. Jabine, M. L. Straf, J. M. Tanur, & R. Tourangeau). Washington, DC: National Academies Press.

National Research Council, Committee on National Statistics, Panel on Incomplete Data. (1983). *Incomplete data in sample surveys* (ed. W. G. Madow, H. Nisselson, I. Olkin, & D. B. Rubin). Orlando, FL: Academic Press.

National Research Council, Panel on Survey Measurement of Subjective Phenomena. (1984). *Surveying subjective phenomena* (ed. C. F. Turner & E. Martin). New York: Russell Sage Foundation.

Nazroo, J. Y. (2003). The structuring of ethnic inequalities in health: Economic position, racial discrimination, and racism. *American Journal of Public Health, 93,* 277–284.

Nelson, E. C., Hays, R. D., Larson, C., & Batalden, P. B. (1989). The Patient Judgment System: Reliability and validity. *Quality Review Bulletin, 15,* 185–191.

Nelson, E. C., & Larson, C. (1993). Patients' good and bad surprises: How do they relate to overall patient satisfaction? *Quality Review Bulletin, 19,* 89–94.

Nelson, E. C., Wasson, J. H., Johnson, D., & Hays, R. (1996). Dartmouth COOP functional health assessment charts: Brief measures for clinical practice. In B. Spilker (Ed.), *Quality of life and pharmacoeconomics in clinical trials.* (2nd ed., pp. 161–168). Philadelphia: Lippincott-Raven.

Nelson, E., Wasson, J., Kirk, J., Keller, A., Clark, D., Dietrich, A., et al. (1987). Assessment of function in routine clinical practice: Description of the COOP chart method and preliminary findings. *Journal of Chronic Diseases, 40*(Suppl. 1), S55–S63.

Nemoto, T., Operario, D., Keatley, J., Han, L., & Soma, T. (2004). HIV risk behaviors among male-to-female transgender persons of color in San Francisco. *American Journal of Public Health, 94,* 1193–1199.

Neudert, C., Wasner, M., & Borasio, G. D. (2004). Individual quality of life is not correlated with health related quality of life or physical function in patients with amyotropic lateral sclerosis. *Journal of Palliative Medicine, 7,* 551–557.

Newby, M., Amin, S., Diamond, I., & Naved, R. T. (1998). Survey experience among women in Bangladesh. *American Behavioral Scientist, 42,* 252–275.

Nicholls, W. L., II, & Groves, R. M. (1986). The status of computer-assisted telephone interviewing: Part I—Introduction and impact on cost and timeliness of survey data. *Journal of Official Statistics, 2,* 115.

Nicol, A.A.M., & Pexman, P. M. (2003). *Presenting your findings: A practical guide for creating tables.* Washington, DC: American Psychological Association.

NORSTAT. (n.d.). *AutoQuest.* Retrieved June 8, 2005, from http://www.norstat.no/en/content.asp?uid=199.

Nova Research Company. (2004a). *HAPI (Handheld Assisted Personal Interview).* Retrieved June 8, 2005, from http://www.novaresearch.com/Products/qds/whatIsQDS.cfm#hapi.

Nova Research Company. (2004b). *QDS (Questionnaire Development System).* Retrieved June 8, 2005, from http://www.novaresearch.com/Products/qds/index.cfm.

Nunnally, J. C., & Bernstein, I. H. (1994). *Psychometric theory* (3rd ed.). New York: McGraw-Hill.

O'Brien, K. (1993). Using focus groups to develop health surveys: An example from research on social relationships and AIDS-preventive behavior. *Health Education Quarterly, 20,* 361–372.

O'Connell, B., Young, J., & Twigg, D. (1999). Patient satisfaction with nursing care: A measurement conundrum. *International Journal of Nursing Practice, 5,* 72–77.

O'Connell, K., Skevington, S., Saxena, S., & WHOQOL-HIV Group. (2003). Preliminary development of the World Health Organisation's Quality of Life HIV instrument (WHOQOL-HIV): Analysis of the pilot version. *Social Science and Medicine, 57,* 1259–1275.

O'Connor, S. J., Trinh, H. Q., & Shewchuk, R. M. (2000). Perceptual gaps in understanding patient expectations for health care service quality. *Health Care Management Review, 25,* 7–23.

O'Muircheartaigh, C. A., Gaskell, G. D., & Wright, D. B. (1993). Intensifiers in behavioral frequency questions. *Public Opinion Quarterly, 57,* 552–565.

O'Neil, K. M., & Penrod, S. D. (2001). Methodological variables in Web-based research that may affect results: Sample type, monetary incentives, and personal information. *Behavior Research Methods Instruments and Computers, 33,* 226–233.

O'Neil, K. M., Penrod, S. D., & Bornstein, B. H. (2003). Web-based research: Methodological variables' effects on dropout and sample characteristics. *Behavior Research Methods Instruments and Computers, 35,* 217–226.

O'Reilly, J. M., Hubbard, M. L., Lessler, J. T., Biemer, P. P., & Turner, C. F. (1994). Audio and video computer assisted self-interviewing: Preliminary tests of new technologies for data collection. *Journal of Official Statistics, 10,* 214.

O'Reilly, M. (2001). PDAs and medicine. *CMAJ, 165,* 938.

Office of Management and Budget. (1997, October 30). *Revisions to the standards for the classification of federal data on race and ethnicity.* Retrieved May 25, 2005, from http://www. whitehouse.gov/omb/fedreg/print/ombdir15.html.

Oksenberg, L., Cannell, C., & Kalton, G. (1991). New strategies for pretesting survey questions. *Journal of Official Statistics, 7,* 349–365.

Oksenberg, L., Coleman, L., & Cannell, C. F. (1986). Interviewers' voices and refusal rates in telephone surveys. *Public Opinion Quarterly, 50,* 97–111.

Oldendick, R. W. (1993). The effect of answering machines on the representativeness of samples in telephone surveys. *Journal of Official Statistics, 9,* 663–672.

Oldendick, R. W., & Link, M. W. (1994). The answering machine generation: Who are they and what problem do whey pose for survey research. *Public Opinion Quarterly, 58,* 264–273.

Oppenheim, A. N. (1992). *Questionnaire design, interviewing, and attitude measurement* (New ed.). New York: Pinter.

Orth-Gomer, K., & Unden, A. L. (1987). The measurement of social support in population surveys. *Social Science and Medicine, 24,* 83–94.

Owens, L., Johnson, T. P., & O'Rourke, D. (2001). Culture and item nonresponse in health surveys. In National Center for Health Statistics, *Seventh Conference on Health Survey Research Methods* (ed. M. L. Cynamon & R. A. Kulka) (pp. 69–74). (DHHS Publication No. (PHS) 01-1013). Hyattsville, MD: National Center for Health Statistics.

Pagano, M., & Gauvreau, K. (2000). *Principles of biostatistics.* (2nd ed.). Pacific Grove, CA: Duxbury Press.

Parasuraman, A., Zeithaml, V. A., & Berry, L. L. (1988). SERVQUAL: A multiple-item scale for measuring consumer perceptions of service quality. *Journal of Retailing, 64,* 12–40.

Parkerson, G. R., Broadhead, W. E., & Tse, C.K.J. (1990). The Duke Health Profile: A 17-item measure of health and dysfunction. *Medical Care, 28,* 1056–1072.

Parkerson, G. R., Gehlbach, S. H., Wagner, E. H., James, S. A., Clapp, N. E., & Muhlbaier, L. H. (1981). The Duke-UNC Health Profile: An adult health status instrument for primary care. *Medical Care, 19,* 806–828.

Parsons, J. A., Johnson, T. P., Warnecke, R. B., & Kaluzny, A. (1993). The effect of interviewer characteristics on gatekeeper resistance in surveys of elite populations. *Evaluation Review, 17,* 131–143.

Parsons, J. A., Warnecke, R. B., Czaja, R. F., Barnsley, J., & Kaluzny, A. (1994). Factors associated with response rates in a national survey of primary-care physicians. *Evaluation Review, 18,* 756–766.

Patrick, D. L., & Bergner, M. (1990). Measurement of health status in the 1990s. *Annual Review of Public Health, 11,* 165–183.

Patrick, D. L., Bush, J. W., & Chen, M. M. (1973). Toward an operational definition of health. *Journal of Health and Social Behavior, 14,* 6–23.

Patrick, D. L., & Deyo, R. A. (1989). Generic and disease specific measures in assessing health status and quality of life. *Medical Care, 27*(Suppl. 3), S217–S232.

Patrick, D. L., & Erickson, P. (1993). *Health status and health policy: Quality of life in health care evaluation and resource allocation.* New York: Oxford University Press.

Payne, S. L. (1951). *The art of asking questions.* Princeton, NJ: Princeton University Press.

Peck, B. M., Asch, D. A., Goold, S. D., Roter, D. L., Ubel, P. A., McIntyre, L. M., et al. (2001). Measuring patient expectations: Does the instrument affect satisfaction or expectations? *Medical Care, 39,* 100–108.

Perneger, T. V., Etter, J. F., & Rougemont, A. (1993). Randomized trial of use of a monetary incentive and a reminder card to increase the response rate to a mailed health survey. *American Journal of Epidemiology, 138,* 714–722.

Peterson, R. A. (1984). Asking the age question: A research note. *Public Opinion Quarterly, 48,* 379–383.

Petrou, S., & Henderson, J. (2003). Preference-based approaches to measuring the benefits of perinatal care. *Birth, 30,* 217–226.

Pettit, F. A. (2002). A comparison of World Wide Web and paper-and-pencil personality questionnaires. *Behavior Research Methods Instruments and Computers, 34,* 50–54.

Pfeffermann, D. (2002). Small area estimation: New developments and directions. *International Statistical Review, 70,* 125–143.

Pierzchala, M. (1990). A review of the state of the art in automated data editing and imputation. *Journal of Official Statistics, 6,* 355–377.

Pitkow, J. E., & Kehoe, C. M. (1995). Results from the third WWW user survey. *World Wide Web Journal, 1*(1). Retrieved July 16, 2004, from http://www.cc.gatech.edu/gvu/user_surveys/papers/survey_3_paper.pdf.

Potthoff, R. F. (1987). Some generalizations of the Mitofsky-Waksberg technique for random digit dialing. *Journal of the American Statistical Association, 82,* 409–418.

Press Ganey Associates. (2005). *Survey instruments.* Retrieved May 26, 2005, from http://www.pressganey.com/products_services/survey_instruments/default.php.

Presser, S., & Blair, J. (1994). Survey pretesting: Do different methods produce different results? *Sociological Methodology,* 73–104.

Presser, S., & Schuman, H. (1980). Measurement of a middle position in attitude surveys. *Public Opinion Quarterly, 44,* 70–85.

Preville, M., Herbert, R., Boyer, R., & Bravo, G. (2001). Correlates of psychotropic drug use in the elderly compared to adults aged 18–64: Results from the Quebec Health Study. *Aging and Mental Health, 5,* 216–224.

Principe, G. F., Ornstein, P. A., Baker-Ward, L., & Gordon, B. N. (2000). The effects of intervening experiences on children's memory for a physical examination. *Applied Cognitive Psychology, 14,* 59–80.

QualityMetric Incorporated. (n.d.). *SF-36.org "community news": A call to establish common metrics for consumer-reported health status measurement.* Retrieved May 17, 2005, from http://www.sf-36.org/.

Quantitative Decisions. (2000). *Sample: Designing random sampling programs with ArcView 3.2.* Retrieved May 30, 2005, from http://www.quantdec.com/sample/.

Quinn, G. P., Jacobsen, P. B., Albrecht, T. L., Ellison, B. A., Newman, N. W., Bell, M., et al. (2004). Real-time patient satisfaction survey and improvement process. *Hospital Topics, 82,* 26–32.

Raftery, A. E. (2000). Statistics in sociology: 1950–2000. *Journal of the American Statistical Association, 95,* 654–661.

Rand Health. (n.d.). *Patient Satisfaction Questionnaire, Long Form (PSQ III).* Retrieved June 6, 2005, from http://www.rand.org/health/surveys/PSQIII.html.

Rao, J. K., Weinberger, M., & Kroenke, K. (2000). Visit-specific expectations and patient-centered outcomes: A literature review. *Archives of Family Medicine, 9,* 1148–1155.

Rao, J.N.K. (2003). *Small area estimation.* Hoboken, NJ: Wiley.

Rao, J.N.K., & Bellhouse, D. R. (1990). History and development of the theoretical foundations of survey based estimation and analysis. *Survey Methodology, 16,* 3–29.

Rapp, C. A. (1998). *The strengths model: Case management with people suffering from severe and persistent mental illness.* New York: Oxford University Press.

Rasinski, K. A., Mingay, D., & Bradburn, N. M. (1994). Do respondents really "mark all that apply" on self-administered questions? *Public Opinion Quarterly, 58,* 400–408.

Rasinski, K. A., Willis, G. B., Baldwin, A. K., Yeh, W. C., & Lee, L. (1999). Methods of data collection, perceptions of risks and losses, and motivation to give truthful answers to sensitive survey questions. *Applied Cognitive Psychology, 13,* 465–484.

Ray, B. B., McFadden, A., Patterson, S., & Wright, V. (2001, Summer). Personal digital assistants in the middle school classroom: Lessons in hand. *Meridian: A Middle School Computer Technologies Journal, 4(2).* Retrieved July 25, 2004, from http://www.ncsu.edu/meridian/sum2001/palm/4.html.

Redline, C., & Dillman, D. A. (2002). The influence of alternative visual designs on respondents' performance with branching instructions in self-administered questionnaires. In R. M. Groves, D. A. Dillman, J. L. Eltinge, & R.J.A. Little (Eds.), *Survey nonresponse* (pp. 179–193). Hoboken, NJ: Wiley.

Revicki, D. A., Osoba, D., Fairclough, D., Barofsky, I., Berzon, R., Leidy, N. K., et al. (2000). Recommendations on health-related quality of life research to support labeling and promotional claims in the United States. *Quality of Life Research, 9,* 887–900.

Rhodes, P. J. (1994). Race-of-interviewer effects: A brief comment. *Sociology, 28,* 547–558.

Richardson, J. L., Lochner, T., McGuigan, K., & Levine, A. M. (1987). Physician attitudes and experience regarding the care of patients with acquired-immunodeficiency-syndrome (AIDS) and related disorders (ARC). *Medical Care, 25,* 675–685.

Richter, D. L., & Galavotti, C. (2000). The role of qualitative research in a national project on decision making about hysterectomy and the use of hormone replacement therapy. *Journal of Women's Health and Gender-Based Medicine, 9*(Suppl. 2), S1–S3.

Ricketts, T. C., III (2002). Geography and disparities in health care. In Institute of Medicine Committee on Guidance for Designing a National Healthcare Disparities Report, *Guidance for the national healthcare disparities report* (pp. 149–180). Washington, DC: National Academies Press.

Rizzo, L., Brick, J. M., & Park, I. (2004). A minimally intrusive method for sampling persons in random digit dial surveys. *Public Opinion Quarterly, 68,* 267–274.

Robine, J. M., Mathers, C. D., & Bucquet, D. (1993). Distinguishing health expectancies and health-adjusted life expectancies from quality-adjusted life years. *American Journal of Public Health, 83,* 797–798.

Rockwood, T. H., Sangster, R. L., & Dillman, D. A. (1997). The effect of response categories on questionnaire answers: Context and mode effects. *Sociological Methods and Research, 26,* 118–140.

Rosenberg, M. (1968). *The logic of survey analysis.* New York: Basic Books.

Rosner, B. (2000). *Fundamentals of biostatistics* (5th ed.). Pacific Grove, CA: Duxbury Press.

Ross, C. E., & Reynolds, J. R. (1996). The effects of power, knowledge, and trust on income disclosure in surveys. *Social Science Quarterly, 77,* 899–911.

Rossi, P. H., Lipsey, M. W., & Freeman, H. E. (2004). *Evaluation: A systematic approach* (7th ed.). Thousand Oaks, CA: Sage.

Rothman, K. J. (2002). *Epidemiology: An introduction*. New York: Oxford University Press.

Rubin, D. B. (1996). Multiple imputation after 18+ years. *Journal of the American Statistical Association, 91*, 473–489.

Rubin, D. B. (2004). *Multiple imputation for nonresponse in surveys*. Hoboken, NJ: Wiley.

Rubin, H. J., & Rubin, I. (2005). *Qualitative interviewing: The art of hearing data* (2nd ed.). Thousand Oaks, CA: Sage.

Rubin, H. R. (1990). Can patients evaluate the quality of hospital care? *Medical Care Review, 47*, 267–326.

Rubin, H. R., Gandek, B., Rogers, W. H., Kosinski, M., McHorney, C. A., & Ware, J. E. (1993). Patients' ratings of outpatient visits in different practice settings: Results from the Medical Outcomes Study. *Journal of the American Medical Association, 270*, 835–840.

Ruspini, E. (2000, Spring). Longitudinal research in the social sciences. *Social Research Update, 28*. Retrieved March 22, 2005, from http://www.soc.surrey.ac.uk/sru/SRU28.html.

Rutten-van Mölken, M.P.M.H., Bakker, C. H., van Doorslaer, E.K.A., & van der Linden, S. (1995). Methodological issues of patient utility measurement: Experience from two clinical trials. *Medical Care, 33*, 922–937.

Safran, D. G., Tarlov, A. R., & Rogers, W. H. (1994). Primary care performance in fee-for-service and prepaid health care systems: Results from the Medical Outcomes Study. *Journal of the American Medical Association, 271*, 1579–1586.

Salant, P., & Dillman, D. A. (1994). *How to conduct your own survey*. Hoboken, NJ: Wiley.

Sale, J.E.M., Lohfeld, L. H., & Brazil, K. (2002). Revisiting the quantitative-qualitative debate: Implications for mixed-methods research. *Quality and Quantity, 36*, 43–53.

Sawtooth Technologies. (2003a). *Computer-assisted telephone interviewing with WinCATI 4.2.* Retrieved June 8, 2005, from http://www.sawtooth.com/products/#cati.

Sawtooth Technologies. (2003b). *Web-only interviewing with Sensus Web.* Retrieved June 8, 2005, from http://www.sawtooth.com/products/#web.

Saxon, D., Garratt, D., Gilroy, P., & Cairns, C. (2003). Collecting data in the information age: Exploring Web-based survey methods in educational research. *Research in Education, 69*, 51–66.

Schaefer, D. R., & Dillman, D. A. (1998). Development of a standard e-mail methodology: Results of an experiment. *Public Opinion Quarterly, 62*, 378–397.

Schaeffer, N. C. (1991). Hardly ever or constantly: Group comparisons using vague quantifiers. *Public Opinion Quarterly, 55*, 395–423.

Schaeffer, N. C., & Presser, S. (2003). The science of asking questions. *Annual Review of Sociology, 29*, 65–88.

Schafer, J. L., & Graham, J. W. (2002). Missing data: Our view of the state of the art. *Psychological Methods, 7*, 147–177.

Schauffler, H. H., & Mordavsky, J. K. (2001). Consumer reports in health care: Do they make a difference? *Annual Review of Public Health, 22*, 69–89.

Schechter, S., & Herrmann, D. (1997). The proper use of self-report questions in effective measurement of health outcomes. *Evaluation and the Health Professions, 20*, 28–46.

Schene, A. H. (1990). Objective and subjective dimensions of family burden: Towards an integrative framework for research. *Social Psychiatry and Psychiatric Epidemiology, 25*, 289–297.

Scherpenzeel, A. C., & Saris, W. E. (1997). The validity and reliability of survey questions: A meta-analysis of MTMM studies. *Sociological Methods and Research, 25,* 341–383.

Schirmer, L. L., & Lopez, F. G. (2001). Probing the social support and work strain relationship among adult workers: Contributions of adult attachment orientations. *Journal of Vocational Behavior, 59,* 17–33.

Schleyer, T.K.L., & Forrest, J. L. (2000). Methods for the design and administration of Web-based surveys. *Journal of the American Medical Informatics Association, 7,* 416–425.

Schober, M. F., & Conrad, F. G. (1997). Does conversational interviewing reduce survey measurement error? *Public Opinion Quarterly, 61,* 576–602.

Schuman, H., & Presser, S. (1981). *Questions and answers in attitude surveys: Experiments on question form, wording, and context.* Thousand Oaks, CA: Sage.

Schwartz, M. D. (2000). Methodological issues in the use of survey data for measuring and characterizing violence against women. *Violence Against Women, 6,* 815–838.

Schwartz, S., Susser, E., & Susser, M. (1999). A future for epidemiology? *Annual Review of Public Health, 20,* 15–33.

Schwarz, N. (1990). What respondents learn from scales: The informative functions of response alternatives. *International Journal of Public Opinion Research, 2,* 274–285.

Schwarz, N. (1999). Self-reports: How the questions shape the answers. *American Psychologist, 54,* 93–105.

Schwarz, N., & Bienias, J. (1990). What mediates the impact of response alternatives on frequency reports of mundane behaviors. *Applied Cognitive Psychology, 4,* 61–72.

Schwarz, N., & Bless, H. (1992). Assimilation and contrast effects in attitude measurement: An inclusion/exclusion model. *Advances in Consumer Research, 19,* 72–77.

Schwarz, N., & Hippler, H.-J. (1995a). The numeric values of rating scales: A comparison of their impact in mail surveys and telephone interviews. *International Journal of Public Opinion Research, 7,* 72–74.

Schwarz, N., & Hippler, H.-J. (1995b). Subsequent questions may influence answers to preceding questions in mail surveys. *Public Opinion Quarterly, 59,* 93–97.

Schwarz, N., Knäuper, B., Hippler, H.-J., Noelle-Neumann, E., & Clark, L. (1991). Rating scales: Numeric values may change the meaning of scale labels. *Public Opinion Quarterly, 55,* 570–582.

Schwarz, N., Munkel, T., & Hippler, H.-J. (1990). What determines a perspective: Contrast effects as a function of the dimension tapped by preceding questions. *European Journal of Social Psychology, 20,* 357–361.

Schwarz, N., & Oyserman, D. (2001). Asking questions about behavior: Cognition, communication, and questionnaire construction. *American Journal of Evaluation, 22,* 127–160.

Schwarz, N., Strack, F., Hippler, H.-J., & Bishop, G. (1991). The impact of administration mode on response effects in survey measurement. *Applied Cognitive Psychology, 5,* 193–212.

Schwarz, N., Strack, F., & Mai, H. P. (1991). Assimilation and contrast effects in part-whole question sequences: A conversational logic analysis. *Public Opinion Quarterly, 55,* 3–23.

Schwarz, N., & Sudman, S. (Eds.). (1992). *Context effects in social and psychological research.* New York: Springer-Verlag.

Schwarz, N., & Sudman, S. (Eds.). (1994). *Autobiographical memory and the validity of retrospective reports.* New York: Springer-Verlag.

Schwarz, N., & Sudman, S. (1996). *Answering questions: Methodology for determining cognitive and communicative processes in survey research.* San Francisco: Jossey-Bass.

Scientific Advisory Committee of the Medical Outcomes Trust. (2002). Assessing health status and quality-of-life instruments: Attributes and review criteria. *Quality of Life Research, 11,* 193–205.

Scott, K. M., Sarfati, D., Tobias, M. I., and Haslett, S. J. (2001). A challenge to the cross cultural validity of the SF-36 health survey: Maori, Pacific, and New Zealand European ethnic groups. In National Center for Health Statistics, *Seventh Conference on Health Survey Research Methods* (ed. M. L. Cynamon & R. A. Kulka) (pp. 91–96). (DHHS Publication No. (PHS) 01-1013). Hyattsville, MD: National Center for Health Statistics.

Scriven, A., & Smith-Ferrier, S. (2003). The application of online surveys for workplace health research. *Journal of the Royal Society of Health, 123,* 95–101.

Searight, H. R., & Gafford, J. (2005). Cultural diversity at the end of life: Issues and guidelines for family physicians. *American Family Physician, 71,* 515–522.

Sensibaugh, C. C., & Yarab, P. E. (1997). Newlyweds' family-formation preferences. *Journal of Psychology, 131,* 530–540.

Shadish, W. R., Cook, T. D., & Campbell, D. T. (2002). *Experimental and quasi-experimental designs for generalized causal inference.* Boston: Houghton Mifflin.

Shafazand, S., Goldstein, M. K., Doyle, R. L., Hlatky, M. A., & Gould, M. K. (2004). Health-related quality of life in patients with pulmonary arterial hypertension. *Chest, 126,* 1452–1459.

Shankle, M. D., Maxwell, C. A., Katzman, E. S., & Landers, S. (2003). An invisible population: Older lesbian, gay, bisexual, and transgender individuals. *Clinical Research and Regulatory Affairs, 20,* 159–182.

Shanks, J. M. (1983). The current status of computer-assisted telephone interviewing: Recent progress and future prospects. *Sociological Methods and Research, 12,* 119–142.

Shannon, D. M., Johnson, T. E., Searcy, S., & Lott, A. (2002). Using electronic surveys: Advice from survey professionals. *Practical Assessment, Research and Evaluation, 8*(1). Retrieved July 16, 2004, from http://PAREonline.net/getvn.asp?v=8&n=1.

Sharma, D. (2004). Health related quality of life and its assessment in GI Surgery. *Indian Journal of Surgery, 66,* 323–335.

Shepard, M. P., Carroll, R. M., Mahon, M. M., Moriarty, H. J., Feetham, S. L., Deatrick, J. A., et al. (1999). Conceptual and pragmatic considerations in conducting a secondary analysis: An example from research of families. *Western Journal of Nursing Research, 21,* 154–167.

Sherbourne, C. D., Hays, R. D., and Burton, T. (1995). Population-based surveys of access and consumer satisfaction with health care. In Agency for Healthcare Policy and Research (Ed.), *Consumer survey information in a reforming health care system* (pp. 37–56). (AHCPR Publication No. 95-0083). Rockville, MD: Agency for Healthcare Policy and Research.

Shettle, C., & Mooney, G. (1999). Monetary incentives in U.S. government surveys. *Journal of Official Statistics, 15,* 231–250.

Shortell, S. M., Wickizer, T. M., & Wheeler, J.R.C. (1984). *Hospital-physician joint ventures: Results and lessons from a national demonstration in primary care.* Ann Arbor, MI: Health Administration Press.

Shrimpton, S., Oates, K., & Hayes, S. (1998). Children's memory of events: Effects of stress, age, time delay and location of interview. *Applied Cognitive Psychology, 12,* 133–143.

Sieber, J. E. (2004). Back to the drawing board: Reactive methodology. In National Center for Health Statistics, *Eighth Conference on Health Survey Research Methods* (ed. S. B. Cohen & J. M. Lepkowski) (pp. 201–207). (DHHS Publication No. (PHS) 04-1013). Hyattsville, MD: National Center for Health Statistics.

Sijtsma, K., & Molenaar, I. W. (2002). *Introduction to nonparametric item response theory.* Thousand Oaks, CA: Sage Publications.

Singer, E., van Hoewyk, J., Gebler, N., Raghunathan, T., & McGonagle, K. (1999). The effect of incentives on response rates in interviewer-mediated surveys. *Journal of Official Statistics, 15,* 217–230.

Singer, E., van Hoewyk, J., & Maher, M. P. (1998). Does the payment of incentives create expectation effects? *Public Opinion Quarterly, 62,* 152–164.

Singer, E., van Hoewyk, J., & Maher, M. P. (2000). Experiments with incentives in telephone surveys. *Public Opinion Quarterly, 64,* 171–188.

Sjöberg, L. (2000). The methodology of risk perception research. *Quality and Quantity, 34,* 407–418.

Smith, T. W. (1987). The art of asking questions, 1936–1985. *Public Opinion Quarterly, 51*(Suppl.), S95–S108.

Smith, T. W. (1999). The polls: Review the JAMA controversy and the meaning of sex. *Public Opinion Quarterly, 63,* 385–400.

Smørdal, O., & Gregory, J. (2003). Personal digital assistants in medical education and practice. *Journal of Computer Assisted Learning, 19,* 320–329.

Snijkers, G., Hox, J., & de Leeuw, E. D. (1999). Interviewers' tactics for fighting survey nonresponse. *Journal of Official Statistics, 15,* 185–198.

Social Science Research Council. (1992). *Questions about questions: Inquiries into the cognitive bases of surveys.* New York: Russell Sage Foundation.

Solomon, D. J. (2001). Conducting Web-based surveys. *Practical Assessment, Research and Evaluation, 7(19).* Retrieved July 16, 2004, from http://pareonline.net/getvn.asp?v=7&n=19.

Spaeth, J. L., & O'Rourke, D. P. (1994). Designing and implementing the National Organizations Study. *American Behavioral Scientist, 37,* 872–890.

Spector, P. E. (1992). *Summated rating scale construction: An introduction.* Thousand Oaks, CA: Sage.

Sphinx Development UK. (n.d.). *SphinxSurvey: The one stop, integrated survey design and analysis solution.* Retrieved June 8, 2005, from http://www.sphinxdevelopment.co.uk/Products_sphinx.htm.

SPSS. (2005). *SPSS Data Entry.* Retrieved June 8, 2005, from http://www.spss.com/data_entry/.

Statistics Canada. (2003). *Joint Canada/United States Survey of Health.* Retrieved June 1, 2005, from http://www.cdc.gov/nchs/data/nhis/jcush_analyticalreport.pdf.

Statistics.com. (n.d.). *Free Web-based software* (compiled by J. C. Pezzullo). Retrieved March 23, 2005, from http://www.statistics.com/content/javastat.html.

Steinberg, L. (2001). The consequences of pairing questions: Context effects in personality measurement. *Journal of Personality and Social Psychology, 81,* 332–342.

Steury, S., Spencer, S., & Parkinson, G. W. (2004). The social context of recovery. *Psychiatry, 67,* 158–163.

Stewart, A. L., & Ware, J. E. (Eds.). (1992). *Measuring functioning and well-being: The medical outcomes study approach.* Durham, NC: Duke University Press.

Stewart, D. W., & Kamins, M. A. (1993). *Secondary research: Information sources and methods.* Thousand Oaks, CA: Sage.

Stone, E. J., Pearson, T. A., Fortmann, S. P., & McKinlay, J. B. (1997). Community-based prevention trials: Challenges and directions for public health practice, policy, and research. *Annals of Epidemiology, 7,* S113–S120.

Stouthamer-Loeber, M., & van Kammen, W. B. (1995). *Data collection and management: A practical guide.* Thousand Oaks, CA: Sage.

Streiner, D. L., & Norman, G. R. (2003). *Health measurement scales: A practical guide to their development and use* (3rd ed.). New York: Oxford University Press.

Stueve, A., O'Donnell, L. N., Duran, R., San Doval, A., & Blome, J. (2001). Time-space sampling in minority communities: Results with young Latino men who have sex with men. *American Journal of Public Health, 91,* 922–926.

Stussman, B. J., Taylor, B. L., & Riddick, H. (2003). Partials and break-offs in the National Health Interview Survey, 2002. In Federal Committee on Statistical Methodology (Ed.), *Federal Committee on Statistical Methodology Research Conference (Proceedings—Wednesday sessions)* (pp. 21–26). Washington, DC: Statistical Policy Office.

Substance Abuse and Mental Health Services Administration, Office of Applied Studies. (2002). *Redesigning an ongoing national household survey: Methodological issues* (ed. J. Gfroerer, J. Eyerman, & J. Chromy). (DHHS Publication No. (SMA) 03-3768). Rockville, MD: Author.

Suchman, L., & Jordan, B. (1990). Interactional troubles in face-to-face survey interviews. *Journal of the American Statistical Association, 85,* 232–241.

Sudman, S. (1998). Survey research and ethics. *Advances in Consumer Research, 25,* 69–71.

Sudman, S., & Blair, E. (1999). Sampling in the twenty-first century. *Journal of the Academy of Marketing Science, 27,* 269–277.

Sudman, S., & Bradburn, N. M. (1974). *Response effects in surveys: A review and synthesis.* Chicago: Aldine.

Sudman, S., Bradburn, N. M., & Schwarz, N. (1996). *Thinking about answers: The application of cognitive processes to survey methodology.* San Francisco: Jossey-Bass.

Sudman, S., Finn, A., & Lannom, L. (1984). The use of bounded recall procedures in single interviews. *Public Opinion Quarterly, 48,* 520–524.

Sudman, S., & Freeman, H. E. (1988). The use of network sampling for locating the seriously ill. *Medical Care, 26,* 992–999.

Sudman, S., & Kalton, G. (1986). New developments in the sampling of special populations. *Annual Review of Sociology, 12,* 401–429.

Sudman, S., & Schwarz, N. (1989). Contributions of cognitive psychology to advertising research. *Journal of Advertising Research, 29,* 43–53.

Sudman, S., Sirken, M. G., & Cowan, C. D. (1988). Sampling rare and elusive populations. *Science, 240,* 991–996.

Sullivan, L. M., Dukes, K. A., Harris, L., Dittus, R. S., Greenfield, S., & Kaplan, S. H. (1995). A comparison of various methods of collecting self-reported health outcomes data among low-income and minority patients. *Medical Care, 33*(Suppl. 4), AS183–AS194.

Survey Sampling International. (2005). *Survey Sampling International homepage.* Retrieved June 12, 2005, from http://www.surveysampling.com.

Susser, M., & Susser, E. (1996a). Choosing a future for epidemiology: I. Eras and paradigms. *American Journal of Public Health, 86,* 668–673.

Susser, M., & Susser, E. (1996b). Choosing a future for epidemiology: II. From black box to Chinese boxes and eco-epidemiology. *American Journal of Public Health, 86,* 674–677.

Szende, Á., Schramm, W., Flood, E., Larson, P., Gorina, E., Rentz, A. M., et al. (2003). Health-related quality of life assessment in adult haemophilia patients: A systematic review and evaluation of instruments. *Haemophilia, 9,* 678–687.

Szende, Á., Svensson, K., Ståhl, E., Mészáros, Á., & Berta, G. Y. (2004). Psychometric and utility-based measures of health status of asthmatic patients with different disease control level. *Pharmacoeconomics, 22,* 537–547.

Taft, C., Karlsson, J., & Sullivan, M. (2001). Do SF-36 summary component scores accurately summarize subscale scores? *Quality of Life Research, 10,* 395–404.

Tanur, J. M. (Ed.). (1992). *Questions about questions: Inquiries into the cognitive bases of surveys.* New York: Russell Sage Foundation.

Thissen, M. R., & Rodriguez, G. (2004). *Recording interview sound bites through Blaise instruments.* Retrieved May 25, 2005, from http://www.blaiseusers.org/IBUCPDFS/2004/34.pdf.

Thomas, L. H., & Bond, S. (1996). Measuring patients' satisfaction with nursing: 1990–1994. *Journal of Advanced Nursing, 23,* 747–756.

Thompson, S. K., & Collins, L. A. (2002). Adaptive sampling in research on risk-related behaviors. *Drug and Alcohol Dependence, 68*(Suppl. 1), S57–S67.

Todaro, T., & Perritt, K. (1999). *Overview and evaluation of AGGIES, an automated edit and imputation system.* Retrieved June 14, 2005, from http://www.fcsm.gov/99papers/todaro.html.

Todorov, A. (2000). Context effects in national health surveys: Effects of preceding questions on reporting serious difficulty seeing and legal blindness. *Public Opinion Quarterly, 64,* 65–76.

Torrance, G. W. (1986). Measurement of health state utilities for economic appraisal: A review. *Journal of Health Economics, 5,* 1–30.

Torrance, G. W. (1987). Utility approach to measuring health-related quality of life. *Journal of Chronic Diseases, 40,* 593–600.

Torrance, G. W., & Feeny, D. (1989). Utilities and quality-adjusted life years. *International Journal of Technology Assessment in Health Care, 5,* 559–575.

Tourangeau, R. (1984). Cognitive sciences and survey methods. In National Research Council Committee on National Statistics, *Cognitive aspects of survey methodology: Building a bridge between disciplines* (ed. T. B. Jabine, M. L. Straf, J. M. Tanur, & R. Tourangeau) (pp. 73–100). Washington, DC: National Academies Press.

Tourangeau, R., Couper, M. P., & Conrad, F. (2004). Spacing, position, and order: Interpretive heuristics for visual features of survey questions. *Public Opinion Quarterly, 68,* 368–393.

Tourangeau, R., & Rasinski, K. A. (1988). Cognitive processes underlying context effects in attitude measurement. *Psychological Bulletin, 103,* 299–314.

Tourangeau, R., Rasinski, K. A., & Bradburn, N. (1991). Measuring happiness in surveys: A test of the subtraction hypothesis. *Public Opinion Quarterly, 55,* 255–266.

Tourangeau, R., Rasinski, K. A., & D'Andrade, R. (1991). Attitude structure and belief accessibility. *Journal of Experimental Social Psychology, 27,* 48–75.

Tourangeau, R., Rips, L. J., & Rasinski, K. A. (2000). *The psychology of survey response.* Cambridge: Cambridge University Press.

Tourangeau, R., Singer, E., & Presser, S. (2003). Context effects in attitude surveys: Effects on remote items and impact on predictive validity. *Sociological Methods and Research, 31,* 486–513.

Tourangeau, R., & Smith, T. W. (1996). Asking sensitive questions: The impact of data collection mode, question format, and question context. *Public Opinion Quarterly, 60,* 275–304.

Tourangeau, R., Steiger, D. M., & Wilson, D. (2002). Self-administered questions by telephone: Evaluating interactive voice response. *Public Opinion Quarterly, 66,* 265–278.

Trivellato, U. (1999). Issues in the design and analysis of panel studies: A cursory review. *Quality and Quantity, 33,* 339–352.

Tuckel, P. S., & Feinberg, B. M. (1991). The answering machine poses many questions for telephone survey researchers. *Public Opinion Quarterly, 55,* 200–217.

Tucker, C., Lepkowski, J. M., & Piekarski, L. (2002). The current efficiency of list-assisted telephone sampling designs. *Public Opinion Quarterly, 66,* 321–338.

Tyson, P., Ayton, A., Al Agib, A. O., Bowie, P., Worrall-Davies, A., & Mortimer, A. (2001). A comparison of the service satisfaction and intervention needs of patients with schizophrenia and their relatives. *International Journal of Psychiatry in Clinical Practice, 5,* 263–271.

UCLA Center for Health Policy Research. (2002a). *CHIS 2001 methodology series: Report 1— Sample design* (ed. I. Flores-Cervantes and J. M. Brick). Los Angeles: Author.

UCLA Center for Health Policy Research. (2002b). *CHIS 2001 methodology series: Report 2— Data collection methods* (ed. W. S. Edwards, J. M. Brick, S. Fry, A. Martinson, & P. Warren). Los Angeles: Author.

UCLA Center for Health Policy Research. (2002c). *CHIS 2001 methodology series: Report 3— Data processing procedures* (ed. J. Rauch & W. S. Edwards). Los Angeles: Author.

UCLA Center for Health Policy Research. (2002d). *CHIS 2001 methodology series: Report 4— Response rates* (ed. J. M. Brick, I. Flores-Cervantes, W. S. Edwards, & R. L. Harding). Los Angeles: Author.

UCLA Center for Health Policy Research. (2002e). *CHIS 2001 methodology series: Report 5— Weighting and variance estimation* (ed. I. Flores-Cervantes, J. M. Brick, R. L. Harding, M. E. Jones, & A. Luo). Los Angeles: Author.

UCLA Center for Health Policy Research. (2005). *California Health Interview Survey (CHIS) homepage.* Retrieved May 9, 2005, from http://www.chis.ucla.edu/.

Ueda, S. (2002, October). *Report of the Study Group on the Subjective Dimension of Functioning and Disability* (Report No. WHO/GPE/CAS/C/02.30). Retrieved May 25, 2005, from http://www.aihw.gov.au/international/who_hoc/hoc_02_papers/brisbane30.doc.

Umbach, P. D. (2004). Web surveys: Best practices. In S. R. Rorter (Ed.), *Overcoming survey research problems* (pp. 23–28). New Directions for Institutional Research, No. 121. San Francisco: Jossey-Bass.

Umesh, U. N., & Peterson, R. A. (1991). A critical evaluation of the randomized response method: Applications, validation, and research agenda. *Sociological Methods and Research, 20,* 104–138.

United Nations International Children's Education Fund (UNICEF). (2000). *End-decade multiple indicator survey manual.* New York: Author.

United Nations International Children's Education Fund (UNICEF). (n.d.). *UNICEF statistics: Multiple Indicator Cluster Survey (MICS).* Retrieved May 23, 2005, from http://www. childinfo.org/mics/.

United Nations Statistics Division. (2005). *Telephone main lines in use per 100 inhabitants: 211 countries, 1986–1990.* Retrieved June 16, 2005, from http://unstats.un.org/unsd/ cdbdemo/cdb_series_xrxx.asp?series_code=13130.

University of California at Berkeley, Computer-Assisted Survey Methods (CSM) Program. (n.d.). *Computer-Assisted Survey Execution System (CASES).* Retrieved June 8, 2005, from http://cases.berkeley.edu:7504/.

University of Michigan Survey Research Center and National Center for Health Services Research. (1977). *Experiments in interviewing techniques: Field experiments in health reporting, 1971–1977* (ed. C. F. Cannell, L. Oksenberg, & J. M. Converse). (DHEW Publication No. (HRA) 78-3204).) Washington, DC: National Center for Health Services Research.

University of Minnesota, State Health Access Data Assistance Center. (2004). *Coordinated State Coverage Survey (CSCS).* Retrieved June 1, 2005, from http://www.shadac.umn.edu/ collecting/cscs.asp.

University of Texas, M D Anderson Cancer Center. (2003). *DSTPLAN: Double Precision Study Planning Calculations.* Retrieved May 12, 2005, from http://odin.mdacc.tmc.edu/bio-math/anonftp/#DSTPLAN.

Urban Institute. (2001). *National Survey of America's Families (NSAF).* Retrieved June 1, 2005, from http://www.urban.org/Content/Research/NewFederalism/NSAF/Overview/NSAFOverview.htm.

U.S. Census Bureau. (1992). *1990 census of population and housing: Alphabetical index of industries and occupations.* Washington, DC: U.S. Government Printing Office.

U.S. Census Bureau. (2002). *Current Population Survey: Design and methodology.* (Technical Paper 63RV). Washington, DC.

U.S. Census Bureau. (2003, July 1). *United States Census 2000: Questionnaires.* Retrieved April 14, 2005, from http://www.census.gov/dmd/www/2000quest.html.

U.S. Census Bureau. (n.d.). *U.S. Census Bureau homepage.* Retrieved June 1, 2005, from http://www.census.gov.

U.S. Department of Health and Human Services, Office for Civil Rights. (2005, April 18). *Office for Civil Rights—HIPAA: Medical privacy: National standards to protect the privacy of personal health information.* Retrieved May 9, 2005, from http://www.hhs.gov/ocr/hipaa/.

U.S. Department of Labor, Bureau of Labor Statistics. (2001, October 16). *How the government measures unemployment.* Retrieved June 1, 2005, from http://www.bls.gov/cps/cps_htgm.htm.

U.S. Department of Labor, Bureau of Labor Statistics. (2005, May 6). *Technical notes to establishment survey data published in employment and earnings.* Retrieved June 16, 2005, from http://stats.bls.gov/web/cestn1.htm.

U.S. Department of Labor, Bureau of Labor Statistics. (n.d.). *Current Population Survey homepage.* Retrieved April 14, 2005, from http://www.bls.gov/cps/home.htm.

U.S. Department of Labor, Bureau of Labor Statistics and Bureau of the Census. (1996). *Testing methods of collecting racial and ethnic information: Results of the Current Population Survey Supplement on Race and Ethnicity* (ed. C. Tucker, R. McKay, B. Kojetin, R. Harrison, M. de la Puente, L. Stinson, & E. Robison). Bureau of Labor Statistics Statistical Note Series, No. 40. Washington, DC: U.S. Government Printing Office.

U.S. General Accounting Office. (2001). *Tobacco settlement: States' use of master settlement agreement payments: Report to the Honorable John McCain, Ranking Minority Member, Committee on Commerce, Science, and Transportation, U.S. Senate* (Report No. GAO-01-851). Washington, DC: U.S. Government Printing Office.

U.S. Public Health Service, Office of the Surgeon General. (1999). *Mental health: A report of the Surgeon General.* Rockville, MD: U.S. Government Printing Office.

U.S. Public Health Service, Office of the Surgeon General. (2001). *Mental health: Culture, race, and ethnicity: A supplement to Mental health: A report of the Surgeon General.* Rockville, MD: U.S. Government Printing Office.

van Campen, C., Sixma, H., Friele, R. D., Kerssens, J. J., & Peters, L. (1995). Quality of care and patient satisfaction: A review of measuring instruments. *Medical Care Research and Review, 52,* 109–133.

van Exel, N.J.A., Reimer, W.J.M. S., & Koopmanschap, M. A. (2004). Assessment of post-stroke quality of life in cost-effectiveness studies: The usefulness of the Barthel Index and the EuroQoL-5D. *Quality of Life Research, 13,* 427–433.

Victora, C. G., Habicht, J. P., & Bryce, J. (2004). Evidence-based public health: Moving beyond randomized trials. *American Journal of Public Health, 94,* 400–405.

Vigderhous, G. (1981). Scheduling telephone interviews: A study of seasonal patterns. *Public Opinion Quarterly, 45*, 250–259.

Waksberg, J. (1978). Sampling methods for random digit dialing. *Journal of the American Statistical Association, 73*, 40–46.

Waksberg, J. (1983). A note on locating a special population using random digit dialing. *Public Opinion Quarterly, 47*, 576–578.

Walker, J. T. (1994). Fax machines and social surveys: Teaching an old dog new tricks. *Journal of Quantitative Criminology, 10*, 181–188.

Wallace, R. B. (1994). Assessing the health of individuals and populations in surveys of the elderly: Some concepts and approaches. *Gerontologist, 34*, 449–453.

Wallman, K. K., Evinger, S., & Schechter, S. (2000). Measuring our nation's diversity: Developing a common language for data on race/ethnicity. *American Journal of Public Health, 90*, 1704–1708.

Wallschlaeger, C., & Busic-Snyder, C. (1992). *Basic visual concepts and principles for artists, architects, and designers.* Dubuque, IA: William C. Brown.

Wänke, M. (1996). Comparative judgments as a function of the direction of comparison versus word order. *Public Opinion Quarterly, 60*, 400–409.

Wänke, M., Schwarz, N., & Noelle-Neumann, E. (1995). Asking comparative questions: The impact of the direction of comparison. *Public Opinion Quarterly, 59*, 347–372.

Ware, J. E. (1986). The assessment of health status. In L. H. Aiken & D. Mechanic (Eds.), *Applications of social science to clinical medicine and health policy* (pp. 204–228). New Brunswick, NJ: Rutgers University Press.

Ware, J. E. (1987). Standards for validating health measures: Definition and content. *Journal of Chronic Diseases, 40*, 473–480.

Ware, J. E. (1995). The status of health assessment 1994. *Annual Review of Public Health, 16*, 327–354.

Ware, J. E., & Gandek, B. (1998a). Methods for testing data quality, scaling assumptions, and reliability: The IQOLA Project approach. International Quality of Life Assessment. *Journal of Clinical Epidemiology, 51*, 945–952.

Ware, J. E., & Gandek, B. (1998b). Overview of the SF-36 Health Survey and the International Quality of Life Assessment (IQOLA) Project. *Journal of Clinical Epidemiology, 51*, 903–912.

Ware, J. E., & Hays, R. D. (1988). Methods for measuring patient satisfaction with specific medical encounters. *Medical Care, 26*, 393–402.

Ware, J. E., Kosinski, M., & Keller, S. D. (1994). *SF-36 physical and mental health summary scales: A user's manual.* Boston: Health Institute, New England Medical Center.

Ware, J. E., Kosinski, M., & Keller, S. D. (1996). A 12-item short-form health survey: Construction of scales and preliminary tests of reliability and validity. *Medical Care, 34*, 220–233.

Ware, J. E., & Sherbourne, C. D. (1992). The MOS 36-item short-form health survey (SF-36): I. Conceptual framework and item selection. *Medical Care, 30*, 473–483.

Ware, J. E., Snow, K. K., Kosinski, M., & Gandek, B. (1993). *SF-36 health survey: Manual and interpretation guide.* Boston: Health Institute, New England Medical Center.

Ware, J. E., & Snyder, M. K. (1975). Dimensions of patient attitudes regarding doctors and medical care services. *Medical Care, 13*, 669–682.

Warnecke, R. B., Sudman, S., Johnson, T. P., O'Rourke, D., Davis, A. M., & Jobe, J. B. (1997). Cognitive aspects of recalling and reporting health-related events: Papanicolaou smears, clinical breast examinations, and mammograms. *American Journal of Epidemiology, 146,* 982–992.

Warner, S. L. (1965). Randomized response: A survey technique for eliminating evasive answer bias. *Journal of the American Statistical Association, 60,* 63–66.

Warren, J. R., Sheridan, J. T., & Hauser, R. M. (1998). Choosing a measure of occupational standing: How useful are composite measures in analyses of gender inequality in occupational attainment? *Sociological Methods and Research, 27,* 3–76.

Washington State University, Social and Economic Sciences Research Center. (1993). *Dental malpractice survey: A nationwide mail survey of practicing general dentists* (ed. T. Tarnai, P. Milgrom, & L. Fise). (Data Report No. 93–10 (MALP No. 0215). Pullman, WA: Author.

Waterman, A. H., Blades, M., & Spencer, C. (2001). Interviewing children and adults: The effect of question format on the tendency to speculate. *Applied Cognitive Psychology, 15,* 521–531.

Weech-Maldonado, R., Weidmer, B. O., Morales, L. S., & Hays, R. D. (2001). Cross cultural adaptation of survey instruments: The CAHPS experience. In National Center for Health Statistics, *Seventh Conference on Health Survey Research Methods* (ed. M. L. Cynamon & R. A. Kulka) (pp. 75–82). (DHHS Publication No. (PHS) 01-1013.) Hyattsville, MD: National Center for Health Statistics.

Weeks, M. F., Kulka, R. A., & Pierson, S. A. (1987). Optimal call scheduling for a telephone survey. *Public Opinion Quarterly, 51,* 540–549.

Weinberg, E. (1983). Data collection: Planning and Management. In P. H. Rossi, J. D. Wright, & A. B. Anderson (Eds.), *Handbook of survey research* (pp. 329–358). New York: Academic Press.

Weisberg, H. F. (2003). *Survey errors in modern survey research.* Thousand Oaks, CA: Sage.

Weiss, B. D., & Senf, J. H. (1990). Patient satisfaction survey instrument for use in health maintenance organizations. *Medical Care, 28,* 434–445.

Wensing, M., & Elwyn, G. (2002). Research on patients' views in the evaluation and improvement of quality of care. *Quality and Safety in Health Care, 11,* 153–157.

Wensing, M., & Grol, R. (2000). Patients' views on healthcare: A driving force for improvement in disease management. *Disease Management and Health Outcomes, 7,* 117–125.

Westat. (2005). *Blaise Overview.* Retrieved June 8, 2005, from http://www.westat.org/blaise/.

White, H. D. (1994). Scientific communication and literature retrieval. In H. M. Cooper & L. V. Hedges (Eds.), *The handbook of research synthesis* (pp. 42–56). New York: Russell Sage Foundation.

White, T. M., & Hauan, M. J. (2002). Using client-side event logging and path tracing to assess and improve the quality of Web-based surveys. *Proceedings of the American Medical Informatics Association Annual Symposium, 22 (Suppl.),* 894–898.

Wilkin, D., Hallam, L., & Doggett, M.-A. (1992). *Measures of need and outcome for primary health care.* New York: Oxford University Press.

Williams, A. (1990). EuroQol: A new facility for the measurement of health-related quality of life. *Health Policy, 16,* 199–208.

Williams, D. R. (1994). The concept of race in health services research, 1966 to 1990. *Health Services Research, 29,* 261–274.

Williams, S., Weinman, J., & Dale, J. (1998). Doctor-patient communication and patient satisfaction: A review. *Family Practice, 15,* 480–492.

Willimack, D. K., Schuman, H., Pennell, B. E., & Lepkowski, J. M. (1995). Effects of a pre-paid nonmonetary incentive on response rates and response quality in a face-to-face survey. *Public Opinion Quarterly, 59,* 78–92.

Willis, G. B. (2004). Overview of methods for developing culturally equivalent methods across multiple cultural groups. In National Center for Health Statistics, *Eighth Conference on Health Survey Research Methods* (ed. S. B. Cohen & J. M. Lepkowski) (pp. 91–96). (DHHS Publication No. (PHS) 04-1013). Hyattsville, MD: National Center for Health Statistics.

Willis, G. B. (2005). *Cognitive interviewing: A tool for improving questionnaire design.* Thousand Oaks, CA: Sage.

World Health Organization. (1948). Constitution of the World Health Organization. In *Handbook of basic documents.* Geneva, Switzerland: Author.

World Health Organization. (2001, November 30). *WHO Multicountry Survey on Health and Responsiveness.* Retrieved June 1, 2005, from http://www3.who.int/whs/P/gpediscpaper37.pdf.

World Health Organization. (2002). *Summary measures of population health: Concepts, ethics, measurement and applications* (ed. C.J.L. Murray, J. A. Salomon, C. D. Mathers, & A. D. Lopez). Geneva, Switzerland: Author.

World Health Organization. (2005). *Global School-Based Student Health Survey (GSHS).* Retrieved June 1, 2005, from http://www.who.int/school_youth_health/assessment/gshs/en/.

World Health Organization. (n.d.). *World Health Survey (WHS) homepage.* Retrieved June 1, 2005, from http://www3.who.int/whs/.

Wortman, P. M. (1994). Judging research quality. In H. M. Cooper & L. V. Hedges (Eds.), *The handbook of research synthesis* (pp. 98–110). New York: Russell Sage Foundation.

Wright, D. B., Gaskell, G. D., & O'Muircheartaigh, C. A. (1997). How response alternatives affect different kinds of behavioural frequency questions. *British Journal of Social Psychology, 36,* 443–456.

Wright, D. B., Gaskell, G. D., & O'Muircheartaigh, C. A. (1998). Flashbulb memory assumptions: Using national surveys to explore cognitive phenomena. *British Journal of Psychology, 89,* 103–121.

Wright, D. L., Aquilino, W. S., & Supple, A. J. (1998). A comparison of computer-assisted and paper-and-pencil self-administered questionnaires in a survey on smoking, alcohol, and drug use. *Public Opinion Quarterly, 62,* 331–353.

Wu, A. W., Gifford, A., Asch, S., Cohn, S. E., Bozzette, S. A., & Yurk, R. (2000). Quality-of-care indicators for HIV/AIDS. *Disease Management and Health Outcomes, 7,* 315–330.

Wu, S. C., Li, C. Y., & Ke, D. S. (2000). The agreement between self-reporting and clinical diagnosis for selected medical conditions among the elderly in Taiwan. *Public Health, 114,* 137–142.

Wyatt, J. C. (2000). When to use Web-based surveys. *Journal of the American Medical Informatics Association, 7,* 426–430.

Wynd, C. A., Schmidt, B., & Schaefer, M. A. (2003). Two quantitative approaches for estimating content validity. *Western Journal of Nursing Research, 25,* 508–518.

Xu, M. H., Bates, B. J., & Schweitzer, J. C. (1993). The impact of messages on survey participation in answering machine households. *Public Opinion Quarterly, 57,* 232–237.

Yammarino, F. J., Skinner, S. J., & Childers, T. L. (1991). Understanding mail survey response behavior: A meta-analysis. *Public Opinion Quarterly, 55,* 613–639.

Yancy, W. S., Macpherson, D. S., Hanusa, B. H., Switzer, G. E., Arnold, R. M., Buranosky,

R. A., et al. (2001). Patient satisfaction in resident and attending ambulatory care clinics. *Journal of General Internal Medicine, 16,* 755–762.

Yansaneh, I. S. (2003). *Construction and use of sample weights (draft)* (Publication No. ESA/STAT/AC.93/5). New York: United Nations Secretariat, Statistics Division.

Yin, R. K. (2003). *Case study research: Design and methods* (3rd ed.). Thousand Oaks, CA: Sage.

Yu, J., & Cooper, H. (1983). A quantitative review of research design effects on response rates to questionnaires. *Journal of Marketing Research, 20,* 36–44.

Zeisel, H. (1985). *Say it with figures* (6th ed.). New York: HarperCollins.

NAME INDEX

SUBJECT INDEX

A

Accuracy of sample design, 134
ADA (Americans with Disabilities Act), 271
Addition (carryover) effect, 304
Administration/monitoring: of attitude questions, 282–283; choosing the most appropriate method of, 241; comparing personal/telephone interviews, self-administered questionnaire, 117–118; of computer-assisted data collection systems, 333–334; considerations for special populations, 335–336; examples of, 337; field procedures, 312–320; guidelines for minimizing errors/maximizing survey quality in, 337–338t; hiring and training interviewers, 320–327; of knowledge questions, 273; managing surveys, 329–333t; questionnaire design and, 217; scale construction and issues of,

76; special considerations for Internet surveys, 334–335; supervising fieldwork, 327–328; of threatening questions, 264–265
Advance notice procedures, 312–314
African Americans: health survey questions on race of, 249–251; weighting sample adjusting for nonresponse/noncoverage of, 189t–190. *See also* Minorities
Agency for Healthcare Research and Quality, 24, 222, 223, 259, 284, 286
Age/sex questions, 248–249, 299
AGGIES software, 333
Aided recall techniques, 258–259
AIDS. *See* HIV/AIDS
AI-SUPERPFP Team, 326
Alameda County Study, 33
Alpha reliability coefficient, 60
Alternative or Ha research hypothesis, 164–167, 165t
Alternative modes of administration, 76

American Hospital Association, 354
American Medical Association, 354
American Psychiatric Association, 66
American Psychological Association, 54, 62
American Statistical Association, 10, 22, 177
Analysis plan: errors related to, 400t, 404; mapping out the, 383–384t, 385–387; written report on, 396, 400t, 404
Analytical designs: comparing descriptive and, 35t–37; comparisons/relationships in, 375–376; computing sample size for experimental and, 164–174; criteria for estimating sample size for, 158e; described, 30; focus on empirically observed relationships, 42; objectives and hypotheses for, 39fig. *See also* Experimental designs; Survey design